Nutricide

the Nutritional Destruction of the Black Race

Llaila O. Afrika

A&B PUBLISHERS GROUP
New York
11238

COVER CONCEPT: *Llaila Afrika*
COVER DESIGN: *A & B PUBLISHERS GROUP*
COVER ILLUSTRATION: *DIMITRIX*

Library of Congress Cataloging-in-Publication Data

Afrika, Llaila O.
   Nutricide:the nutritional destruction of the Black race/Llaila O. Afrika
            p.   cm.
   Previously published1994
Includes bibliographical references and index.
   ISBN 1-886433-30-5 (pbk.: alk paper)
   1. Nutritionally induced diseases. 2. Blacks--Nutrition. I. Title.

RA645.N87. A36 2000   00-058611
613. 2'089'96073--dc2111

                              Published
                                 by

                      A&B PUBLISHERS GROUP
                        1000 Atlantic Avenue
                        Brooklyn, New York,
                              11238
                          (718) 783-7808

                 97 98 99 00 01 6 5 4 3 2 1

          Manufactured and Printed in the United States

Acknowledgment

There are many seen and unseen Godly Forces that caused me to write this book. It is impossible to acknowledge all of them.

Godly Forces were instilled within me by our living and dead ancestors. There have been many people in countries such as Germany, America, Holland, France, Israel etc., that would walk up to me and tell me that I had something special to do for my people. There was a little African girl who walked up to me and asked me to please teach her how to know whether she was healthy or not. There was the musician Maurice Williams who taught me to know structure and form and the principles that allow you to change forms. There was my wrestling teacher Mr. Robinson who taught me to use whatever the enemy gives you to destroy them.

I acknowledge and respect all of those who have contributed to my life especially my wife Aseelah, daughter Naima and son Maideah. I bless those who dislike, scorn and actively discredit me. My special thanks to Dr. Gloria Peace who coined the word "Nutricide" and to Ricardo Battle who encouraged me and told me "Black Folks need a book that is totally raw so they won't have any excuse for eating junk food and getting sick." I thank Dr. Otis Williams who encouraged me to keep focused.

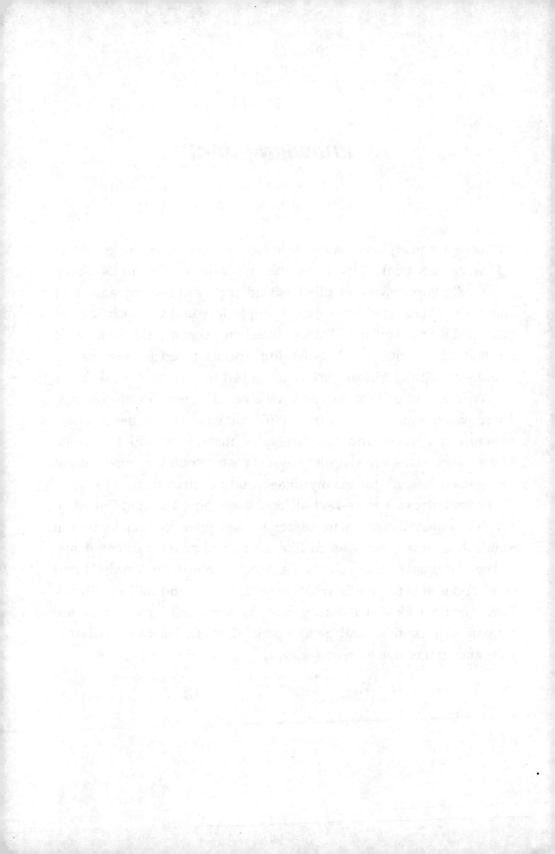

Dedication

This book is dedicated to my sisters Paula, Carolyn (deceased), Beatrice (deceased), Patricia and Kathleen, and my brothers William and Richard. They loved me and cared for me. My father also provided me with additional sisters (Terry, Donna, April and Latisha) and a brother (Cecil, deceased) who I was not raised with and never got to know. God has allowed us a life together.

This book is especially dedicated to my oldest sister Paula Ann Brown. She spent countless hours discussing our race, politics, racism and revolutionary movements with me. My mother calls her "Blacker than Black." She always saw something in me that I could not see myself. One day after I finished a lecture, she turned to me with tears in her eyes and the biggest smile. She said, "My Llaila, My Brother, My Prince!" She then gave me a big hug that felt like a reward. It was then that I realized my mission in life. I "love myself some" Paula Ann, because she is my big sister. Her African name is Amatulla. She says that you have to be deep into African culture to use an African name. I must be truthful to you about my sister Paula. I didn't like her too much when I was a little boy because she would spank me for doing bad things. Paula told me that I did not talk until I was almost three years old. My mother would get angry with me and scream, "Boy, why don't you say something?" Paula would tell mamma, "Leave him alone, maybe he don't feel as if there is anything important to talk about right now." I love Paula and all of my sister and brothers with a spirit that could shake the world.

Contents

Foreword

This book is a brief look at the state of African American health and Nutricide. In this book, I may refer to African Americans as Africans. Basically, the health of all Africans (Diaspora included) is controlled by diseased Caucasians. Nature has provided Africans with the most superior physiological structure and the gift of melanin dominance. It is our responsibility to take proper holistic care of ourselves. We must use Caucasian medical technology and diagnosis with caution. Unfortunately, too many Africans do not understand the far-reaching disease effect of Caucasian medicine and nutrition, nor do we have the slightest idea of how to develop or maintain our health. We must become healthy so that our children can become healthy. We cannot expect the Caucasian to do what we will not do ourselves. We are created by God to be Goddesses and Gods. A healthy body is the only vehicle that will make us realize our Godliness. Hopefully, this book will help us become more focused on our date with God's destiny.

This Africentric book includes reports about the Caucasian's mind and behavior. Unfortunately, many Africans believe that if you honestly report about whites, you hate whites, are putting them down or being negative. It is absurd to hate someone for having a disease such as diabetes, cancer or White Supremacy.

It has always irritated me to use Caucasian references when I write, it is as if an African cannot have an idea unless a Caucasian had it first. This Caucasian information control creates a "Scientific Plantation" and "Information Colonialism." I used some Caucasian references within the text for those Negroes still on the "Information Plantation." However, the only books that I suggest or recommended as references are books written by Africans, and those books are the Ancient Papyrus and those listed at the end of this book. Aside from this, Caucasian references are full of White Racism, Caucasian norm values and weird superstitions that make them too mentally, spiritually and emotionally painful to use. I also must follow the Slave Master's "Information Plantation" rule of disclosing and disqualifying everything written in this book, so that the Caucasian capitalist pig will not sue me and or have me incarcerated for practicing medicine without a Caucasian medical license. Therefore, this next sentence is written. "No statement in this book should be construed as a claim for a cure, treatment or prevention of any disease or should take the place of a Caucasian trained, certified, licensed or accredited medical practitioner."

It is important that you should know that the African community has always had traditional natural Healers. These Healers use many different techniques, methods and systems. I find that it is a mistake to compare them as each has a special talent granted by God. The vast majority of Healers are dedicated to making all of us healthy. I greatly honor the countless ancestors who passed this tradition on. I greatly respect the African Healers, Herb stores and/or Health Food stores that keep traditional medicine alive.

To be African is a blessing from God. To be a holistically healthy African is wonderful. The only other choice is disease. There is nothing more restrictive than a disease. It is best to be strict and restrictive with your diet than to let a disease like arthritis, fibroid tumors, high blood pressure, herpes, hypertension, PMS or constipation cause your life to be restricted. There is plenty of health information but very little on the subject of African ethnomedicine and the unique biochemical nutritional status of Africans. I see many Africans in bookstores, health food stores, at lectures and at Caucasian health conferences trying to make Africentric sense out of the information. They usually end up more miseducated and frustrated than informed.

In this book, I have simplified and concentrated vast amounts of information to provide the reader with knowledge that will help them become more Africentrically health focused. I have carefully explained the Caucasian mentality. The fight for our holistic existence can be won only if we understand our enemy. I have reported descriptions of the Caucasian mind and behavior many times in this text because they need to be familiar to our ear. We are an ancient people from an ancient civilization and we do not always use the ancient authority that melanin and our higher spiritual and mental status grants us. We are not humanistically on the same level as the Caucasian. We are biochemically and electromagnetically superior to them. Therefore, we must examine the inferior Caucasian from the superior African status. It may take some getting used to, but we are the chosen race from the spirit world and the race blessed by the Sun. We must take our position of world leadership on this planet or have no planet because the Caucasians' will destroy it. I beg of you, *do not let the Caucasian junk food diet or diseases make you a prisoner in your own body*. African social life, marriages, relationships, children, health, families and communities are under siege. We are in a nutritional combat zone. We must fight for the sake of our children and the Motherland. We are in a military situation. The food industry is controlled with military logic. The Caucasians' are military, aggressive and violent people. Military people use tactics to seize the advantage in order to dominate and control others or destroy others. We can not use social science (marching, singing and voting, money etc.) in a military science situation. There is no such thing as peaceful coexistence or compromise with military people. It is either victory or defeat. Africans are the only race capable of defeating the Caucasian. However, a junk food diet clouds our vision to see and accept our victory.

Repeat this affirmation daily so that you can change your Caucasian junk food diet to a natural diet. "*I will no longer be part of the nutritional ignorance of my race.*" This affirmation, along with herbs that cleanse the organs, blood and colon will help us. A raw juice diet and any other Africentric healing systems will help change the health. We have got to get the white man out of our stomach. Remember that Nutricide is very deadly because it is a combination of menticide (extermination of the African mind), genocide (extermination of the body by violence. cloning or drugs) and spiriticide (extermination of the African spirit). I wrote this book because I *had* to write this book. When I would sit down to relax. I would feel the earth tremble beneath my feet with the bones, groans and pain of our murdered African ancestors. I hear them telling me to write the nutritional truth. My spirit will not be allowed to rest until I tell this truth to you. Holistic health is my language; it is how life communicates to me and how I communicate to life. It is my voice in this life.

This is a photograph of the inside of the human brain. The cells of the brain are magnified to the size equivalent to the size of a car. The electromagnetic galaxy-like cloud in the center is the Eye of Horus. It is inside the brain in a fluid filled space called the Third Ventricle. The Eye Horus is alive and active and floats above the Pineal Gland and is influenced by melanin and the spirit world (unseen).

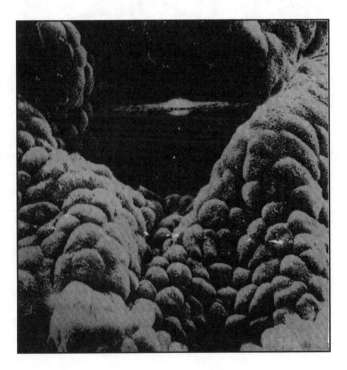

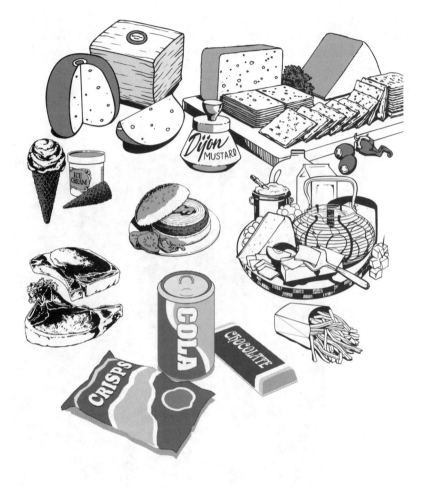

Chapter One
Nutricide

"If a person (*Caucasian*) would send another (*African*)
into bondage (*slavery*), he would, it appears to me,
be bad enough to send him to hell, if he could."

Harriet Tubman

Nutricide

The nutritional genocide of African people, which is called Nutricide, is a reality that must be faced by Africans. Nutricide is the deliberate and systematic alteration of foods in order to cause physical and mental dis-eases, genetic mutations and/or death.

African children are deprived of vital nutrients, which cause attention span disorders, learning problems, behavioral disorders and hyperactivity. It is typical to find a zinc deficiency in boys and iron deficiency in girls. Iron deficiencies in boys are ignored. African boys in Philadelphia Public Schools were having conduct problems, disruptive behaviors, restlessness, irritability and learning problems. They were found to have an iron deficiency. Iron is the nutrient needed by the left hemisphere of the brain. The part of the brain used for cognitive skills is in the area of the brain that manages reason and logic. This is the region needed to do well on standardized tests. When an African girl or boy has an iron deficiency he/she perceives information differently and does not respond well.

African children fed on Caucasian junk food and cooked foods aside from having an iron deficiency also have a deficiency in a vitamin called Thiamine. Thiamine deficiency causes the child to be sensitive to criticism and to have poor impulse control, to be easy to anger, aggressive, hostile, depressed, and have headaches and/or sleep disturbances, (Institute for Bio-social Research, Tacoma WA).

The child's mind and behavior is destroyed by MSG (Monosodium glutamate) found in fried foods, fats, and Chinese foods. MSG can cause heart problems, brain and nerve damage, infertility, bone damage etc. Added to this, Aspartame, (i.e. Nutra Sweet) can cause brain tumors, seizures, constipation, tiredness and cloning in children and adults.

The public schools (educational plantations), books (Caucasian media) promote junk food, cooked food and a high white sugar diet. The American Academy for Pediatrics reports that the average child spends more hours watching television than he spends in school. The child eats a sweet snack for every two hours of television viewing. The African American child watches more television and eats more sweets than the Caucasian. Children, especially in poverty and so called minority children (African American), eat more junk food, fast food, sodas and snack foods than poor Caucasian children. The majority of African children and 22% of Caucasian children do not eat breakfast. They usually eat snack junk foods (Citizens Pubecy Center in Oakland CA). Junk foods are nutrient deficient and addictive and do not have natural B complex vitamins, B_6, Niacin. Folic Acid, Riboflavin, Iron, Potassium, Chromium, Vitamin C, Beta-Carotene, Phenylalanine, Lysine, Glutamic acid and the nutrients the brain needs to function. The junk food business is deliberately processing out nutrients and not giving the child the vitamins, minerals, trace elements, fiber and amino acids that they need. They are deliberately placing the child in a Nutricide status. This is done deliberately because milling or processing grains such as brown rice, corn, whole flour and sugar cane increase its shelf life, which increases the Caucasian profits. Shelf life is the ability of a food to stay on the store's shelf without spoiling. Processed foods have become manure in the stomach and colon and have a long shelf life while whole foods do not. Whole foods (whole wheat, brown rice, yellow grits etc.), have plenty of vitamins, minerals, proteins and fiber, spoil very easily, and have a short shelf life. Selling natural foods would decrease the Caucasian business profits. Consequently, the African child is mutilated and sacrificed for Caucasian business profits, which are used to support White Supremacy. (A book such as *Psycho-Nutrition* by Carlton Fredericks can be a resource.)

Children's brains also suffer from allergic reactions from junk foods. They cause learning and behavioral problems. There are various types of plants processed and refined to make white sugar such as beets, corn and sugar cane. Any one of these processed sugars can cause a reaction in the brain. However, the Truth and Labeling Law protects companies. A company only has to report an ingredient such as sugar and not the synthetic chemicals added to that ingredient. For example, common table salt contains close to 32 synthetic chemical ingredients in it that the original wholesale manufacturer put on his label when sold to the second manufacturers. However, the second company only has to put on the retail label that the ingredient is salt. The Caucasian junk food companies, with the government's help, are able to practice Nutricide and to put harmful synthetic chemicals into foods that destroy the human body. Children are mentally, nutritionally, and physically abused by such government institutions as the National Institute of Health's Genetic Factors in Crime. They label them genetically violent and use chemicals to alter the brain and drugs to genetically modify and control the behavior of nutritionally deprived children. C. A. Frazer M.D explores allergic reactions in children in Parent's Guide to Allergy in Children.

The Nutricide of African Americans continues despite the fact that the 1988 Surgeon General's Report on Nutrition and Health reported that diet influences and causes diseases. The diseases destroy the body's ability to function, to protect itself, and to be African. Junk food companies are in business to stay in business. Their foods deplete the children of energy and lead them to a life of diseases until one of the diseases places their body in a cemetery. African Americans are victims of the junk food industry.

Disease and death are a by product of poor nutrition and a Caucasian weapon designed to commit Nutricide against Africans. Allowing Africans ethno-nutritional natural foods diet is in no way a part of the government's design or purpose for Africans. This information is published in "The Food Gap, Poverty and Malnutrition in the United States"(Washington DC. Government Printing Office 1969) and in N. Kotz's Book, *Let Them Eat Promise: The Politics of Hunger in America*.

It is a total illusion to rely upon Caucasian junk foods or allopathic disease causing medicines to save Africans. Caucasian nutritionist, doctors, dietitians, and health practitioners are just as infected with junk food and White Supremacy as the general public. If one of their science disciplines (gangs) decides to be humanistic or allow Africans to use their culture's herb medicine or Africentric hygienic health treatment system or natural diet, then one of the other disciplines (science gangs) will attack them. They attack each other in order to keep the African caucus alive long enough to drain more economic profit from it.

The Caucasians do not have an intelligent brain that supervises White Supremacy or divide and conquer techniques or selfish individualism or violent wolf pack attacks upon African peoples. They use thought, political and military instinct. Historically, the basic unit of their society is the dysfunctional family. The Caucasian family structure is divided. Basically, their normal dysfunctional family is a loose collection of individuals that will betray and deceive each other. In their distant past they would sell bricks that were cracked to each other. They would hide the cracks in the bricks with wax and sell them as good. Eventually a house built with cracked bricks would fall apart. They have a saying left over from their deceitful behavior and we sign letters with it, "sincere." Sincere means my bricks are not sealed with wax. The deceit and divided characteristics of their family, spirit, minds and countries is still present.

Caucasian dysfunctional families and mixtures of families called clans were blood related and fought each other. Then after a battle against a common enemy they would fight amongst each other. Individuals in their families would betray, deceive and abuse each other violently and sexually, so that by definition they were dysfunctional families. Caucasian dysfunctional broken homes would unite, and then break up their unity. Then the cycle of dysfunctional families, clans and tribes would continue. This led to dysfunctional kingdoms and governments. This cycle of dysfunctional governments was repeated in America when dysfunctional European families separated from dysfunctional governments, then came to America to escape the violence with their blood relatives. Then, they fought their blood relatives over ownership of the government, money, resources (Africans and Africa), and land that belonged to their European relatives and called this the American Revolution. Then, they loosely united again to later fight their own relatives and clans over control of the dysfunctional economy which was the War of Northern economic aggression against the South (so called Civil War). It is inherent in Caucasian civilization to be dysfunctional and divided and to behave like an animal pride.

The ingredients for dysfunctional families are a Caucasian product that was combined with a dysfunctional diet and diseases then passed along to African people. Any race that has the ungodly misfortune to have to associate with White Racist diseased Caucasians will become divided and conquered, inferiorized, use group sex, use violence upon itself, use homosexuality, have dysfunctional families, dysfunctional dis-ease producing diets, have dysfunctional economics (i.e., inflation, depression, recession, etc.), use drugs, abortions and won't know their history (Europeans do not know their history). They would have reproductive failures, rotten teeth, suicides, rape each other, have White Gods and Saviors, and commit wild wolf pack dog attacks upon each other (gang warfare) which they call wars.

The synthetic foods are addicting and biochemically help to support addiction to Caucasian behavior. Biochemically the brain nourished by junk food has a predisposition for addiction, which means it can become easily addicted to other things.

Melanin participates in addiction by bonding the harmful chemicals to it. It is a self-defense mechanism of the body for melanin to attach to the synthetic harmful chemical or harmful thoughts. Melanin then waits for an opportunity to eliminate these harmful chemicals and thoughts from the body. This melanin reflex holds the addiction in the body. The constant consumption of synthetic Caucasian foods (chemicals) with addictive chemicals makes Africans more addiction prone than Caucasians. Caucasians who are melanin deficient and lack melanin's free radical chemical bonding ability. They are chemical people (caffeine, sugar, alcohol, chocolate, salt etc.).

It must be remembered that foods (synthetic or natural) are chemicals. All chemicals influence the body, mind, mood, and consciousness either positively or negatively. The body reacts to chemicals, cooked foods (inorganic) and cooked herbs (inorganic). This reaction is called nutrition. Biologically, foods either have a sympathetic or parasympathetic nervous system response.

Africans' melanin makes their nervous system more sensitive by responding to the electromagnetic force of foods and nutrients. A harmful food would cause the melanin to turn on the sympathetic response (defense reaction). The sympathetic defense reaction sends melanin out to attach to the harmful food or drug. This inadvertently makes Africans more prone to addiction especially if they stay on a junk food diet. The junk food diet stops the melanin from releasing the addictive drug or food. A natural diet would stop the addiction and cause melanin to get rid of the harmful addiction instead of bonding with it. A strictly Caucasian level of drug detoxification would leave the African still addicted, as detoxification would be based on the low level of Caucasian melanin. Therefore a so-called detoxified African with melanin dominance would still remain attached to a drug, food, social or spiritual Caucasian disease.

African Americans suffer due to the nutritional level set by Caucasians African American women and girls' diets are the most nutritionally deficient. For example, Africans and African Americans have the highest level of malnutrition, stress, degenerative diseases, birth defects, venereal dis-eases and even the most headaches. Johns Hopkins University's research reports that the poor have 60% more headaches. Added to all Caucasian research must be the additional dis-eases caused by White Racism and Melanin deficiencies, which their science totally ignores when evaluating African Americans health.

Food is used to destroy African's health while at the same time that same constipating synthetic Caucasian food makes an abundance of profit for food companies. The dis-eases the food causes make profits for hospitals, doctors and drug companies (disease industry). Incidentally, aspirin and laxatives are the two largest selling chemicals of drug companies. The cooked junk food causes the headaches (aspirin use) and constipation (laxative use). Africans are indoctrinated (so-called educated) to believe that they are born to be sick or born in sin. Indoctrination teaches you what to think while education teaches you how to think. African people are indoctrinated until they believe that they are going to get sick no matter what they eat or do not eat. They think that you must die from disease and often say, "You gonna die from something, so why should

I eat health foods." The Caucasian society reinforces this nutritional mis-educational thinking.

There are many countries, (United States of America, Canada, England, France, etc.), that have hospitals with drug stores, emergency medical services, clinics and ambulances everywhere. They sell drugs for dis-eases at gas stations, grocery stores and amusement parks and everyone buys them including doctors, nurses and morticians (undertakers). African people are carefully taught to be junk food addicts. They are merely permanent hospital outpatients with some type of walking dis-ease believed to be caused by a bacteria or virus instead of the Caucasian. Because of the manmade (Caucasian) synthetic foods, Africans walk around with a fear that their own body will fail to be healthy or that their body will fall apart or self destruct from a mysterious germ that has attacked them. It is the Nutricidal actions of the Caucasians that have attacked all African people. Furthermore, Nutricidal "certified Negroes" reject health food and will say that they are not dietary extremists like the African health food and vegetarian dieters. Consequently, they eat in 'moderation' which means their diet is a mixture of Caucasian junk food and health food. 'Moderation' is used as an excuse to stay addicted to Caucasian junk food, junk culture and junk religions.

Junk culture is a mixture of Caucasian culture in a superior position and African culture in an inferior position. These "certified Negroes" can be seen wearing European tuxedos and African Kente cloth bow ties, high heels and straightened hair with an African gown; celebrating Christmas, Thanksgiving, Valentine's Day or St. Patrick's Day or other Caucasian holidays. They pledge allegiance to Caucasian cultural perversions of religions (Jews, Christians and Muslims) with the use of books written by and for Caucasians such as the *Torah, The King James Version of the Bible and the European Arabic Koran*. These religions refer to African religion as sinful, inferiorize women and Africa. In any case, junk food, junk culture and junk religions addicts may call themselves "moderates." However, the deadly effect of all junk is Nutricide, spiriticide and genocide = death.

There are many alibis (excuses) used by junk addicts. For example, the addicted Negroes say that all Caucasians are not racist or that some Caucasians are nice. There are also "nice" alcoholics, drug addicts, thieves' homosexuals, rapists, cancer patients, diabetics' etc. Being "nice" does not stop white folks from having the disease of White Supremacy just as being nice does not stop diabetes. "Nice" Caucasians accept the benefits of their white skin (White Supremacy) and do not actively or militarily stop other whites from being racist. They are guilty of White Racism by passive participation and association. They live in a cracker (white racist) house and accept the economic benefits and social advantages from supporting the cracker (White Racism). If they were truly "nice" they would move out of the cracker house or stay in the house (work within the system) and destroy it without any African participating or telling them to do so. "Nice white folks" is another Negro excuse used to stay addicted to Caucasian junk food, junk culture and junk religions. Nutritionally, Caucasian junk food is twice as deadly to Africans.

The Caucasian uses African's history to force their dietary ignorance upon Africans. In history reportage writings Africans never read about the historical impact of foods upon themselves or the Caucasians. In fact, Africans never view themselves as a holistic part of the history that they read. In any case, omitting nutrition and food as a holistic moving force of history causes the reader to assume that all people basically eat the same as Caucasians and use Caucasian allopathic medicine. Racist Caucasians have distorted history and made it non-rhythmical (non-melanated). Caucasian historical events, dates and adventures type history reportage is static. In other words, it lacks holistic "hue-man" rhythms and does not emphasize the spontaneous changing melanated creative (Godly) African. It is the same as the Caucasian diet with cooked food (static energy), junk food (static energy) and food combining based on static (inorganic = dead) food chemistry and superstitions. Food combining is a lively African art based on the electromagnetic aura, color, rhythm and spirituality, Nutrient Male/Female Principles, cyclical laws, plant communal families and living nutrition of raw foods.

African civilization is a rhythmical communal life force of peoples in motion with nutrition and spirit. It is constantly cyclic, rhythmic, cultural, organic, balancing, changing and does not move from one static event to another stationary event like Caucasian culture. Caucasian culture and White Racism is static based on a cemented disease idea of White Supremacy and Black Inferiority. Consequently, if an African studies the Caucasian mind and behavior once then there is no realistic reason to study it again. Be that as it may, the ever changing African melanin driven social, spiritual, medical, dietary, and holistic health events are unified communally by an Elder, Drummer, Health Practitioner, Story teller, Council of the Wise member or Priest/Priestess. The melanin electromagnetic Third Eye senses the total unity purpose, harmony and beginning and end of the energy collective and unites the Africans into a singular family movement. For example, the Elders' primary purpose is to holistically censor, synchronize and balance the spontaneity of all the different cultural, spiritual, mental and emotional forces that simultaneously occur in the community before, during and after a social event. The Caucasian myth about Africans creates the image that Africans are frozen in static (inorganic) traditions (ceremonies and rituals) that move from one ceremony and ritual to another ceremony and ritual. The subtle and electrical movements that Africans have in relationship to universal changes (cycles) and universal change impact on melanin is too fast an energy exchange for Caucasian albino historians to note. The power of the melanin force can remove White Racism disease within Africans. Africans can never completely lose their true Africanity, ethics, aesthetics, morals, Godliness, communal approach to life, drumming, science, diet, dance, health, herbs, discipline, order and identity despite Nutricide.

There are a few words that hide the crimes of Nutricide. The Caucasians use the words "Western Science," "Modern Man," 'The Western Countries," "manmade," "Modern Medicine," "Scientific Proof," "Statistics," "Education," "Professional License," "Certified" etc., all of which means Caucasian. It is not "Modern Man" that has polluted the earth, it is the Caucasian man/woman. It is not "Western Medicine," it is Caucasian medicine. It is not an "Education," it is a Caucasian approved "Indoctrination." It is not junk food; it is Caucasian scavenger foodstuff. It is not "degenerative diseases." It is Caucasian dis-eases. It is not a world full of wars and violence; it is a Caucasian world of war and violence.

African peoples everywhere must eat natural foods to be healthy. Caucasians are the ones producing these natural foods for other Caucasians to eat because a Caucasian with a natural foods diet is still a White Racist. It is the natural foods industry that believes that they will always be in control of the natural foods and Africans will always be consumers never producers. In the past the Caucasians have had control over health food movements and perverted them. For example, Dr. Kellogg was a pioneer in the health food industry. He started the use of fibrous and nutritionally rich whole corn flakes. Today, Kellogg's corn flakes are a junk food. There are more nutrients and fiber in the box than in the flakes. He performed many surgical removals of part of the colon to adapt it to junk food. Dr. Graham started the use of nutritionally rich and fibrous cracked whole-wheat crackers. Today his "graham" crackers are junk food. Of one of the early Caucasian health food movements only the mealtime salad remains. It is reduced to a junk food with synthetic salad dressing. The Caucasian health food movements usually ruin themselves. They eat health foods in order to run from diseases not because it is a part of their spirituality. In African culture, health food keeps you spiritual and African.

Caucasian health food industry usually ruins itself because it is part of their diseased mentality. The natural foods industry is still an unnatural Caucasian racist industry. They manufacture supplements and herbs for themselves without African ethno-medicine or ethno-nutritional or ethno-food consciousness. These Caucasians are becoming physically fit with a diseased White Supremacist dysfunctional mind. They are totally capable of continuing Nutricide on another level. It must be historically noted that it was Caucasian Arabs on health foods that had Eastern Africans in the most vicious evil form of chattel enslavement in East Africa for over 1,000 years. Then the Caucasians called Eastern Europeans and Western Europeans (these are Caucasians that do not live in China or India) were on cooked natural foods when they started the Western African slave trade. This slave trade forcefully brought Africans to North and South America. Slavery and colonialism contributed to the mass murder of at least 200 million Africans.

The Caucasians label any Caucasian that has killed 5 people or more as a mass murderer and mentally ill. They then look into the history of the mass murderer and identify the ingredients that created the killer's insane mind. If an African should use Caucasian standards then by definition the Caucasian race is one of a mass murderer (killed over 200 million Africans) and is mentally ill. Examine the Caucasians history and it will reveal the ingredients that shaped their insanity. Ironically, any African that truthfully labels and identifies the Caucasian race as a race of mass murderers that are biochemically and mentally insane, will be classified as angry, hostile, full of hate and/or a Black racist. An African with a "slaves mentality" will verbally attack and character assassinate any African that speaks truthfully about the dis-eased mind, spirit, biochemistry (melanin albino) and behaviors of Whites.

Caucasians on health foods murdered, raped, enslaved and destroyed African land. Again, a physically fit Caucasian is still a white supremacist. The only thing that an African can gain from a healthy Caucasian is more Nutricide. A book such as *How the White Man's Diet Affects Natives of Africa* by Albert Schweitzer can give some insight. The extent of the crime of Nutricide is far reaching. Nutricide not only occurs before birth but during birth as well. A natural delivery, which is drug free, allows the umbilical cord to stop pulsating before being cut. The baby's delivery is in the squatting position. Relatives, extended family and a midwife are present, and Africentric rituals and ceremonies are used. The natural birth allows the normal contractions to help drain the fluid out of the lungs, stimulates the lymph fluid, cerebral spinal fluid and helps send nourishing blood, oxygen, and nutrients to the child's brain. Drug induced contractions nutritionally rob the brain, causes a sympathetic response in the child while a parasympathetic response is normal, weakens the immune system, pollutes the liver, pancreas and thyroid, and reduces the electromagnetic and biochemical responses of melanin. A Cesarean Section (C- Section) interrupts the synchronic cyclic rhythm of mother and child, and causes lung diseases, behavioral problems, slow growth and/or retarded growth. Instead of nutritionally solving this problem Caucasian doctors add to the problem with their interruption and interference with the Bonding and Nutritional Rites of Passage of birthing.

There are psychological aspects to Caucasian interference with African births. For example, the Caucasian indoctrinates Africans to believe that a baby has a birthday. This logic is used to inferiorize women and de-Africanize Africans. In African culture the mother (Isis) has a birthday as she gives birth to the child. The child cannot birth itself. The child has a day of "emergency" as it emerges from the mother's womb. The only true emergency occurs at a child's birth. It is part of Caucasian diseased individualism to think "I had my own birth" or "all for me" or "me for me." It helps to affirm their White Supremacy, which says they are the center of the world. They believe that their scientific drugs are the solution for all things. They proceed to solve the medical problems they created by creating a synthetic chemical (drug) problem.

Caucasian medicine defines any problem the child has after their drug and surgery interference with natural birth as a bio-chemical problem of the baby. They use drugs to torture the African child's entire body combined with the torture of the C-section surgical operation. What awaits the child as a consequence of a C-Section are drugs for asthma, bronchitis, behavior problems, colds, learning problems, hormones and melanin problems which the Caucasians created before and during birth. Books by R. S. Mendelsohn MD, titled *Confessions of a Medical Heretic and Male-Practice*, document the Nutricide crimes.

The Nutricide problems that are started at birth are never corrected. In fact, the Caucasian junk food diet compounds the problems. They proceed to classify Caucasian created problems as a genetic brain illness that causes violence, and learning problems. Ritalin or similar type drugs are given in addition to Genetic altering drugs. Ritalin is a narcotic that is in the same category as cocaine. It retards growth, increases blood pressure, attacks melanin, weakens immunity, and is toxic to the brain and nerves. The use of drugs such as Ritalin has not been documented to increase intelligence or performance. They simply make the African child a dope robot, alter the normal biochemistry and give the child a predisposition for mental, physical and spiritual addictions.

Ritalin is a chemical solution for a Caucasian indoctrination problem called education. The mental and physical chemistry between the African child and the Caucasian educational system is the problem, not the chemistry of the child. Aside from this, drugs that are given to African children by the public schools are actually based on money. It is profit motivation that causes the schools to drug African children. The schools, hospitals, medical science, and food companies run a cash and carry business. They receive cash money for every child that swallows drugs. Schools get more money from the federal government if they can qualify children for certain problems. The federal government offers more money to schools that have children with mental or behavioral problems. The federal money given to schools to treat children with special problems is used for salaries (extra pay), supplies, books and other items the school needs. The schools desiring the money can conveniently find that 40% of the children have behavioral and/or mental problems or brain damage. The drugs are given to the children despite the unscientific diagnosis for their use. They give African children such narcotics as Ritalin or other behavioral drugs such as Toframil, Cylert, or Dexedrine. African children are basically drugged because of the nutritional problems Caucasians created before, during and after birthing.

Drugging the child covers up teacher's failure to educate, psychologist failure to counsel and parent's lack of parenting skills. The Black parent tries to be the village in order to educate the child. However, a parent is not a village. Consequently, the parent compensates for not being the village by giving the child expensive clothes, or cable TV, X-rated shows and movies to watch and allows computer games to parent the child. This further dysfunctionalizes the addicted child and co-dependent addicted child.

A co-dependent child is an non-drug-addicted schoolmate of an addicted child. Non-addicted school children are forced to socialize with the addicts. This causes the Ritalin addicts classmates to develop distorted emotions, feelings, thoughts and behaviors in order to survive the addict and socialize with the addict. A co-dependent creates a dysfunctional personality. This once mentally healthy classmate of the addict recreates themselves into a distorted personality in order to maintain a relationship with the addict. The co-dependent playmate of the addict changes into a personality that can complement, maintain and feed off the dis-eased Ritalin addict. The addict's entire classroom of children becomes affected and infected with forms of mental illnesses. Co-dependents will have dysfunctional relationships and dysfunctional children in order to feel normal.

A dysfunctional African is by definition a "seasonin" African (a slave) an economic benefit to Whites. Whites earn money (capital, profits) from all types of African dysfunction. Dysfunctional African children and adults buy material goods to be comfortable in their oppression-slavery. White Supremacy can only be successful if and only if Whites create and maintain dysfunctional Blacks.

Once a disease (Dysfunctionality, AIDS, Cancer, Hyperactivity, Crime, Homosexuality, White Racism etc.) becomes an industry it never dies. The disease industry moves to protect itself by periodically coming out with a new model. This means new signs and symptoms for disease, new research findings, new crimes (hate crimes), new treatments and drugs therapies. They must constantly redefine the disease, create a new disease within the old disease so that the industry can expand its market share and profits. Dis-ease no longer functions as a disease; it functions as a business—a Nutricide business.

The Nutricide of African people has many dimensions. It is not seen or acted upon by African scientists, militants, freedom fighters, social activist, teachers, preachers, entertainers, parents, professionals, writers, historians or prisoners because most of them are already nutritionally dead. They are so infected with Nutricide that they only dance to the drum of McDonalds, Swine, Alcohol, Coca-Cola, KFC, coffee or some other Caucasian food chemical company. They can no longer dance to the rhythm of natural food. Natural foods that enhance the rhythm of the pineal gland are the same foods that African ancestors used to create the first university, civilization and nutritional science of the world. African junk food addicts are involved in spiriticide because they use Caucasian written religious books and pray to the Caucasian idea of Allah, God, Jesus, Jehovah, Yahweh, Ra or any other assortment of saints and ask that their Caucasian food be blessed. They join in a Caucasian conspiracy against their own health. These Negroes are taught to ignore that the melanin deficient Caucasian mind is nutritionally dysfunctional, unstable and non-rhythmic. This causes Caucasians to have unstable personalities. An unstable Caucasian bonds to fear, superstitions and self-hatred very strongly. Stability or rhythm in thought and life is a specific melanin dominate African characteristic. In the book, *Biological Rhythms in Human and Animal Physiology*, Gay Gaer Luce, stresses the importance of rhythm (the more melanin the more rhythm).

The African junk food addict arrogantly defends junk food. "Arrogance" is a learned Caucasian characteristic. Arrogance occurs when a White Supremacist exaggerates their fantasized superior self-worth in an overbearing manner and defends it with pride. This Caucasian disease of arrogance is exhibited when Africans arrogantly assume that their group is the only group that is aware and conscious. For example the African Christians, Jews, Moslems, Khemetics, Vegetarians and/or Health food dieters and history, political and social activist groups assume that their individual groups are the only group that is aware or conscious of the proper way to be African or obtain freedom. They will arrogantly state that other groups are not conscious and holding back the race from progress. All Africans, regardless of their level of consciousness or awareness, are working to uplift the race unless diseased by White Racism. Arrogance is a type of slave or colonial mentality. Arrogance is another tool given Africans to destroy themselves and their children. It is the children that need nutritional salvation and not some group's ideological plantation. Nutricide has slowly distorted the thinking and dis-eased the body of all arrogant Africans.

Nutricide is a slow degenerative disease process. It is disguised because Africans are trained to think that constantly getting sick or being sick is normal. They are trained to think that the habitual taking of non-prescription and prescription drugs is normal. It is normal for Caucasians to be sickly but not Africans. Drugs, medical procedures, cooked foods and junk foods cause diseases.

Nutricide is further compounded by Africans blind religious belief in Caucasian science, a science that solves nothing and cures nothing. Caucasian science is totally designed to create and support White Supremacy. Science means to "know" and melanin is the organic bodily substance that makes one "know." The more melanin the more "knowing." Historically, it has been the Africans that "know" astrology, Dogon Star, Sirius, Galaxies, cycles, God, architecture, nutrition, acupuncture, human relationship, biology and chemistry. Melanin albinos (Caucasians) copy the knowers (Melanin Dominant Africans). The Caucasians do not know and have to search, research and then write fantasy superstitions in a science language, which only Caucasians have the stupidity to call science. The basis for all science is melanin. For example, biology is the study of how melanin within cells directs energy. The melanin nucleus is the brain and control center for all life activities in cells. Chemistry is the study of the interaction of melanin with melanin. Scientifically speaking, if Africans flushed all the Caucasians science books down the toilet, it would be the worst thing to happen to the sewer and the best thing to happen for the African science students.

Nutricide is scientifically disguised and misdiagnosed. For example, the Caucasians non-cyclic control of light and dark in hospital infant nurseries can cause pineal gland immaturity. Light manipulation weakens the pineal, immunity and predisposes the child for junk food Nutricide. Nutricide is the most democratically distributed form of death among all Africans and reaches into the future by nutritionally destroying the yet to be born. This demonstrates how Africans have been taught to be disconnected to the spiritual purpose of food.

Food that has been irradiated, rodenticided, synthetically fertilized, insecticided, herbicided, cloned with human/insect/animal cells, and processed with synthetic chemicals is in need of godly prayers and protection from Caucasians. It is not the Caucasian pollution of plants that are the greatest health fear. It is the minds of the Caucasians. In other words, Africans should not be afraid of the created monster Frankenstein. It is his creator Doctor Frankenstein that is to be feared. In any case, protection and reparation to "nature" are the spiritual right of plants, air, water, soil and Africans. Reparation for Nutricide is beyond the comprehension of the practicing insane (Caucasians). Africans that benevolently ask the Caucasians to voluntarily pay reparations might as well ask white people to stop having white skin. A new standard of reparation must be developed to meet the requirements demanded by Africans, as the white standards are for "Whites Only."

The standard for reparations is entrenched in Caucasian superstition and psychosis. For example, Caucasian science, nutrition, medicine and social science uses the belief that the natural existence of life is confusion, antagonistic, a conflict, and contrary to nature then becomes confused, chaotic and die. This linear logic justifies their continued psychotic need to dominate and Nutricide Africans. In Caucasian allopathic medicine (medical doctors) the fundamental belief concept is that "contrary cures opposite." This means that to be against nature cures nature of disease and confusion. If reparation is left to the devices of Caucasians it will follow the concept that contrary to reparation solves the reparation problem. Reparation will be another tool of destruction used against Africans just as nutrition is a tool for destroying Africans.

Reparation obtained from mentally ill Caucasians is in itself a crazy concept. Sane people can pay reparations to sane people. However, any demand of reparations made against the mentally ill is questionable. In other words, African people would have to decide how much the thief (Caucasian) should keep of what they have stolen. This is what Africans call reparations. No thief has any rights to claim any part of what they have stolen. The Caucasians will never accept themselves as being insane thieves that warrant punishment or habilitation. Reparations mean that all of the Caucasians, countries, and religions must pay money for killing over 200 million Africans during colonialism and slavery. Added to this, they must pay for Africans lynched via drugs, by police, in jails, as a result of drug experiments, medical treatments, eating junk foods, mis-educated mental deaths, alcohol, cigarettes lead poisoned, syphilis, killed fighting in Caucasian wars and abortion victims. They (Caucasians) must pay for the direct death of potential offspring of those murdered. Aside from this, the Caucasians must give back the economic profits they got from 450 years of free slave labor, the money and profits of the over 10 million dollars in gold and jewels given to the U.S.A. for distribution to ex-slaves by Emperor Menelik in 1865. Pay for the patents stolen from George Washington Carver and many other inventors. Pay for the stolen music copyrights of Fats Waller and other musicians. Pay for the stolen resources of Africa such as gold, diamonds, books, tin, wood, land, uranium, plutonium, trees, ivory, oil and treasures looted from ancient cities and Egyptian tombs. Again, no thief has any rights to claim what they have stolen. Therefore, the Caucasians must give back what they have stolen, and then reparations can begin. Anything else would be an insult to our ancestors. Only a sane people can be punished or pay reparation. Caucasians would have to be habilitated. Habilitation means they must learn to live in holistic harmony with themselves, nature and then other races. After habilitation the Caucasians should be holistically balanced (reparations) and then rehabilitated. Reparations in Caucasian linear logic means punishment while with Africans it means healing and harmony with God. Reparations for Nutricide are part of the reparations that the Caucasian must confront in order to gain some form of sanity.

African Woman Nutricide/Cultural Genocide

African men and women are faced with one reality and that is to rid African culture of nutritional and cultural genocide. Male sexism against the African American woman obviously exploits, oppresses and denies the African woman her human rights. Currently, the African woman is assumed a "slave of a slave" (African man). "Seasonin" during slavery caused the mental enslavement of men and women. It needs to be eliminated. A holistic balance requires new words and deeds of behavior from the African man. Reparations for years of African relationship, spiritual, mental, physical and cultural genocide are necessary, yet risky. Risky because a new definition for the African man's mental, spiritual and social cleansing has not yet been defined. This cannot be defined until the woman/man unity effort puts holistic cleansing in motion. A spiritual dis-ease that caused the African man to act upon himself and upon the African woman with mutilation called infibulation, excision, hair relaxers, circumcision, earnings, bleaching cream, nose rings and high heels makes the African woman's physical body a sacrifice. Black male sexism as well as female feminism requires the power to have human rights. Human rights and civil rights can only be guaranteed by a group that has control over resources and land. There are no individual or relationship rights and freedom without a group to protect the rights and freedoms.

The African male and female can only imitate Caucasian relationship problems and assume they are their own problems. It is the same as a slave saying "Master we are sick." Sexism and feminism are merely former slave individuals and relationship methods of coping with and confronting racism and slavery trauma in each other and in the relationship. It is a mechanism to divide and conquer. Typically, the relationship is based upon confusion (love). Love defined by Caucasians is a mysterious feeling, an accidental falling in lust (love), a battle of the sexes and a heavenly confusing thing. Caucasian love used by Africans creates confusion resulting in divorces, adultery, destroyed children and destroyed culture. All social customs, rituals, ceremonies, dance, music, make-up, artifacts, clothes, monogamy, polygamy and current Africentric values must be disrupted, lives upset and a new holistic order enacted.

The African woman and man's current spirit was not Maat or mother bonded. They were not breast fed 3 to 5 years. The man was not married to the African woman by the family or the elders' decision process. He was not fed natural foods. He was not trained in the rites of passage. He *has* been under Nutricide. He does not use sexual regeneration. He erotically looks at her buttocks' where manure evacuates, her cellulite legs and milk feeding breasts and uses Caucasian romance instead of spiritualized unity. He demands that women wear makeup and high heels and allows the woman to be abused by PMS as a norm. The African man today can not behave as he did in the past. The African man must defeat his acts of enslavement of the African woman. Furthermore, the African man must live and act according to a new woman/man order whose Maat definition is yet to unfold.

The White Supremacy of the Caucasian has a total effect upon the African man/woman relationship. The relationship is not normal because it is under Caucasian siege with psychosocial battlefield conditions. The African man suffers from the side effects of racism and Nutricide, which impacts the African woman with enslavement. He lives in a culture that alienates him and his mate from adulthood; in turn he alienates the African woman from her womanhood. The African man suffers from the effects of being inferiorized by the Caucasian man. He has withdrawn from the traumatic emotional, mental and spiritual impact of slavery. In this distortion the African man suffers from Nutricide.

The African woman's intellectual and emotional partnership with the African man is believed to be controlled by the moon instead of Maat. The use of the moon as a timing device of the galaxy can indicate changes. The moon's sunlight reflection has an impact on water, tides and menstruation. Ironically, the African man's body has 10% more water than the woman does and the woman has 10% more fat (earth attribute) than the man does. So it would follow that the man's body would respond to the moon with equal if not greater force than the woman's does. It must also be taken into consideration that the man's body is half female in hormonal and anatomical structure. The role of the woman as an equal partner against racism is defined by whites as a sort of "slave of a slave." This is based on Caucasian religious beliefs, superstitions and mainly chauvinism.

Historically, it is documented that African women were soldiers, presidents of countries, Supreme Court judges (Chief of the Council of Elders). Men equally parented and raised children, wore dresses (gowns), make-up and mutilated their bodies with earrings. The African man's Caucasian created image is that of being an irresponsible parent. The Johns Hopkins Children's Center, of Baltimore, Maryland, study (1992-1993) of married, separated and single

parents indicated that over 74% of the African fathers were active
in parenting and during pregnancy. The paternal instinct is media
controlled and depressed in today's African man. His attributes of
being a "gentle-man" or having a Female Principle are depressed. It
is part of his depressed Female Principle that allows the African
woman's nutritional exploitation to go unchecked. Nutricidal diseases are added to her oppression. Africans are forced to be poor
under Caucasian domination which makes all disease rates the
highest. Diseases decrease the quantity and the quality of life. Diseases in African Americans are caused by Caucasian social and environmental factors. The Department of Health and Human Services Task Force on Black Health reported this information from its
research.

The effects of Nutricide are brutal assaults against the African
woman. The disease of Premenstrual Syndrome (PMS) is being
used as a Caucasian weapon to distort the woman/man relationship. PMS causes at least 15 days of each month to be emotionally
and intellectually hostile for men as well as women. This hostility
can result in arguments, negative feelings, divorces, fights, crimes,
and promiscuous sexual behavior and child abuse. PMS goes untreated because it is chauvinistically defined as normal.

The Caucasian junk food diet creates PMS because it does not
have vital nutrients. The body and mind react to being nutritionally starved to death with PMS or fibroid tumors. For example, the
junk diet is low in Riboflavin, which affects memory, low in Beta-
Carotene, which decreases cognitive skills, low in manganese,
which results in low pineal, pituitary and thyroid functions. Low
manganese decreases the mother's instincts and is related to diabetes, high blood pressure, hypoglycemia, epileptic seizures and myas-
thenia gravis, while low dietary potassium is related to hypoglycemia, high blood pressure, heart problems. Low selenium is related
to sudden infant crib death; low copper is related to postpartum de-

pression and hyperactivity; low manganese is also related to irritability, muscle tremors, depression; and low vanadium is related to decreased birth weight and high death rates. These are just some of the nutrients lacking in the African woman's diet when she eats Caucasian junk foods and cooked foods. This diet causes the African woman to be weak and not fully nutritionally in control of her life and health. African women are not tested for nutrient deficiencies. If tested, it is by the normal standards of the Caucasian woman. These Caucasian standards for normal indicate a subclinical form of malnutrition in African women, because Africans have a higher mineral level, lower protein level and higher Vitamin D level related to melanin metabolism of ultra-violet rays and starches.

When an African's health is reduced to a low Caucasian nutrient state the Caucasian science reads it as normal. No ethno- medical steps are taken to improve African health using African nutrient levels as the standard Instead they wait until the level falls Africentricity low and is viewed simply as normal for Caucasians. In other words, the African woman is twice as sick as the Caucasian woman is. Therefore, the African woman's PMS, and other dis-ease states, disease reactions and recovery is twice as horrible. Added to this, the Nutricide continues and multiplies the dis-ease beyond the scope of the Caucasian.

A natural foods and raw foods diet could stop the dis-eases of premature births, birth defects, spontaneous abortions, menstruation difficulties and holistic disease attacks on women's bodies. *Nutrition Against Disease*, by Roger Williams reviews these problems. Aside from these Nutricidal dis-eases, eclampsia is a dis-ease of poor nutrition which strikes the poor severely. Africans are forced to be poor and undernourished under Caucasian domination. This makes all disease rates the highest.

Eclampsia is a toxic convulsive condition of late pregnancy. Hypertension is usually a contributing factor and statistically higher

African Americans suffer from hypertension. The woman with eclampsia will have swollen feet and legs, spots before the eyes, severe headaches, and dizziness which if untreated leads to a coma and death. There is mild eclampsia and just as in any disease, there are various degrees of torture. Eclamptic behavior can be present and unnoticed. The American Medical Association has offered no cure for eclampsia, or the common cold for that matter. African women fall prey to all of the Caucasian woman's diseases by eating what Caucasians eat. The white male supremacist, medical profession does not acknowledge melanin. They do not consider White Racism, biochemical differences or the fact that women exhibit disease symptoms differently from men. They do not evaluate the nutritional factors of dis-ease.

The Nutricide of the African woman starts early. A life of dis-ease is believed to be normal. The Caucasian anti-melanin diet causes hormonal imbalances in African women. Hormone imbalances cause cholesterol to accumulate. For example, high cholesterol and low bile acid in the liver's gall bladder can cause gallstones. The gall bladder holds about two cups of bile. However, the junk food diet exhausts the liver, pineal, pituitary, thyroid, pancreas and sex glands. The liver is not able to emulsify fats or get rid of excess estrogen. Thus, cholesterol is not emulsified and it sticks together and forms stones. Women are at a higher risk for stones because estrogen imbalances can increase the cholesterol.

Other waste accumulates in the body causing arteriosclerosis, varicose veins and atherosclerosis. The arteries get blocked or clogged and in the case of varicose veins, the legs cramp and become painful. This varicose condition is inside the body as well. In any case, clogged or blocked vessels give Caucasian medicine a chance to profit from the Nutricidal diseases that they have created. Coronary artery bypass surgery is used to replace constipated, blocked or clogged vessels. Coronary bypass replaces 2 to 3 inches of a vessel while leaving the other 99% of the artery clogged with liquid manure called plaque. In other cases, long pig veins or plastic veins are surgically used to replace clogged veins, which eventually get clogged from the junk diet.

The University of California Medical School has increased nutrition, lowered fat and cholesterol and removed 70% of the plaque from clogged vessels by diet. However, hospitals and doctors operate a business and are paid over $50,000 per operation. The Medical Review Board cannot prove that the operation is medically feasible. After the bypass the patient develops plaque in the new arteries within 5 years. Nutricide causes the disease. Mutilation of the woman's body for beauty reasons or godly reasons is not only physically destructive, but has mental and historical aspects as well.

The mutilation of the body can be subtle, such as earrings, circumcisions or overt; such as during slavery Africans' tongues were cut out (removed). Tongues were removed to prevent Africans who spoke the same language from communicating. Front teeth were knocked out with hammers so that Africans who protested slavery by starvation protest could be forced fed. Furthermore, Caucasians would remove (amputate) feet, legs, hands, arms, lips, ears and other body parts, or cut open a pregnant woman's stomach and cut up the unborn child as punishment for attempting to run away, talk back, fight or in any way demand human rights. Slaves that attempted to hit a white would be mutilated (whipped) in the face until the flesh hung from the face.

The Caucasians started scalping the heads of Africans to serve as evidence that a slave was murdered. Scalping was believed to disconnect the silver cord, which is the pineal gland electromagnetic connection with higher forces (God). Scalping mutilations are not an American Indian (Native) custom, but a Caucasian custom which natives used in retaliation against the Caucasian scalpers. Scalping is connected to Caucasian cannibalism ceremonies. Incidentally, mild forms of cannibalism are practiced when Caucasians give their children candy lips to eat or human-shaped vitamins to eat (Flintstones vitamins). It demonstrates that they are still attached to the Ice Age mentality, violence, self-hatred, cannibalism and a melanin deficit dysfunctional mind.

A melanin dominant African, who has been breastfed, bonded and raised on a natural foods diet has a nutritionally nourished pineal gland, and has a chance to be holistic. The pineal gland's melanin acts as a coordinator, clock, interpreter, receiver, and transmitter and storage center of holistic information. It is not the primary clock in the body. Clock-like cycles of cells, enzymes, organs, blood, minerals, smell, taste, sight, vitamins, pressure, organ systems tend to be independent of rest, exercise, darkness, light and nutrition. The above factors can influence rhythmic cycles and do so electromagnetically, and have female and male attributes. The female and male attributes can stop the mutilations.

Africans who still mutilate the African woman are totally unholistic as well as those who give bloodletting and animal sacrifices spiritual significance. The woman's vaginal lips and clitoris are removed. A spiritual ceremony is used to justify this cannibalistic behavior. Excisions, or removing the clitoris and infibulation, the removing of the vaginal lips' which leaves the uterus exposed is done and was done among the Dogon, Mandingoes, Tukolor, etc. This practice is performed today in hospitals such as Gabriel-Toure, Hospital Bamako, Mali and is still performed in Niger, Somalia, Egypt, Yemen, Jordan, Benin, Southern Algeria, Syria, Iraq, Ethiopia, Saudi Arabia, Sudan, Senegal, Guinea, Burkina Faso (Upper Volta), Ivory Coast, etc.

Mutilation is a physical act that is first created in the mind and spirit. In other words, it is a crude symbolic representation of a need to damage God's creation in order to appease damage within. If the mutilation was just, (and it never is) a man would remove his own foreskin completely and his scrotum (exposing the testicles) because of the need to satisfy self-hatred and betrayal within him. But instead, the man uses the woman's body to mirror his own misadventures in spirit and mind. A holistic cleansing ritual for the man and child in harmony with the woman/child bonding could resolve this age-old excision and infibulation. This could help restore the African woman back to her drone of Goddess and "She-ro" (i.e., female hero).

African women were praised as the most holistically beautiful women in the entire world. Great African women such as Queen Hatsheput, Nefetari, Ty of the Egyptian 18th Dynasty, Queen Candace of Ethiopia and Queen Katabla, 16th century Queen Nzingha who defeated the Portuguese, 18th century Queen Aora Poku, leader of the Baule of the Ivory Coast, Queen Zenobia, Queen Ngokady, Pyann, Ngeede of Kuba Kingdom and the queens who ruled Cush for 600 years.

There are numerous unsung contemporary queens such as Harriet Tubman or Mary Seacole (the real Florence Nightingale), Charlotte Ray the first African American lawyer (1872), Rebecca Lee, M.D., (1864) first African American woman doctor and Pigs Foot Mary (Lillian Harris) 1901, first African American woman to accumulate a large fortune etc.

The Caucasian man, woman and homosexuals have a great fear of the African woman's superiority, so they inferiorize her. Ironically, Caucasians at the same time are imitating her by making their limp fur (so called hair) kinky (curly), wearing brassieres, wearing buttock pads, wearing Egyptian (African) clothes to sleep in (night gowns), using cosmetics to darken skin, eyes and lips, using earrings, doing lip enlargement operations, wearing girdles to imitate Africoid hip development, sun tanning, buying sex manuals to imitate Africans, trying to dance like African women, and attempting to have an Africoid rhythmic walk (so called switching). The

African woman is represented by ancient paintings and statues of the Black Madonna (Isis) which are found in countries such as Italy, Germany, Poland, France, Spain, Guatemala, Greece, etc. The mutilation of the African woman's beauty with hair relaxers, bleaching creme, high heels, Nutricide, hospitals, and drugs is profound. Mutilation not only maims and cripples; it deprives women of an essential part of holistic life such as bonding and sexual regeneration.

Sexual regeneration is also the nutrient reabsorption of injaculatory fluids by the lymphatic tissue. Some of those nutrients are selenium, methionine, glycogen phosphorus, zinc, lactic acid, lecithin, calcium, choline, histidine, vitamins C and E, trace elements, melanin hormones, electromagnetic energy etc. The nutrients are not ejaculated out of the body of the woman or man. Instead, these nutrients are injaculated (recycled) and serve to fertilize the pineal gland, melanin centers of the brain, chakras (melanin centers of the body), and the cells within the body. The brain has high amounts of the same nutrients as the seminal fluids. Consequently, injaculation excites and enhances the brain. Excessive ejaculatory sex (nongenerative) causes an excessive loss of vital nutrients which degenerates health, immunity, and melanin centers while depleting nerve reception, storage and transmission. This causes mood swings, outbursts of violence, unstable personalities and memory storage difficulty. The sudden climatic ejaculation of vital nutrients causes shaking, a climax of tension, tension release and fatigued relaxation erroneously called an orgasm.

The mucous lining of the woman's uterus absorbs the nutrients in the ejaculated seminal fluid. These fluids can be found present in the woman's blood an hour or more after sexual intercourse. The sex glands injaculated release of nutrient fluids can be caused by sexual spiritualization, trance or physical sexual excitation. Normal injaculated internal secretions excite the cerebral fluid, fluid filled ventricles of the brain, and the sympathetic and parasympathetic nervous system. A highly acidic diet (junk food, drugs, cooked food), excessive ejaculation and sexual excitation (movies, dance, videos, games, music) weakens the vital trace nutrients, electromagnetism, and Ankh Force supply. This perverts the body's biochemical balance. Furthermore, this can cause children to be born with a deficient nutrient biochemistry, have a predisposition for drugs, junk foods, white culture and an inadequate melanin supply.

Bonding reinforces the Creator within the woman, child and man. It also reinforces the bond of marriage to a mate, nature, God, ancestors and Africanity. Bonding also cultivates and helps to develop holistic languages (verbal, spiritual, mathematical, astrological, dance, etc.), with God, nature the Godhead, and is basically a part of the Melanin Rites of Passage. Melanin Rites of Passage are growth cycles in which Melanin is holistically recharged. The Melanin Rites of Passage help the African child to very easily understand melanin or Caucasian so-called science.

The only science is the science of melanin. The living action of melanin in the cells of humans, animals and plants is called biology. It must be noted that the nucleus of each cell is made of melanin, and particles of melanin called electrons, protons, neutrons, and photons. They are melanin particles (family) that orbit the mother/father (nucleus). The interaction of melanin and other forms of melanin (inorganic and organic) is called chemistry. The measurement of melanin such as distance, time, cycles and cluster cloud particles are called aerodynamics, radar, clairvoyance, astrology, chakras, extrasensory perception, spirituality, etc. Again, the only science is the science of melanin.

Melanin is truly a holistic energy concentrate that harmonizes the body. Melanin should be utilized to recharge the regenerative cycle of sexual intercourse. Regeneration requires that sexual intercourse is stopped just before orgasm and the energy is recycled to the pineal gland (injaculation). In regeneration no sperm is ejaculated, it is injaculated. The orgasm energy is sent to the pineal gland in order to regenerate. The gonads, (testicles, ovaries) pineal and other glands harmoniously stimulate each other. In bonding, the pituitary, mammalian, and pineal glands synergistically rekindle each other, which increases biochemistry and the electromagnetic life force. The Trance (meditation) is a Melanin-driven event, which utilizes the Third Eye's electromagnetic cloud that vibrates above the pineal gland and sends holistic energy through all of the ventricles (holy waters).

This Melanin rite of passage is another necessary ingredient in shaping the African woman, child and man. The Caucasian melanin albinos mention none of the melanin cycles since it is not important in their life. In fact, the issue of melanin cycles is overlooked, but melanin dominated Africans can see the importance of it by looking at their Black melaninated skin. Caucasians have destroyed the melanin bond between mother/child, man/woman, and man/child and are forcing "self-centered," competitive, conflict, and "non-family centered" relationships. This does not allow melanin to be utilized in spirit, mind, psychic, nutrient absorption, higher consciousness and immune defense. It makes Nutricide more effective. African men who in any way contribute to the mutilation of the African woman cannot be called anything but diseased by White Supremacy. It is not something an African man or woman addicted to mutilation can singularly solve. Solutions and thinking are holistic to African people and not a single individual idea solution but a family and community (group) process.

The Caucasian white racist uses a thought (thinking) process and has the ability to memorize ideas in a step by step manner-process. Caucasian non-melaninated thinking is linear and adds one word to another word to make an idea. In other words, Caucasians do not conceptually spiritualize thought like an African but

merely follow thought order which they call thinking. To think
you have to be creative. Creativity is a cyclic melanin force in motion. In order to be creative one has to allow the "Creator (God)" to
enter the mind. Thinking is a spiritual process. It is not in the body,
it is of the body; it is not an activity done solely in the brain, it utilizes the brain's ventricles (holy waters), melanin centers in the
brain and body (chakras), and is rhythmic. Caucasians are not utiliz-
ing the spirit to think, so rhythm is not a part of thought for them.

African women should not be forced to mutilate (deprive)
themselves of Bonding, disfigure body parts (clitoris, labia) or cut
out holes in the skin or any other ungodly activity in order to
please a dis-ease social custom. In a cosmetic effort to appear
healthy, the African woman tries to stay slim. Staying slim on a
Caucasian junk food diet is contradictory to health and can result in
under-nutrition. The junk food diet is very poor nutritionally and
at the same time fattening. Junk food puts the woman in a weight
gain, then weight loss and then weight gain cycle. It is truly designed to keep the weight loss industry rich while mentally and
emotionally assassinating the woman. Additionally, it weakens
immunity and melanin and gives the cosmetic appearance of
health.

Nutricide and cultural genocide holistically attack every child,
woman and man. Additionally, African marriages are attacked and
restrained. Consequently, marriage is forced to be under a new holistic definition whether that marriage is monogamous or an extended family type called polygamous is inconsequential. Most African marriages are diseased. This results in diseases of African
women by holistic spiritual definitions. Whether the African man's
spirit caught this enslavement attitude of the African woman from
Caucasians or whether the African woman caught her self-mutila-
tion (earrings, nose rings, high heels, PMS, fibroid tumors) from
Caucasians or granted this illness religious approval or Karmic ap-

proval, still results in destroying the African child and family. African marriages that place romantic love which is "self-centered" above African "family centered" Maat unions, are diseased.

Africa's gift to the world is "Human Relationship" based on Maat. African women/men must give this humanistic spiritual gift to each other in order to cleanse the emotional trauma of enslavement. Despite the obstacles of this cleansing, nothing can take place without a holistically healthy body. If you are dead due to Nutricide you have no chance of being spiritually enlightened, Africentrically focused, and culturally aware of having a family centered life. You must have a living body to participate in life. If you are on a Caucasian diet, you will be a part of the White Racism/White Supremacy disease and not a part of the Africanity. Liberation of the African woman is a family effort, not a single-minded effort of African women or men. The purpose of marriage and any relationship between African peoples is to serve Maat.

Family—The First Technology of Africa

The first technology (science) of Africa is the family. In traditional European terms, technology means a scientific way to achieve a practical purpose. However, technology is a method (holistic) used to create a family, a community and a civilization. The family, holistically (body, mind, spirit) was used as the basis for all the growth and development of ancient African science and technology. The family was nourished on a diet of natural foods free of additives, dyes, synthetics, artificial ingredients and preservatives. Herbal medicine has no synthetic "medi-sins." It was a life defined without European influences or Nutricide.

In chattel slavery, slaves were forced to breed like animal livestock. Any attempt of slaves to have African cultural-type marriages and have children by God's will was met by the European slave-masters' chemical weapons (alcohol, drugs), biological warfare (diseases such as syphilis) or physical brutality. A child of an African cultural marriage was cut from the pregnant woman's belly in full view of the plantation slaves, the man's testicles were cut off and the child cooked and given to the dogs. Today, the child is allowed to be born and then attacked by the chemical warfare (synthetic foods, drugs), biological weapons (Aids, TB, cancer), and psychological weapons (miseducation, jail, recreational sex, abortions, homosexuality, selfishness) and taught to be religious, not spiritual.

One of the primary European weapons is the psychology of sexism. Sexism teaches the African man to love and have sex with the African woman as if she were a white woman (slave and master). The African woman is taught to have sex and relate to the African man as if he were a white man (slave and master). Holistic sex starts with a spiritual sharing in communion with Mother/Father God and ends with both partners sharing in communion with God. Thus, holistic sex is for procreation or regeneration, not as the European believes, for recreation. A slave's sex starts with lust and ends with a real or imagined physical climax instead of a spiritual climax. The purpose of an African couple's marriage, offspring and procreation is to strengthen and uplift the culture and family structure. In contrast, European sexism teaches Africans to marry for the ego, which is called romantic, love (lust) and family is a secondary concern. This psychological sexist weapon divides the African from the technology of the family.

The African family structure (technology) was built around the Mother/Father God concept. In this structure, each child views all adult family members as mother, father, sister or brother. For example, the child's father's brother would be called Father Uncle. The child's father's sister would be called Father Aunt. The child's mother's brother would be called Mother Uncle, and the mother's sister would be called Mother Aunt. There are Male Mothers and

Female Fathers in the African family. The child's grandparents on the father's side would be called Father Grandfather, and Father Grandmother, while the grandparents on the mother's family side would be called Mother Grandmother and Mother Grandfather. All children relate to each other as sisters and brothers, which makes all children relate to all adults as Mothers and Fathers. The adults have the same parenting responsibility to the child as the birth mother and father. If the child is disobedient, the Elders punish the parents and family and then the parents punish the child.

In the African family structure, an adult (single or married) must have their parents' permission before engaging in any social or personal activities. This family technology does not allow arguments, verbal abuse or physical violence. A husband or a wife who has a disagreement about a social, economic or parenting activity will not argue about the issue. For example, a wife will talk about a disagreement in a joking manner to the husband's brother in the case of the woman or the wife's sister in the case of the man who is in disagreement. Then the sister of the wife will confront the wife with the disagreement or complaint that was reported by her sister's husband. The wife's sister may try to resolve the conflict or disagreement between the couple. If the disagreement cannot be resolved on that level, then it is taken to the sisterhood group (age grade) leader or priestess. If the sisterhood group leader cannot resolve the disagreement, it is then taken to the parent of the mother of the wife. If that does not resolve the conflict then it is taken to the wife's grandmother. Usually the disagreement is resolved before it reaches the Council of Elders' Queen Mother.

This African family structure makes every member of the family directly responsible for every member of the family. In the pure sense of African family technology and the ancient African language, there is no such thing as an aunt, uncle, cousin, stepmother, stepfather, stepbrother, stepsister, half sister, half brother or in-laws.

Additionally, there are no adoptions because you cannot adopt a child into your family that is already in the family. There are no orphans or out-of wedlock children, called bastards. A child is born with a mother and father and is part of a family. The African family structure is holistic while the Caucasian family is fragmented. The use of the Caucasian family structure creates individualism, selfishness, dysfunction and destruction. It may sound oversimplified, but a Caucasian couple (male and female) gets married and has a family while two African families get married and have a couple (male and female union). The contemporary Caucasian practice of African men and women choosing to get married without the families' permission, control or discipline is an outgrowth of slavery and colonialism.

Slavery was started because the Europeans needed to act out their psychosis and needed technology. The European looked at the African buildings, urban cities, mathematics, chemistry, religion, industry, commerce and thought that this technology built Africa. The Europeans were completely ignorant of the fact that African technology is based on the family. The chattel slaves carried the technology in their brains stored in melanin. Melanin stores memory and intelligence. It was intelligence that guided the first cowboys in American-Africans from Gambia. They were forced to herd cattle on the Sea Islands off the East Coast of North America. The first contemporary American deep-sea divers were Africans who possessed these skills learned in Africa. Many technological skills were raped from the African family. Europeans used the profits (money) from over 400 years of free slave labor (European welfare) to build past and present wealth and empires. Europeans first destroyed the African family technology by divide-and-conquer and/or by selling family members to different plantations. The family concept is clear in African culture, science and art.

Ancient African procreation, regeneration, health, art and science were viewed from a holistic communal or family perspective. The African science of nutrition is a family-based technology. It views the relationship of the family of vitamins, family of minerals and family of proteins as a communal nutrient community. Each nutrient family has ceremonies for inter-relationship (chemical reaction) and must work in harmony with other nutrients. This electromagnetic harmony is a melanin energized Godly union. Organic (living) Gods create living (organic) nutrients. Living nutrients are designed to speed up, slow down, maintain, and stimulate energy already within "hue-mans." Living people can only use living (organic) energy to stimulate energy within. For example, a cooked apple (dead) cannot get nourishment from a live apple nor can people get positive stimulation from dead (cooked and junk) foods.

It is Caucasian superstitious science that declares that dead food is healthy and assumes that a live tree can get nourishment from dead soil. They actually believe that plants eat dirt (inorganic dead matter) for food. Food is passive and the body's action upon it is mistaken for energy in the food. The body rushes its own energy towards the food and this feeling from the body's energy is mistaken for the food's energy. Human beings at birth have all the energy they ever will have; nothing can add to it; it can be stimulated or junk food, drugs, cooked food and animal flesh as food can destroy it. Again, food is passive, people must chew it, digest it with enzymes, push it along the digestive tract with muscles, use muscles to distribute it into the body, and push it out the body as bowel movements.

The need for food is the excuse to be destructive. It is a Caucasian superstition that humans, animals and plants can only live by destroying something. They created the myth that destruction is natural in nature. Therefore, Caucasians believe that it is natural for them to destroy Africa and Africans in order to be powerful and supreme. In contrast, African nutrition is based on the communal family concept that sharing nutrient synergistic interactions for the good of all creates power. Disease is caused by holistic disobedience to Imhotep's health system. Following the health laws allows the body to cure itself of disease by nutrient family interactions.

The African holistic health system has the following principles and requirements:

- Spiritual Regeneration

- Disease and Death are abnormal

- The Body is self-healing

- Live foods for live people; herbs for medicine

- Sunshine daily, deep breathing, exercise, trance (meditation)

- Cyclic laws must be followed (i.e. eating, birth, exercise, male/female principles, etc.).

- Communal life

- Clean (unpolluted) air, water, soil, food, people (vaccinations) etc.

- Maat (means living according to Truth, Justice, Propriety, Harmony, Balance, Reciprocity and Order) in relationships with nature and people.

- African focus

The holistic family concept is applied to dimensions of life. For example, in art the colors were combined in a family. The color "Black" consists of the "color family" of indigo, violet, blue, black and red. In African music, a musical sound (note) consists of a family of sounds of partial tones (sounds). For example, the musical note "A" natural has a family of partial tones that were also called the musical note "A." On the piano, these tones are found in between the black and white keys. In nutritional science, the vitamins and minerals are a family. For example, the Vitamin "C" family also has extended family members in a communal network. The nutrient family concept was too difficult for Europeans to understand so they called the Vitamin "C" family, the Vitamin "C complex" (B complex). In ancient African universities, this advanced family science concept was in all fields of knowledge and was too difficult for Europeans to understand so they called an African college a mystery system.

The African family colossal (large stone-carved statues of African families) of men and women united by holding hands or interlocked arms standing or sitting side-by-side to show family unity, were destroyed. The female companion statue was destroyed by cannons or explosives and/or cut off by invading European armies. These invading European states did not come into existence until the fall of the Mediterranean countries of Rome and Greece. These Europeans tried to destroy the "hue-man" (human) family concept.

The word "human" (hue-man) comes from the word "hue" which means color (black, melanin) and "man" which means "thinking" the "hue-man" family or Black thinking family. Melanin (Black pigment and hormones of the pineal gland) is produced in the center of the brain. Melanin controls the internal clock (cycles) of all organs, the growth from childhood into adulthood, the time of day you sleep, the growth of hair, electromagnetic energy, spirituality and rhythm. The more melanin in the body the more rhythm and the more an individual is connected to nature, the galaxy and the sun's cycles. The Melanin/Solar connection is clear in African science, religion and physiology.

The solar (sun) cycle is obvious in African civilization. The childbirth cycle of African women having a baby every three years is a solar cycle. The newborn child's umbilical cord is connected to the solar center of the child (abdomen) and the child is carried in the solar center of the mother (abdomen). Amon Ra, a religious faith, is solar-based and the yearly calendar is of solar African origin. The African metric (meter) measuring system is solar-based. Eating food was solar-based as the heaviest meal eaten was before the sun is perpendicular (high noon) and the last meal was eaten before the sun is horizontal to the earth (sunset). African games had solar-bases such as the card games (52 cards, 52 weeks in a year, total points in the deck, 364 plus the joker an extra point for the 365 days of the year). The 4 cardinal points of the directional compass are of African solar origin. The breast-feeding of children lasted 3 to 6 years and is solar-cycled. Melanin is highly responsive to the solar cycles and electromagnetic energy of the sun and has significance in African "sexuality."

Black (African) "hue-man" nature is totally different from White nature. The digestive system processes a higher amount of nutrients, buttock muscles are more highly-developed, bone mass is 10 times greater, the White Blood Cell count is lower, the ears hear more sound (due to high melanin content), protein is recycled and the calcium requirement is lower. Africans have more fast twitch muscles, non-electric brain and nerve messages are sent via water, the body has a lower salt content and the brain processes brain waves faster and the hair has more color bands than animals. This means Africans have hair and Europeans have fur (identical to color bands of animals) which is erroneously called hair.

Africans who ignore the melanin factor in family and community (communal), fall victim to the slave mentality and go against the genetic code of their hue-man race. Africans who ignore that they evolved from God accept the Caucasian theory (fantasy belief) that they evolved from an ape. If there is an evolutionary "missing link" between man and ape it is the Caucasian. It is Caucasians who anatomically are partial ape and perhaps partial "hue-man" (black men?). It is Caucasians who have white skin, short legs, thin lips, limp hair and flat buttocks, like the ape.

The evolutionary theory is merely a fantasy idea used to justify Caucasian primitive barbaric behaviors towards Africans and other colored people. This racist evolutionary theory suggests that Caucasian have to be excused for their crimes against Africans because Caucasians are simply growing towards humanism (evolving) and are part of the African races "hue-man" family. European Nutricide, racism and sexism are destroying the African "hue-man" family.

The African woman is the direct victim of medical sexism, hysterectomies, abortions, fibroid tumors, rape, petty rape, chemical castration, birth-control pills, poor synthetic diets and scientific racism. The African woman is unprotected and denied her "hue-man rights and is given civil rights. Civil rights can be taken away by Congress or the Supreme Court. They are privileges given by Whites (Europeans) to former slaves. Hue-man rights are granted by God and cannot be given by Whites or voted upon or taken away.

The African American man makes up a large percentage of the military and police forces. This makes him the most highly armed, technologically skilled and combat-trained African soldier in the world. Militarily, he has free access and knowledge of a variety of weapons and tactics to protect and liberate his women, children, family, community, nation and himself. Yet, he stands in awe and fear of white soldiers with the same training.

The male African singers and rappers record music that popularizes sexual lust instead of marriage and family. This promotes the White Racism that is destroying the woman, child and family technology. He is also a victim of a White racism that has mentally destroyed his "hue-man" manhood and given him a slave mentality. Ironically, he makes enough money from Black-exploitation music videos, records, sports, acting, commercials, and television to sponsor Freedom revolutions in Africa, America and the world.

The ignorance of the great nutritional science of ancient Africa is destroying the family's future–children. The Nutricidal European diet has destructively replaced natural foods with cosmetic foods that look and taste good and are nutritionally valueless (junk food). This modern processed "food" is usually dyed, preserved, bleached, salted and sugared. White sugar harms the pancreas, while artificial sweeteners harm the liver. Feeding the body poorly with synthetic food also feeds the brain poorly. An undernourished brain causes learning problems, depression, violence and fatigue. High amounts of sugar cause irritability, schizophrenia, uncontrolled emotional explosions, confusion and addiction. High amounts of salt can cause waste to stay in the body, depression and mood swings. Junk "foods" are low in vitamins which can cause paranoia and personality problems. These European processed foods are a weapon used against our children. An over abundance of valid research has proven this Nutricide to be a weapon.

In New York City, a ten year study was conducted on 803,000 children (over 60% Black) by the University of California, at Berkeley, School of Nutrition. This research was presented at The International Conference on Nutrient Brain Functions hosted by the American College of Nutrition at Scottsdale, Arizona. In the study, the school children who ate school breakfast and lunch on a natural diet got the highest Achievement Test scores at all grade levels and had the highest intelligence gain in United States history. Aside from this, disruptive behaviors and dropout rates decreased dramatically. Additionally violence, learning problems, short attention spans, suicides, rape and drug addiction had a 45% decrease in 25 studies with over 20,000 juvenile prison inmates (over 70% Black) in 7 different states. Virginia Wesley University, Southern Mississippi University, Johns Hopkins University and California State

University conducted this research. Basically, the nutritional research returned the African children to the natural foods diet of ancient Africa. These studies made three basic changes in the diet. Bleached white flour was taken out of the diet, white sugar in food was reduced by 3 to 5% and all preservatives were removed (including dyes. flavorings). Sodas were eliminated and fruit juices were substituted. Ironically, private schools in Connecticut and New Jersey saw the results and started buying natural food from the New York Public Schools.

There are natural supplements available to prevent mental (learning) and physical diseases of children. Profit-motivated companies are allowed to mask the nutritional starvation and death of African children. This means no future for the African family. The food industry has no moral concern for African children. Added to this, the National Academy of Sciences has lowered the recommended daily allowance of vitamins, minerals and other nutrients. This information can be used to lower the amount of money spent on school lunch programs, federally sponsored food programs, and food stamps. This is a strategy used to aid in the deterioration of African children and senior citizens' health and will increase disease. This is done at a time when the number of children and adults with physical impairments (handicap) and birth defects has been increasing steadily at 10% per year because of junk foods and drugs (World Health Organization Survey).

Nutritional suicide is prevented by the family technology. A holistic family–a family built on the foundations of spiritual, physical and mental unity will always seek whole (holistic) foods to nourish itself and guarantee a future. It will no longer be diseased by nutritional white racism. Charles Darwin, who founded the theory of evolution, wrote *The Next Million Years* and pointed out that the least creditable feature of White Supremacy is [that] it is criminally foolish. It is foolish to allow the diet to be contrary to nature (processed) which makes it contrary to "hue-mans" and the African family.

The African community in America of the past had a family structure and ate a natural food diet. The first contemporary Africans in America (also called Gullahs) were born in 1526 on St. Catherine's Island off the coast of Georgia. The Gullahs and many others had independent family-structured communities in Florida, Alabama, Georgia, and North and South Carolinas in the 16th, 17th, 18th and 19th centuries. They traded with each other and threatened to end slavery because they attacked plantations, destroyed plantation crops and had armies (called runaways by Whites) that freed slaves. General Andrew Jackson used the War of 1812 as an excuse to attack these independent communities. He also attacked them again in 1816 and 1818. Finally, in 1842, General Jesup of the United States War Department told Congress to make no mistake about it: "This is a Negro and not an Indian War." Thus, he declared "The Negro War." He told the War Department that the runaway Negroes were able and willing to defeat America. If they were not destroyed, they would Africanize the South. The U.S. military attacked and murdered those African Americans, destroyed their families, communities and defeated their armies. The survivors of the "Negro War" were driven off their land and marched at gunpoint to reservation-type areas in Mexico. Some moved to Seminole County, Arkansas or Brakettville, Texas or moved to Indros Island and other areas. In any case the survivors of slavery and "The Negro War" still legally have their own land in America.

Ironically, European power elite whose economic purpose was to capture states and resources financed the Civil War (War of Northern Aggression). The power elite capitalists have never been interested in democracy or government. They are motivated by power to feed their psychotic needs. They did not want the African prisoners of war (so-called slaves) to be aware that they (Africans) could fight and gain control of states. Consequently, the Europeans created the lie called the Civil War. The British and Confederates emancipated slaves before the Union did. This allowed them to use the slaves to fight for the Caucasians (caucrazians) civil rights. Emancipation kept the slaves unconscious of the fact that the European criminals were fighting over what they had stolen (America, Africa and Africans). Emancipation means transfer of ownership. Slaves were no longer property of individuals. They became property of the federal government (U.S.A.). Emancipation and the Civil War were political devices used to keep the slaves from uniting to form an all-African army. This army could have fought and defeated the flea-infested, homosexual, violent, cannibalistic, bed wetting, criminal Europeans and gained states, resources, reparations and Africa's freedom.

In 1848 the United States versus Henry Turners' Heirs court hearing ruled that the "Neutral Strip" of 2,961,983.5 acres of land in Louisiana, Arkansas and Mississippi belongs to African Americans. In 1940 the neutral strip of land was again verified to exist as not belonging to the United States. The Louisiana Department of Transportation acknowledged the Neutral Strip on its survey. Historically, it is neutral because it was not included in the sale of the land by the Spanish to the French and it was not a part of the 1803 Louisiana Purchase of land by America. The African communities legally have land and possess the skill, ability and technology to be free.

Also, the 13th Amendment to the U.S. Constitution calls for the elimination of slavery and all incidents of slavery. Therefore, African Americans not allowed a reparational economic base, land or to maintain African citizenship suffer from an "incident of slavery" and have the legal rights to file claims and pay no income tax. The African community first must use the family technology to build positive communities, relationships and diets in order to be "hue-man."

The technology of the family is not the only thing for freedom; it is everything in freedom. The family is the root from which the strong tree of Africa grew. The African family tree gave the world fruits such as science, religion, civilization, nutrition and community. What the ancient African ancestors have done can be done again. What they achieved can be achieved on a higher level if the family technology is used. It is African people who must save the future and world from Caucasian holistic destructive behaviors. It is stupid for Africans to wait for mother nature's revenge—major changes in the galaxy, saviors, destruction of the ozone, millennium, collision of planets or stars, spiritual cleansers, diseases, climatic changes, etc., to do the job that Africans must do themselves. It is the world's change agent (melanin dominant Africans) that must discipline and correct Caucasians' holistic toxic behaviors. It is a human issue that must be solved by humans. The African family must stop Nutricide and meet its date with destiny.

Eternal African Family Relationship

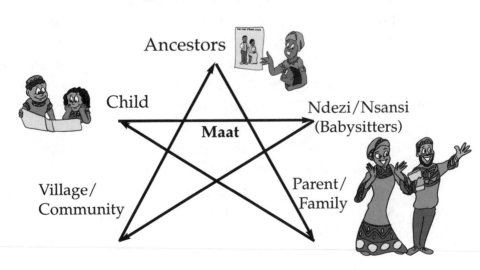

The Family is Medicine

The African American family is the central holistic force that nurtures, loves and develops the African child and nation. The family, which consists of grandparents, aunts, uncles, cousins and adopted members, is a politically activist, self-policing, healing institution, a government unto itself, a religious center, a savings bank, a judicial and militant organization. However, one of the primary functions of the family is to protect, maintain and build the health of its members. Family holistic health consists of the spiritual, mental and physical well being of each member. An illness or sickness of an African person was automatically considered an illness but belonged to each member of the family institution. In a communal sense, each family member shares in the health, wealth, problems, child rearing, success, food supply and dis-ease of each member. Ironically, today the communal life-style is forced upon Africans when a family member such as a father, is an alcoholic, cocaine (crack) addict or AIDS victim. In such a case, the family begins to recreate their emotions, thinking, behaviors and feelings in order to cope with the psychological effect of the dis-ease. They adjust their entire life-style to protect their feelings or hide their feelings or hide money in order to cope with the violence, arguments, sexual abuse and drunken behavior of the alcoholic. Alcoholism, like all dis-eases, is a family dis-ease that only a family can solve. If the family does not solve it, another family will in some way be a victim of it.

African rituals and ceremonies were used as a type of education in conduct and behavior and as preventive medicine. Therefore, ceremonies as a preventive medicine were used during births, marriages, deaths, meetings and illnesses. The health practitioner (Shaman, Juju, Root Doctor, and Witch Doctor) used psychology, spirituality and rituals along with medicinal herbs in the treatment of the ill person.

Medicinal herbs were always available in Africa. There were many herb stores in ancient African cities. They sold live medicinal and spiritual herbs and herbs used to decorate altars, schools, mummies, candles, homes, stores, temples, animals and those to be worn with clothing. Sennufer, the Mayor of Thebes during the 18th Dynasty under Pharaoh Amenophis II (1425 BC), required medicinal herbs in gardens. Inemi, under Pharaoh Tuthmosis I (1425-1510 BC), was the herbalist who maintained the herb garden and fruit orchard. Akhenaton maintained a medicinal herb garden at Kawa near Dongola. The herb extracts stolen from Tutankhamen's tomb had labels that list the ingredients, dosage and schedule to be taken. There are carvings of herbs in ivory on the panel of Tutankhamen's Sarcophagus (18th Dynasty). An herbalist such as Kakht who was director of the Amun herb gardens of Amenophis III (1375 BC), used many medicinal herbs and foods such as chamomile, mandrake, fig, cornflowers, peppermint, myrtle, juniper berry, wormwood, anise, licorice, fennel, myrrh, black cumin, willow, plantain, fenugreek, purslane, marjoram, basil, rue, flax, rosemary, carob, fleabane, pomegranate, etc. The herb stores also sold herbs for use as packing-type material, and for storing utensils, clothes, food, bread, baskets, and dried fruit and vegetables.

The health practitioner and his store were a functional part of the society. The health practitioner participated in the family's rituals and ceremonies as an extended family member. Any health practitioner who came to an ill family member's community or house was under the guiding control of the family. The practitioner was basically a technical tool of the family and gave healing advice and treatments.

The family itself actively cured the illness. The family was the medicine and practiced family medicine. The family provided natural foods and used foods as medicine. Aside from this, the family would have at least one herbalist of its own that gave dis-ease care. If it was necessary for the ill person to quit work until he was cured, then the family provided holistic and economic support. Families took care of all its children, elderly, ill or handicapped.

Basically, the family and community of families were the home of hospitality—a hospital. The true measurement of a civilization's superiority or inferiority is judged by the family's treatment of the sick, elderly, children and handicapped. If the civilization leaves the care of the blind to a dog (seeing-eye dog), puts its elderly in prisons called nursing homes, puts its children in jails called Youth Detention Centers, or uses abortions to kill children, then it will be judged as an inferior civilization.

Caucasian medicine stops the African family from functioning as a hang team. It stops the holistic family from being a medicine for the sick. They do this by not building hospitals for the African family members to sleep overnight and stay during the day in order to be participants in healing. Hospitals, clinics and doctors' offices do not have healing rooms that are circular, which would be similar to family rooms in compounds (communities). Further, Caucasian hospitals isolate the ill and do not allow community support of the ill. Caucasian medicine and health insurance will not economically, socially, dietary, herbally, or ethnomedically support an ill African family. An Africentrically ill family is one that has one family member sick.

Caucasian hospitals stop African family medicine because they do not let children participate in the cure of an illness. They usually demand that a child be over 12 years old before they can visit the ill. For some superstitious reason Caucasians believe that when a child becomes 13 years old he is declared germ-free and unable to give an illness to the ill or catch an evil death-causing germ from the ill. Why Caucasians believe the child at 13 years of age is suddenly immune is hidden in Caucasian ignorance. In any case, a sick African in the hospital's Intensive Care Unit's prison rooms are usually allowed visitors at designated times, and children may not be allowed to visit no matter what their age. Families cannot sleep in the room or use holistic remedies. In fact, holistic remedies such as Dance, Herbs, Drums, Natural foods, Juice Therapy, Psychic Healing, Ancestors, Curative Oils, Sunlight or any African spiritually based treatments are forbidden in Caucasian hospitals.

The hospitals are another White Supremacist tool used to divide, conquer and destroy the African family medicine. Families are viewed negatively by Caucasians. Caucasians refer to the family as a "nuclear family" as if it is a nuclear bomb that will explode and destroy itself. They also refer to the African family as an "extended family" as if African families are not the "normal" Caucasian size. The Caucasian "normal family," is a fragmented family in which members must go to others for spiritual support (church), for economic support (unemployment insurance stipends), for sickness (hospitals), for cultural education (schools) and for protection from each other (police, courts, government, medicine and food policing agents). This Caucasian social order makes the African family dysfunctional, Nutricidal, fragmented and not Africentrically holistic.

Caucasians have a conflict with the understanding and the acceptance of the African Divine Kinship of families. For example, when a Caucasian man and woman decide to get married, it is a "self-centered" individual decision. They, of course, make the decision without the guidance, spiritual support of the elders or ancestors. They do not allow elders or deceased ancestors to have the final decision on the mate choice. The Caucasian couple gets married and believes that they will have a family. In direct contrast to this, two African families get married and have a couple. It is a marriage of families, ancestors, elders, spirits and a community of Africans. It is a holistic spiritually healing medicine.

The married couple has individual training and marriage couple training called "Rites of Passage" rituals and ceremonies. They learn that the family nurtures, heals and spiritualizes the community and is more or less a medicine. Medicine simply means balance or harmony with God and the ordained laws of the body, diet and herbs. The family is a vehicle of balance–a medicine. Whenever there is an imbalance (dis-ease) the family moves to re-establish balance holistically with herbs, food and other natural remedies. It is family medicine.

Family was and is important medicine to Africans. An African Prisoner of War (so-called slave) would be stolen and put on slave ships such as the good ship "JESUS." It was common knowledge that if a man were captured, his wife and children would often follow him into slavery in order to preserve the family. On the ship the slave would be supported by educational societies (secret societies such as Prono and Sando) and elders world use the family-created organizations to protect themselves and from slave rebellions. Once the slave arrived at the Caucasian plantations, he would be put into a family. For example, a slave child would arrive at the slave compound (community) and would be instantly adopted by a family and given a stepmother and stepfather.

Divine kinship assigns everyone a family, ancestor, history and health practitioner. Divine Kinship means that all Africans are related by God's Will. The family was structured to enforce and be in harmony (medicine) with God. Consequently older spirits such as grandparents and elders are considered divinely important. Health practitioners were considered as having a calling by God's Divine Will to heal others. In any case, if one of the parents of the slave child were sold, then a new "step-parent" was selected.

Marriage was important to African slaves and considered an act of God. They believed that marriage vows were commitments made similar to tying the tongue into a knot that could not be taken a loosened. Marriage was the Divine will of God and necessary for the community and the children. Even after slavery, the misplaced and scattered slaves, first action was to find their family. They would wander all over America looking for family members. Family unity and communal life-style and herbal medicine have always been the primary force in African society. A family is protective of its ill, heals its ill, and all family members totally share in the ill person's healing process. As the African family's usage of natural foods and herbal medicine decreased the Caucasian dis eases of the family increased.

Family Medicine provides the healing, nurturing, bonding and socializing. Family is an essential part of African science. Family concepts are African governments, laws and the understanding of health. The cleansing of the body is a process performed by the family of organs (organ systems). However, Caucasian superstition has it that the skin can singularly (individually) cleanse the body. Thus, they believe that "sweating" cleanses the entire body. Consequently, they take herbs or drugs that cause sweating and do exercise work-outs that cause sweating with the belief that sweat cleanses the internal organs of the body. Sweating primarily helps to keep the body temperature normal (98.6) and cools the overheated body. If a person would sweet 4 gallons of water, less than 4 of an ounce would be solid matter (minerals, urine-type waste, dead cells, and oil) and w of that would be salt. Salt holds the sweat to the skin and increases the cooling action. A long walk (4 miles) would be more cleansing for the body's family of organs than making one's self sweat with herbs or drugs. However, ignorance prevails in Caucasian science and gossip theories, and sweating remains popular.

Further, "hearing" is a family-influenced sense. Hearing does not create itself. Family consciousness helps create mental, physical and spiritual reactions to sound images. Family members tend to hear the same quality and quantity of sound as hearing is cultural, psychic, a state of consciousness and a melanin however influenced sense.

The Caucasians believe that hearing is an individualistic (self-centered) event. They assume that all people hear the same quality of sound as they do and that all people hear sound as individualistic vibrations. Africans are taught by media (school textbooks) to hear as whites. Africans hear clusters of sounds with overtones (communal). Hearing like white folks causes a diseased type of hearing. Africans who hear as whites must disregard the Africentric psychic, spiritual, divineness and mental consciousness of sound information that comes to their brains. Diseased hearing and disease junk society laws are anti-family, Nutricidal, and self-centered for Caucasians.

African Laws are family based. Africans' natural behavior starts with Bonding, a natural foods diet and family. Africans naturally behave holistically in harmony with each other and scribes (writers) wrote down the observed rules of human relationship. Africans observed the behavior, then wrote the laws. Caucasians wrote the laws, then tried to get the behavior. Caucasians have many laws and are too diseased to understand that people make the laws, laws do not make the people. They constantly disobey their own laws. They have a violent, chaotic, immoral, sexually perverted, anti-family, anti-children and Nutricidal society. Caucasian societies' foundations are based on an anti-family and individualistic government.

Caucasian governments of democracy typify giving the "Individual" (self-centeredness) more importance than the elders, ancestors, the council of the wise and family consensus. Individualism reinforces the belief that an individual vitamin, mineral or amino acid has more importance than its activity in nutrient groups (family). This causes the African to believe that Caucasian dead organic and inorganic chemistry can answer living questions. Oddly enough, organic (living) chemistry also is the science of dead nutrients. Whether the democratic government votes to give power to an elite group (party) or to share the government management power in ratios based upon the proportion of votes received it is still a "self-centered" concept. Democracy with an open election in which age is used to determine eligibility to vote is Caucasian self-centered as opposed to "family centered."

Caucasian democracy destroys the African council of the Elders and the family as a political cultural force. No African people can be free under the Caucasian democratic, socialistic, communistic or feudalistic governments. Caucasian governments are conceived and designed to support, promote and perpetuate White Supremacy. Medicine and health are the governments' form of media that voices white cultural imperialism.

Caucasian government is not "family centered" nor is Caucasian health "family centered." They believe an individual nutrient (specific) causes a specific disease. They constantly search for a specific individual cure for a disease by totally disregarding that each organ family (system), mental state; emotional mood and spirit force expresses the same disease differently. The organs, and organ systems, different symptomatic expressions of disease are erroneously viewed by Caucasians as separate individual diseases. Caucasian-based science, government and disease rely upon self-centeredness (individualism)" instead of "family centeredness (communalism)." Consequently, Caucasian government is anti-family, anti-African, anti melanin and causes diseases.

Caucasian medicine and governments combine to serve as a tool of White Supremacy. The economic profits from medicine are symbols of an individual's ability to be a successful white racist. Caucasian money is the symbolic way that the mentally ill reward the mentally ill for being mentally ill. Caucasian money has no economic value. It can represent success at being mentally ill, dysfunctional, self-centered, culturally imperialistic, physically ill, spiritually diseased and happy (self-actualized). Caucasian governments (empires, countries) are failure prone and disease producing. Historically, none of their governments lasted over 300 years and all exploited the poor.

The Caucasian peasants (poor) under communism, socialism, feudalism or democracy (hypocrisy) have been on welfare, homeless, sickly, criminals, orphans, thieves, liars, mentally ill, beggars, addicted, violent, hungry, whores (male and female), rapists, murderers, etc. They have reflected the behavior of the upper class (rich), except they did not have the decorations of luxury and money.

Caucasian's collective mental illness causes the body to be ill by blocking electrical flow, hampering digestion, decreasing blood circulation, weakening immunity, degenerating all bodily functions plus adding depression to the mentally ill state. This is called a psychosomatic (mind-caused bodily disease) illness, which results in a somatic psychic illness (bodily caused mental disease). Added to this double illness condition is the mental and physical diseases caused by the flavorful undiluted garbage called junk food. Caucasian governments cause disease and destroy the "Family Centeredness of Africans. A return to the political family, council of elders' natural foods, Africentric science and Rites of Passage is the family medicine needed for healthy Africans. Family first, family last and family always is Africans' strength and key to the mother continents' survival.

Health is an African family Spiritualized Art. Without the family as a medicine, Africans will die from Caucasian-created diseases. It must be recognized that the dis-eases of Africans can only be solved by the African Family. The family is medicine. In order to be a healthy African, you must see, understand or accept the African in your own brothers sisters, mothers, fathers and the family before you can see Africa in yourself. You must first accept them as Africans no matter how distorted they are. Your family members may not wear African clothes, claim an African name, be African centered, eat natural foods, use herbal medicine or speak with an African philosophy as a base. However, they still have fragments of family medicine, African mannerisms, behavior, thoughts, spirituality, rituals, ceremonies, habits and speech that the effects of White Racism, slavery and colonialism cannot erase.

Your family (Africans in the diaspora and in Africa) is the closest you will ever get to Africa, being African and family medicine. It is through your family that you obtain the vision to accept yourself as an African, Africa's holistic medicine and future. Your health is Africa's health. Your family is Africa's family. They reflect the seen and unseen affects of White Supremacy, White Racism and point to the holistic solution. Oddly enough it is within the family medicine system that the spiritual technology exists that can destroy the holistically–diseased white race that started the Race War in the 14th century. The Family is medicine and the key to ending Nutricide.

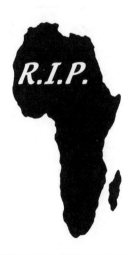

Chapter Two
Health

"The most difficult thing to get people to do is to accept the obvious"

Dick Gregory

White Racism: Nutritional Causes

A ll past behaviors are current behaviors, just as the study of history is the study of current events. The Ice Age era of Europe helped to produce the mental illness of White Supremacy/White Racism among at least 99% of the Caucasians. Large mountains of glaciers melted at the end of the Ice Age. Melting glaciers resulted in massive floods and soil erosion. Massive flooding and erosion caused the soil to be stripped of water soluble nutrients such as iodine, sulfur, zinc, manganese, copper, selenium, magnesium, etc. Aside from mineral-depleted soil caused by melting ice, Caucasians used the soil nutrient depletion technique of cultivation farming. Today, Europeans continue to rob the soil of nutrients by their farming methods. In addition to this, the totally unnecessary cooking of nutrient-depleted fresh fruits and vegetables further depletes the nutrient value of plants and makes the nutrients left in plants raised on nutrient-depleted soil less valuable. Further, cooking of animal flesh destroys nutrients.

Nutrients have an effect on the mind, mood, and state of consciousness, spirit and physical body. Ironically, Caucasians assume their nutrient deficient race and civilization are normal. They use their nutrient-deficient biochemical make up as the standard for Africans and all races. Caucasians further assume that their moods, thoughts and behaviors are normal. The Caucasian psychotic mental illness of imagined White Supremacy diseases their mind and they assume this is normal. The scientifically documented nutrient robbed plants from poor soil and historically documented worldwide behaviors of violence, ruin, destruction, rape, dysfunctional families, and dependence upon Africans on the continent and elsewhere on the planet contradicts their assumption of supremacy.

Glaciated soil lacks many minerals. For example, Selenium is a vital mineral lacking in certain types of soils. Caucasians have established a normal biochemical standard, which is an abnormal deficiency of selenium. Selenium deficiency causes premenstrual symptoms, hot flashes, breast cancer, infertility, birth defects, crib death, and liver damage and alters the rhythm and cycles in the body. Cow's milk is deficient in selenium. A diet high in saturated fat causes selenium drain.

Another mineral deficiency the Caucasian race suffers from is sulfur. Lack of optimum sulfur causes depression, rhythmic imbalances, irregular nerve impulses and retarded growth of egg and sperm. Sulfur is denatured or destroyed by cooking.

Zinc depletion is also harmful as it causes schizophrenia, infections, retarded growth, fatigue, digestive problems and sterility. Zinc is denatured or destroyed by cooking food. It is drained from the body by ingesting cow's milk, alcohol and contraceptive pills.

Further, Europe's iodine-poor soil can cause nervousness, irritability, toxins in the brain, low energy, obesity, melanin deficiency and growth problems. It is destroyed by heat, cooking and processing.

Manganese is lacking, which can result in pineal irregularities, muscle problems, brain and nerve difficulties and digestive problems. Caucasian women with this deficiency also can lose their mother instinct (Mother Love) and ability to protect their child. This may allow them to let their human baby suck the breast of a lower animal (cows, goats, etc.). Excessive sex and high amounts of cow's milk, calcium, iron and phosphorus can destroy manganese.

Additionally, other minerals were lost by the many floods of the Ice Age. The absence of nutrients for plants to biologically transmute imbalanced soil nutrients causes copperless soil. Soil that grows plants with very low levels of copper results in depression and easily imbalanced brain and nerve responses such as hyperactivity. Inadequate levels of magnesium in the soil can cause irritability, depression, tremors, muscle, nerve and brain problems. A loss of the mineral vanadium can cause low birth rates and high death rates.

Soil with inadequate phosphorus levels can result in feeble minds, mental and physical inability to coordinate muscles, brain problems and increased aging. Soil with potassium depletion causes high levels of physical and mental stress, aging, nerve problems, arthritis, rheumatism and heart problems. Potassium can also be destroyed by processing foods, cooking, salt, white sugar, alcohol, coffee, bleached white flour and stress.

The ancient Africans and contemporary Africans came in contact with mentally ill Caucasians raised on soil robbed of minerals from the Ice Age. These mentally ill Europeans were also physically imbalanced because of their glaciated, nutrient-drained diets. This biochemically diseased and mentally ill Caucasian believes himself normal, believes himself humanly evolved, believes himself capable of understanding the nutritionally and culturally superior African. The Caucasian psychotic mind feels that what his nutritionally inadequate brain thinks is correct and perfect. This abnormal mind has become a victim of its own imagination. An imagination that has been mentally ill and nutritionally deprived for centuries assumes that it is not ill when, in actuality, it is mentally ill. A nutrient-deprived mind hallucinates about reality and its intelligence.

Whatever the insane mind creates is believed to be sane. Added to this, when their melanin is stimulated it causes them to see or sense Black images in their imagination. This is a mild trance that melanin stimulation can induce. However, their melanin albino mind, emotions, subconscious, senses and spirit cannot cope with this stimulation. Therefore, they associate fear with melanin stimulation and Black (melanin) as evil. The conscious and subconscious mind becomes an insane complementary pair which reinforces its own insanity and labels it sane.

The Caucasians' cooked animal flesh diet is depleted of nutrients, which cause mental problems and disease. Cooking destroys the amino acid, Glutamic acid. A loss of Glutamic acid results in learning and behavioral problems, schizophrenia, senility, rhythmic loss, poor memory and stress. Cooking meat also destroys the amino acid lysine, which regulates the pineal gland, growth, activates breast milk, and monitors acid and alkaline balance. Without lysine, infections are common. Tyrosine is an amino acid that can be deficient, causing an unstable mind, irritability, and irregular rhythm of the organs, glands and melanin deficiency. The amino acid histidine is necessary for proper child growth and organ rhythm. It is inadequate in Europeans, who were raised on cow's milk. Africans came in contact with these unstable personalities from dysfunctional families with mental problems and the psychosis of White Racism.

The social climate of the mentally ill Caucasian race was diseased. Many (perhaps all) of the mental problems of their race have never been therapeutically treated. This may be caused by their inability to see or admit that they are a mentally diseased race. Their documented behavior in history points to maladjustments with reality. In the 9th Dynasty of Egypt 3000 BC, Caucasians were described as a miserable race living with a shortage of food, a shortage of plants, a shortage of water (it was frozen) and always in search of food, be it plants, animals or another Caucasian (cannibalism). Additionally, long periods of food shortages (human flesh and plant foods) added to massive diseases caused by nutritionally lacking soil and plants.

The Caucasian was/is a violent animal. In fact, when the Caucasian was first recorded in history, he was recorded in acts of violence. The Palettes and Mace heads found at Hierakonopolis, an area near the upper Nile River, reported that the Africans were fighting uncivilized groups of Caucasians around 4000 BC The Palermo Stone reveals that Africans were fighting the barbaric, pagan Caucasians who were trying to invade Africa. It was King Menes who drove out the savage Caucasians and stated the First Egyptian Dynasty. Since that time in world history, the mentally ill Caucasians have been using violence, war, peace and White Racism to rule, ruin, criminalize and inferiorize Africans.

Caucasians have a deep sense of insecurity about nature and themselves. Currently, they still have barbaric hordes (gangs) which they call alliances. These alliances (barbaric clans) attack African people all over the world and inferiorize Africans so they can have imagined superiority. Caucasians believe that money is the root of evil. Money is a symbol of Caucasian power and is used to make them feel secure. It is a sense of human worth that Caucasians try to achieve with White Racism and money.

Usually, after a Caucasian wolf-pack type attack upon Africans, they soon start to attack each other over the human and resource carcass. The anthropology of Caucasians documents gang attacks, gang sex (orgies), as well as gang chaos. Chaos seems to follow their insecurity. Caucasians only feel secure when they use violence to control. They tend to only unite for violence; then afterwards they fight among themselves. They are cultural, historical, religious, natural and human resource thieves who fight over what they have stolen. W.E.B. DuBois summarized Caucasians fighting in World War I as a fight between pirates over the spoils—Africa.

Caucasians are not consciously aware of themselves as a primitive group. Their primitive Ice Age genetic heritage causes them to still eat frozen food such as ice cream and to use ice cubes to make drinks very cold. Drinks cannot be used by the body unless they are 98.6° F and within African normal temperature range of 97.5° F to

98.6º F normal for Caucasians but a low-grade fever for Blacks. Therefore, a cold drink retards digestion and is a form of nutritional violence.

They disregard their religious differences (Jews, Muslims, Christians), political differences, (democrats, republicans, communists), ethnic differences (Irish, Slav, Russian) and will unite to watch violent sports such as football, boxing, ice hockey, wrestling, racing cars, movies with violence or violent threats to life, such as circus acts with tight rope walkers, lion tamers, knife throwers, or violent activities, such a, skiing, roller coaster riding, sky diving, Ferris wheel riding and hunting.

After the violence is over they separate, mistrust, abuse, lie, steal and use each other in a chaos that they call society. This chaos is their superstitious, socialized system of rituals and ceremonies that they alone call European "culture." Their culture is a White Supremacy psychosis. It is democratically shared by each Caucasian gang called an ethnic group. The Caucasians psychotically label their inferiority as superiority. If the European uses a wooden club to kill a person this is called primitive. If the European puts on a suit, shirt and tie and uses a gun to kill a person this is called modern or civilized. The behavior is still primitive, and the tool, be it a wooden club or a gun, is simply another way to be primitive. White Supremacy is simply a tool of an inferior, primitive people that is used to make them feel human worth. They are a chaotic collection of adult delinquents who have children who are also delinquent.

The current cannibalistic, animal flesh consumption, dairy and junk food diet of Caucasians causes them to be mentally, physically and biochemically imbalanced (perverts). Perverted biochemistry causes abnormal behaviors, thoughts, spirit, sex and relationships with other races. A biochemically imbalanced Caucasian with a high protein diet and junk foods has a high acid content of blood.

Acidic blood will cause high blood pressure and will allow too much blood to fill the uterus and prostate (engorge) causing the prostate to weaken and degenerate. This can result in premature ejaculation. A constantly engorged uterus results in endometriosis and menstruation. The combination of an acidic uterus and an acidic prostate together with high blood pressure may cause excessive sexual stimulation.

Animal flesh eaters have toxic, poisonous uric acid blood that irritates the brain, nerves, muscles, digestion, and especially, the reproductive organs. This abnormal, acidic biochemistry irritates the sex organs causing wet dreams (ejaculation while asleep), masturbation, homosexuality, violence, perversions and a need for sexually stimulating music, dance, movies, videos, games, clothes, religious books, etc. The uric acid and acidosis from junk foods irritates the mucous membrane of the uterus and prostate. This acid condition is compounded by food irritants, such as cocoa, alcoholic beverages, sodas, cooked foods, caviar, condiments, coffee, onions, vinegar, oysters, chocolate, caffeine, tea pepper, wheat, salt, oats, mustard and garlic. The naturally alkaline African vegetarian diet biochemically balances the body, mind and spirit.

The Caucasian mental illness of overeating (binges) causes acidic biochemistry. Overeating constipates, resulting in an increase in sexual activities. In a constipated state, the body is toxic and acidic. This irritates the reproductive organs. Irritated sex organs become engorged, accompanied by a rise in blood pressure. This acidic biochemistry triggers sexual excitation. Biochemically perverted Caucasians consider their abnormality as normal. Their sick normal is called the natural sexual instinct. Caucasian White Racism uses their diseased body and diseased sexual behavior as the normal standard for all Africans. The Caucasians' behavior is the behavior of biochemical imbalances, which perverts their social activities and mind.

Caucasians with nutrient-caused mental illness added to their psychotic White Supremacy are too diseased to recognize or ad nit to their mental illness. However, a Caucasian scientist, such as Albert Einstein, inadvertently admitted to their mental illness when he said, "we (Europeans) live in a world of problems, which can no longer be solved by the levels of (European) thinking, which created them." In other words, their state of mind cannot and will not solve their mental illness. If they could, they would not be mentally ill. This White Racism psychosis is so deeply implanted in their minds that it escapes contact with reality. Reality is African civilization, is the superior civilization. Africans are the superior race by all biological and chemical analyses.

All Caucasians participate directly or indirectly in maintaining their White Racism. White Racism is democratically distributed to all Africans. Benjamin Franklin once said, "If everyone (Caucasians) is thinking alike, then no one (Caucasians) is thinking. White Supremacy does not have to be thought about or purposely acted on; it is a disease that feeds on itself. They have an acceptable level of mental illness, which they call the normal mind, and they have unacceptable mental illness, which they call mental disease. The mental disorders that were present in the Ice Age, Dark Ages and Feudalism are present today. They are weaved and mixed in every aspect of their social, moral, religious, family, sexual and violent behaviors. All past behaviors are current behaviors, just as the study of history is the study of current events. They are psychologically protected and reinforced until these mental disorders are no longer visible to their mind.

Additionally, they have a melanin deficiency. Their pineal gland has 60 to 80% calcification (dead) or inactivity. Their pineal glands' inactivity causes nutritional and mental imbalances resulting in obsessive compulsive thoughts and behaviors. Melanin deficiency causes a need to control and limits the range of thinking. Africans have 12 melanin centers in the brain, while Caucasians have only 2 melanin centers. Limited melanin centers make them mentally incapable of evolving thoughts holistically. They are trapped in a nutritional-and melaninated-deficient body.

Caucasian neurohormonal development is poor and has limited responsiveness. This causes their nerves to slowly grow to muscles at age 2 while Africans' nerves grow to muscle within 6 months of age, allowing toilet training. The complete adult neurohormonal growth occurs at 12 years of age in Africans, and between 18 and 21 years of age in Caucasians. This slow development limits the amount of emotional and mental flexibility Caucasians can have. Consequently, Caucasians lack the melanin ability to voluntarily accept holistic therapy and free themselves of White Supremacy's illusions and mental illness.

The continent of Africa provided Africans with nutrient-rich soil, vast varieties of fruits and vegetables, which supplied all the amino acids, minerals and vitamins for a normal mind and body. The European soil was nutritionally robbed. Additionally, Caucasians lack nutritional science and proper food combining knowledge have a melanin-deficient biochemistry and are civilized in an immature infant culture, which nourishes their mental illness of White Supremacy. They are historically and scientifically a racial and culturally inferior race that could be helped and developed if they wanted to change. However, Caucasians do not recognize their disease and enjoy the status it gives. Caucasians entered recorded history after all other colored cultures had been in existence over 10,000 years. They also entered history violently attacking Africans.

Traces of their cultural immaturity and violence still exist today. The vast majority of their amusements and activities are focused in violence such as violent children's fairy tales, movies (murders, rape), or stealing, lies, word trickery, marriage and relationship conflicts, cops and robbers, one group overpowering another, deception, etc. Because they were raised in an uncivilized culture infected with murder, dysfunctional families, rape, fear, anger, violence, homosexuals, conflicts, wars, threats to life, sex orgies, cannibalism and social wolf-pack behaviors, they have difficulty communicating within themselves and to others.

The Caucasians, due to nutrient-depleted soil and food, are mentally and physically ill. Chronic undernourishment is more dangerous than the diseases of rickets, anemia, kwishikora, and beriberi, because it causes personality disorders, violent behavior and mood swings. The victims of undernourishment have slowly gotten the disease state and do not recognize themselves as ill. When this condition (nutrient deficiency) has occurred over centuries and the vast majority has it, the majority believe themselves normal. The correction of chronic undernourishment takes place slowly over a period of 5 to 6 weeks. This is too slow to show an immediate change in nutrition status. This also makes it difficult to be recognized. In obvious diseases such as beriberi, a vitamin B hypodermic needle injection will immediately help the tongue and lips feel less sore, the digestive disorders and thinking will clear up. Centuries of chronic undernourishment from glaciated land have been erroneously scientifically documented as normal. Their abnormal behaviors and thinking are erroneously documented as normal by Caucasian civilization, and their religions verify their abnormal behaviors as normal. The study of Caucasian history is actually the study of mental illness and asocial behavior. The nutritional and historical behaviors validate their psychosis (White Racism) as an illusion reinforced by nutritional deficiencies. Their culture, religions and nutritionists are too nutritionally deficient to recognize this. It is similar to this: in a land where everyone has one eye (Caucasians), a person with two eyes (Africans) is considered a freak. It is a nutritional trap with no escape.

Destroy the Pineal Gland

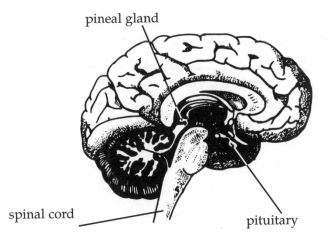

pineal gland

spinal cord

pituitary

A healthy pineal gland secretes melanin. Melanin makes highly melaninated African people superior to all races. So it follows, an unhealthy pineal would have an effect upon the Africans' health, mind and spirit. There are many ways to deteriorate, weaken and/or destroy the pineal gland. This destruction can occur without the knowledge of the victim. In the vast majority of Caucasian health, mind and spiritual sciences, and psychic books, the pineal gland is omitted and no mention of its health status is even vaguely discussed. It is medically clear that all glands can get diseased. Medical White Racism ignores the dis-eases and nutrient-deficiencies of the pineal gland, because in the Caucasians, the gland has the lowest activity or is usually inactive (dead), so it is not diagnosed or treated for illnesses.

The pineal gland is highly sensitive, nutrient-dependent, oscillates, and is biochemically and electromagnetically very active. AD drugs and nutrients cross the so-called "blood brain barrier" and get into the pineal gland's tissue. Drugs such as cocaine, alcohol, cough syrups with codeine or with iodine, X-ray, low radio waves, ultrasound waves, caffeine, Librium, microwaves, nicotine, antibiotics, Demerol, Tylenol, morphine, Ergotamine, toxic fumes, marijuana, antihistamines, decongestants, amphetamines, aspirin or Tagamet, can have an effect on melanin and the gland. This includes lye and lye-like chemicals (hair relaxers) skin bleaching agents and hair depilatory chemicals. Toxins in the pineal gland can result in degenerative diseases such as arthritis, senility, cataracts, cancer, Alzheimer's, diabetes, Parkinson, menopause (and in men impotence), glaucoma, osteoporosis and arteriosclerosis.

The Caucasian myth of the "blood barrier" serving as a form of liquid protection against toxic substances is an excuse used to stop pineal diagnosis. Synthetic toxins such as Caucasian-made drugs, white sugar, saturated fats that lodge in cells, viruses, genetic drugs, free radicals, bleached white flour and mucus congestion can interrupt the pineal gland's cycle and ability. This can result in degenerative diseases, abnormal growth activity, altered moods, spirit and consciousness.

The sensitivity of the pineal gland on many levels is unique. The nutrients stored in the pineal, such as indoles (tryptophane and natural indigo chemicals), histamines; dopamine and norepinephrine (noradrenalin), monitor and direct holistic energy. Synthetic chemicals destroy these nutrients. Many chemicals and foods made by the Caucasian are dangerous even to themselves. Public drinking water is basically deodorized toilet water. It can irritate the pineal gland because the toxic, synthetic water is chemically recycled sewage water. Fluoride in drinking water, toothpaste and all related chemicals such as chlorine and iodine are harmful. Hay fever, allergy or cold medicine with antihistamine can result in slowing down the secretions (melanin) of the pineal gland.

Additionally, the junk food diet with animal fats, fried foods, sugar, and heavy-metal toxins are dangerous. Many of the dangerous junk foods are hidden in foods. For example, animal fat is found in cream, peanut butter, salad dressing, butter, whole milk, cheese, potato chips and other snack foods. Aside from this, animal fat and white sugar are in bread, medicine, doughnuts, pizza, cakes, pies, candy, pastry, catsup, mustard and mayonnaise.

African people, especially those in large cities, can have a sunlight deficiency. This can result in an under-stimulated pineal gland, which for Caucasians is called "seasonal affective disorder (SAD), but for African people it can be an "all-seasonal affective disorder." This illness results in depression. Low energy, metabolism problems, cravings for sugar, drugs or other stimulants and a vague sense of feeling ill.

The stressing affect of White Racism can lead to cravings. Stress causes the pineal gland to be over-stimulated and exhausted. This can result in a vicious cycle of eating and taking drugs for cravings, which can further exhaust the pineal gland. Ironically, this causes the African to seek security and avoidance of fear by using Caucasian values. For example, an African person with a "slave plantation servitude mentality" will not visualize economic success unless it includes Caucasian values or a Caucasian high-paying job, Caucasian College degree, Caucasian expensive junk food and/or the Caucasian dollar. In other words, success is being in some way white and a part of the slave master's plantation.

The under-stimulation of the pineal with inadequate sunlight, junk food and a polluted environment can be destructive to the gland. Drugs can cause low energy and reduce pineal gland activity. The African's desire to combat the low pineal activity can cause a craving for junk religions (white God. white Jesus. white Moslem culture) or physically a Caucasian energy lift (drugs. white sugar). This nutritionally leads to another cycle of low pineal energy production. The pineal gland becomes weaker and weaker by this cyclic destruction. This lowers the quantity of melanin available and weakens or Nutricidally destroys' the Africans' ability to be African.

The pineal gland directly or indirectly controls many functions in the body such as the cyclic behavior of organs, growth and development states of children, catecholamine production, sleep patterns, energy storage, information storage, (memory), genetic information; regulates body temperature, carbohydrate metabolism, bone growth, cellular respiration, collagen synthesis, hair growth, skin growth, extrasensory perception, etc. Melanin also stimulates the repair of cells, tissues and organs. It acts as an antibiotic, enhances immunity, converts sunlight energy (vitamin D), stimulates DNA synthesis and influences lymphocyte production and increases sound and light absorption.

In Africans, the melaninated galaxy is connected to their holistic melaninated "inner space." In Caucasians with melanin albinism, the galaxy is "outer space" to them. Without optimum melanin production Africans self sabotage any effort to use their holistic genius for freedom from Caucasian White Supremacy. White Supremacy inherently emphasizes Caucasian nutritional values and destroys melanin and the pineal gland. This directly destroys African people. Without the full use of the pineal gland Africans can become puppets for White Supremacy and Nutricide.

The pineal gland masterminds the control of the pituitary, hypothalamus, gonads, and adrenal glands. An African person under Caucasian caused tension, stress, White Racism and the stress caused by a Caucasian-created dis-ease diet has a weak immune system and a weakened pineal. The pineal gland as a defense reaction to dis-ease will stimulate the adrenal glands to produce adrenaline. This leads to adrenal and pineal gland exhaustion. The pineal gland's ability to switch the sympathetic and parasympathetic nervous system off and on is weakened. The systems cannot harmonize and all bodily activities become imbalance. The pineal stimulates the release of prostaglandin, which defends the body from heart and circulatory disorders. Therefore, an undernourished pineal gland can cause heart disease and circulatory problems. African people are not taught about the pineal gland or melanin because it is a way to control and destroy them through "information colonization." They may vaguely know that Caucasians use melanin-stimulating hormones for suntans without sunlight. But, they are neither taught that pineal gland extract stops cancer or tumor growth, nor are Africans taught that the life span of animals is increased by 25% when given melanin extract. This type of Caucasian melanin research acknowledges the power within an African with a healthy natural foods diet that feeds a healthy pineal gland. Without a natural foods diet, the pineal gland is basically non-functioning. The African becomes easier to control, rule and ruin. The African is educated to use the food in his mouth as a tasty way to die. However, the escape from Nutricide will awaken the godly gift of the Sun–Melanin.

Caucasians and their running dogs and puppets (i.e., Japanese) are constantly researching melanin. The melanin information is used militarily, dietetically, medically, for drugs, computer science, sex, genetic breeding and outer space. It is mostly classified as top secret and not given to Africans. Their public and secret melanin organizations of information pirates and thieves publicly has the European, Pan American and Japanese societies for Pigment Cell (Melanin) Research. They have held fifteen International Pigment Conferences between 1946 and 1993. The Africans have held five Africentric International Conferences through the KM-WR Science Consortium, Inc. However, they lack the economically fueled research organizations that can bring massive social and nutritional changes to Africans.

The natural defenses of the body use energy conservation. If tissue, cells, organs, or glands are not being used, then the body will not give energy to the unused tissue or gland. It is a "don't use it, you lose it" philosophy. In some cases the unused tissue or gland will become calcified (turns to stone). A gland can be damaged by toxic poison from drinking alcohol. If it is continuously abused by alcohol, it will turn to stone (cirrhosis). The prostate gland can get damaged or diseased and will become hard like stone (calcified). Many toxic residues from junk food or toxic drugs will inflame tissue, organs, or glands causing disease reactions such as appendicitis, pancreatis, vaginitis, hepatitis, nephritis, prostatitis, and pelvic inflammatory disease. The pineal gland, like any other gland, can suffer the same type of inflammation. This can contribute to calcification. For example, Caucasians with low pineal gland secretion and melanin albinism cannot fully utilize the pineal gland and it is mostly calcified in them.

Caucasian diets, drugs, psychic ability and spirituality do not take into account the utilization of the pineal gland. The highest amount of pineal inactivity and pineal gland calcification is 60% to 80% among Caucasians. African people have the lowest amount of pineal gland calcification. This low calcification indicates the effect of the dietary abuse the Caucasians have caused in African people, (5% to 15%). This calcification can increase as African people continue to use Caucasian drugs, junk food, junk culture, junk religions and sexual abuse. A weakened pineal gland aids in the control and destruction of Africanity. Africans with dull weakened or partially destroyed pineal glands are waiting for Caucasian science to scientifically tell them that they are killing the pineal gland. Scientists will use Nutricide to destroy the pineal gland and tell you nothing.

White Out

Black culture

"White Out," a white liquid used to "correct" **black** (ink) mistakes made on paper is symbolic of Nutricide. Nutrition, or the science of how to nourish the body, mind and spirit is an African science. However, the majority of Africans are eating a Caucasian disease-causing diet and they are dying from it. This may make them a "healthy" White person but never a healthy Black person. It is ironic that nutrition is an African-derived word, which comes from the Egyptian word "Menat." Menat means to nourish or nurse. In recorded history, one of the earliest uses of nutrition was recorded in the Egyptian 6th Dynasty. The Amulet of Menat, worn by Osiris in pyramid paintings verifies this fact. Colorful (Melaninated) Africans should eat colorful food.

Color is very important in nutrition–especially for African people. Nutritionally, "white-out food" that has been conjured up in synthetic chemical factories–called "food" companies–is diseased. The Caucasian chemical foods and drugs factories are solely interested in profit–not nutrition–and least of all the correct nutrient level for the melaninated, biochemically unique, Africans. It is no accident that most grocery stores sell "food" that "makes you sick" and incorporate a "drug" store section with drugs that suppress one's sickness while adding other sicknesses (dis-eases).

Caucasians have not learned how to eat, what to eat, when to eat, how to prepare food or how to combine foods. For example, combining sugar and starches; meat and potatoes; sugar and milk; oil and starch; oil and protein; fruits and vegetables; drinking and eating at the same time are all nutritionally wrong, Caucasian cave man food combinations. Correct combinations would be starches and vegetables; vegetables and proteins; fruits eaten separately; grains and cereals eaten separately; and never drinking while eating.

Nature's naturally colorful food is not as valuable to Caucasians as the constipating and disease causing bleached white flour, white sugar, white salt, fried and drugged foods. The Caucasian superstition that white (food) is supreme is because the white race is viewed as supreme. Processed white foods are very dangerous and Nutricidal.

Africans should avoid processed foods and try to avoid plants that Caucasian have bred; for example, wheat, oats, say, white rice, grits, lima beans, chickpeas, black-eyed peas, pigeon peas, carrots, celery, cauliflower, beets, peanuts (bean), pistachios, cashews, walnuts, pecans, and sunflower seeds. Nightshades, such as eggplant, tomato, bell peppers, asparagus, potato, etc., should be avoided. The African diet should be less than 5% wheat instead of the over 50% wheat diet of Caucasians. Africans are not used to this mucus-forming, anti-melanin, high wheat diet. Africans should always eat natural foods, wild rice, short grain brown rice, string beans, collards, mustard greens, okra, avocado, cho cho, kale, squash, bananas, oranges, papaya, plum, mango, passion fruits, cantaloupe, limes, plantain, red yams, water-melon (eat rind), honeydew, pears, and whole wheat flours, such as rye, masaltarina, amaranth, Quinoa, spelt, Kamut, buckwheat etc.

The main object is to eat as natural as possible and as much raw food as possible. Follow the rules of food combining and do not mix protein with starch [i.e., meat and potato, meat and bread (sandwich), or sweets (sugar) with starch (i.e., breakfast cereals, cake, pies)]. Combine vegetables with starch, protein and vegetables, eat fruits alone and never drink and eat at the same time (drink one-hour before or after a meal). Caucasian food combining ignorance creates diseases and their grocery stores promote faulty scavenger food-combinations.

The "White" food area in the grocery store includes cakes, pastry, pasta, bread, pizza, snacks, ice cream, milk, cookies, dyed liquid/white sugar (pop, soda), potato chips, etc. White "food" can remain on the shelf much longer than colorful natural foods. Natural foods are alive and will spoil. Therefore, they have a short shelf life, which decreases the storeowner's high profit margin. Grocery stores sell processed "foods" which must be embalmed with preservatives. Africans who eat embalmed foods are getting sick and are themselves becoming embalmed with dangerous toxic chemicals. The "food" store is, in reality, a funeral home.

Grocery stores also have a "pink" area which is, perhaps the most dangerous and is anti-melanin. The pink color of the dead animal flesh is caused by their blood. Blood—be it red, clear or gray—is usually 50% sewage waste of the animal (this includes fish, seafood and fowl). Animal and animal's flesh is the most processed food and has toxins (poisons) such as arsenic, genetic mutants, radiation, DDT, sex hormones, nitrites, deodorants, herbicides and pesticides. The Caucasian diet is high in animal protein and fats which prevents Africans from recycling proteins. High amounts of protein are related to cancer, soft bones and sickling of cells.

The "green" area of the store, the vegetable produce and fruit area has chemicalized, lethal, gas-sprayed, radiated and plants cloned with human and animal cells. Plants mixed with animal flesh can cause genetic changes are toxic. Fortunately, vegetables cannot hold concentrations of toxins as high as meat. Boiling vegetables (which should only be steamed) causes the nutrients to be washed away in the water which will "white out" (dilute) the nutrients. This "white out" causes disease and is anti-melanin (anti-color).

Color is essential for foods and Africans. Nutritionally valuable foods have color. For example, natural oils (olive, corn, canola, vegetable) have a brownish color. Caucasian "food" companies destroy nutrients with bleach, antifreeze, radiation, deodorants, heat, and filter out the nutrients in brown color, rendering the oil clear.

Food that lacks natural color also lacks nutritional value. If the food is "whitened" (processed), it is nutritionally worthless. If it is white, don't eat it. It will "white out" your "hue-man" life and replace it with disease, death and a Negro mind.

Cooking alters the color of food. Cooking has become an accepted way to denature, devitalize, clone and process food. This causes food to become a synthetic poisonous concoction that destroys "hue-mans" to the same degree that it has been destroyed. In other words, you destroy the food and the food destroys you. It is nature's revenge. Cooked food was never an accepted dietary tradition in ancient Africa. Cooking allowed the war mongrel Caucasian armies to carry their own food supply. This increased their mobility. Cooked foods have the lowest nutrient content and contain toxic inorganic irritants. Eating devitalized dull colored cooked foods caused African armies to become holistically weak and sick from food-caused diseases. Africans who eat dysfunctional, degenerative cooked foods are unable and nutritionally raped to use their melanin to fight White Supremacy and diseases.

The Caucasians forced the practice of cooking foods upon Africans. This food cooking habit started during colonialism, slavery and the societal disruptive invasions (wars) of Africa. Caucasian invasions destroyed crops, farmers, irrigation and the agricultural trade system. This caused fresh and ripe foods to become scarce, and dried foods, such as legumes had to be cooked or sprouted in order to be eaten. Ripe beans, rice, millet etc. are partially green and should be eaten when ripe, not when unripe. Unripe dried beans are basically half protein and half starch in nutrient content. When cooked while unripe, they are an improper nutrient combination of starch and protein. Cooked unripe beans ferment and rot in the stomach causing stomach gas (flatulence).

The Caucasian Information Age began with the "Race War" (invasion) against Africa. The Race War caused Africans to lose control of land, food transportation routes, resources, agriculture and their diet. Caucasians developed the cooked food habit to preserve food. Cooking enabled them to eat rotten and partially spoiled foods. Cooking food has caused Caucasians to be mentally sick, physically ill, spiritually perverted and to have degenerative diseases.

Cooking food destroys the quality and quantity of life. Over half the life expectancy is totally lost by cooking foods. Ancient Africans consumed an over 90% raw food diet, and were free of disease. Adults had the constant energy of a child, required less sleep, had no rotten teeth, heart trouble, sex organ diseases, mental illness, colds, childhood diseases, diabetes, high blood pressure, arthritis, and lived to be over 150 years of age. Africans with high blood pressure believe they get disease from, picking up paper all day (i.e., paper work, administrations, etc.,), while their enslaved ancestors on a mostly raw food diet did not get hypertension, high blood pressure or stress from picking acres of cotton every day. The Caucasians' evolutionary ape-like cousin, the Orangutan monkey, lives on a raw food diet and is free of disease and has a long life span. The Orangutan's human cousin the Caucasian, eats cooked food and is continuously diseased, with a short life span.

There is no safe cooked food, be it an apple or spinach. All cooked food is anti-melanin and anti-life. Added to cooked foods are drugs such as salt, white sugar, cooking oil or animal grease, vinegar, alcohol, synthetic dyes, preservatives and toxic spices that irritate the digestive tract. Cooked food perverts the taste buds and chemistry of the body. This perversion causes the African to crave more dead, flavorful garbage, which erroneously is called cooked food. Cooking destroys the live enzymes, vitamins, minerals, proteins, fats, fibers, water, and carbohydrates within the food. The heat from the cooking process causes food nutrients to become inorganic, addictive, coarse, harsh, abrasive, poisonous toxic irritants, which are deadly. For example, cooked organic calcium turns into a coarse inorganic (dead) type metallic crystallized sand, which makes it indigestible.

Africans who eat cooked food turn into a Caucasoid-animated cesspool of walking liquid manure. Cooked proteins stick together in broken particles of acid. Acid accumulates in the body and weakens all tissues, cells and bones. Cooked starches turn into an inorganic crystallized sugar and charcoal. Cooked oils turn into acid, transoils, and coat the internal organs with slime, causing cells to stick together. Cooked starches and sugars ferment in the stomach while cooked protein putrefies. They are not metabolized but are absorbed as irritants. Dead (cooked) food feeds bacteria. Bacteria create more ammonia, acids, toxic gases, alcohol, vinegars and poisons. Ironically, cooked food junkies season their food with the same addictive irritants the foods makes in the intestine produce such as vinegar and acids (white sugar and white flour make vinegar and acids) and ammonia (animal flesh makes this).

Digestion is slowed down, hampered, constipated and suspended by cooked food, Melanin deficiencies, malnutrition, stress, worry, anger, tension, fatigue, fear, White Racism, anxiety and frustration. Cooked food basically stops melanin utilization and helps to keep the African biochemically addicted to Caucasian food and culture. The Caucasian culture and White Racism experience is a record of what has been. Their history is a record of the past and past experience. Experiences are merely a record and teach nothing. Experience teaches the Caucasian nothing other than to repeat the past. Wisdom teaches Africans not the trials and errors of experience learning but the learning through wisdom and melaninated ancestral genes. A solution to past experiences is part of the past event. The future belongs to the teachings of melanin's wisdom, not the teachings of experience's learning. A healthy African who eats naturally colorful raw food and health food can stop Nutricide.

Catch AIDS, Catch A Cold, Catch an Infection or Catch Ignorance?

Colds, AIDS (Acquired Immune Deficiency Syndrome) and Vene-real Disease (VD) are not contagious but cleansing processes of the body. Sores, warts, bumps, blisters, mucus draining of the nasal pas-sage and lungs, rashes, inflammations, lesions, ulcers or mucus drainage from the genitals are the body's way of getting toxic waste and dead cells out of the body. This is called a cleansing process or healing crisis. The body will use many different varieties of cleans-ing until it is free of toxins. Once the cleansing process is over, the sores, lesions, ulcers and blisters will heal the nasal passage and lungs will be clear of mucus free and cellular waste.

The body uses lesions, bumps, rashes etc., to cleanse itself only if the bowel movements, kidneys, urine and breathing action cannot eliminate liquid manure (mucus) Bodily cleansing is what Cauca-sians erroneously call catching a contagious viral or bacterial dis-ease.

Bacteria of all types are generally present in the body at all times. Contagious bacteria are found in people without diseases as well as those with diseases. The various bacteria populations increase in numbers when they have a fermented or putrefied, constipated food supply of uneliminated waste and dead cells. The bacteria growth increases as a defense reaction of the body. They are acti-vated when toxins and waste accumulate at a speed faster than the kidneys, intestines, liver, lungs and bowel movements can keep pace with. Specific bacteria have a favorite fermented and/or putre-fied waste that it likes to eat. The Caucasians label the garbage dis-posal action of bacteria as the disease instead of labeling the cause of waste accumulations as the disease. They therefore treat the bacteria instead of eliminating the waste.

Africans can die from Caucasian treatments of the disease rather than the disease itself. Drug treatment of a "cold" is estimated to kill over 20,000 annually. A natural remedy for colds is to get bed rest, keep warm and drink plenty of water. Usually within 2 days the cold (bodily cleansing) is over. However, most Africans have more belief in Caucasian superstitions than the Caucasians. It is necessary that Africans stop trying to blame scapegoat such a virus or bacteria for illnesses they themselves cause. Viruses and bacteria are not in conflict with the body. They mythologically demonstrate that disease is abnormal and that Africans Nutricidally use food to destroy themselves.

The African adoption of the Caucasian superstitious belief that a virus, bacteria or germ causes a disease instead of the Caucasian diet is Nutricidal. This belief forces the Africans to deny their hygienic health science, a science that teaches that your food is medicine and medicine is your food. Food in Caucasian society is a cooked synthetic, chemically polluted concoction put together to honor-perverted taste buds and crazy superstitions rather than health. The African acceptance of the contagious germ belief denotes faulty reasoning. Africentric common sense tells you that a contagious virus or bacteria is in the blood and can freely travel all over the body. If a so-called contagious disease such as athlete's foot were truly contagious it could travel to the eyes, genitals, stomach or brain causing Athlete's Foot Brain disease. It could start as athlete's foot brain disease then travel to the feet. Contagious diseases can travel freely. Contagious diseases are given names based on their visible location, such as Venereal Disease.

Colds, AIDS, Infections, Venereal Disease and the fear of germs are all part of the contagious disease superstitions of Caucasians. It is apparent that a person cannot Catch Healthy, Catch Bad Breath, Catch Ugly, Catch A Cold, Fibroid Tumors or Bumps. The Caucasian medicine science classified cancer, asthma and pneumonia as contagious and then removed them from the contagious disease list. Lies change, but truth never changes.

The United States Navy proved the contagious disease superstition a lie. At the end of World War I, the U.S. Navy had several venereal diseased (VD) infected persons have sexual intercourse with non-infected people. The contagious VD did not infect those free of VD. The Rockefeller Institute of New York City sponsored Dr. Noguchi's experiment whereby he had contagious, infected people attempt to infect others. The results were that the disease-free people were not infected. Historically, Doctor David Livingston (1813-1873), an invader of Africa, noted that Caucasians with syphilis could not sexually transmit the disease to Africans.

Despite the overwhelming scientific evidence and simple use of Africentric common sense, Negroes continue to believe in White medicine and die for it. They also believe that the White Man's ice cubes are colder than the Black Man's ice cubes. These Africans are competing with Caucasians in destroying themselves. Contagious diseases are a Caucasian superstition, because if you cannot catch healthy" then you cannot "catch sick" or AIDS. It is illogical for a person to be healthy enough to get a "cold" (contagious disease) and then become sick enough to get rid of the Colds. You cannot catch the weather—Colds, Hot, Partly cloudy, Storms, snow etc. The so-called contagious diseases of Flu (influenza), chicken pox, mumps, measles, polio are still called contagious and occur among people with and without immunization shots. They recur year after year because the same diseased dietary practices are used year after year. A close look at a contagious disease such as AIDS can give clarity to this Caucasian superstition.

An AIDS virus is a particle of a dead human cell. It cannot eat, reproduce, grow, move, attack you or be attacked. It is not a plant or animal, and it is not alive. A virus is not active one month and inactive (sleep) the next, nor does it sleep between 2 to 5 years before it attacks the person. A virus is neither retrogressive (retro = within) or progressive. A virus is dead cellular particles. Dead cell particles come in all sizes and can pass through the pores of condoms. The body's cells are constantly being produced and constantly dying. Therefore, it is easy to find a particle from a dead cell and label it a virus that caused a disease. The cells are composed of many organs (called organelles) which are similar to the human body's digestive, excretory, respiratory, immune, circulatory, nervous and reproductive systems. The cell has a melaninated nucleus (brain). The cell's genetic code is within a cell organ called the mitochondria. Genetic information is stored on the mitochondrion DNA (Deoxyribonucleic Acid) and RNA (Ribonucleic Acid). It is the DNA and RNA of dead molecule particles that are labeled the AIDS virus. What is called AIDS is a cleansing process of the body and what is called a virus is a dead cell particle.

Sores, bumps, blisters that burst, pus, mucus, and open sores that drain fluids are the body's cleansing process. The cleansing process is called a contagious disease by Caucasians. They chemically try to cure, remedy, stop or suppress the cleansing with drugs or surgery. The body gets overloaded with toxins, waste and dead cells and drains them out via the lungs, nasal cavities, skin and genitals. If the kidneys and intestines fail to get rid of waste and toxins, the body cleanses by using pustules, rashes, vesicles, diarrhea, lesions, fevers, colds, sweats, yeast, tumors, etc.

The continuous eating, drinking or smoking of toxic chemicals, meat, white sugar, bleached white flour, salt, drugs (legal and illegal), cooked food, and the taking of vaccinations and immunization chemicals destroys the immune system. Eventually the immune system collapses and it is called AIDS and blamed on a dead cell particle labeled a virus. Ironically, Kaposis Sarcoma has the same sign and symptoms as AIDS, just as syphilis has the same sign and symptoms as Herpes.

The change of labels for diseases is based on the Caucasian economic profits gained from the treatment of sick people. Caucasian businesses make large profits by selling synthetic drugs, selling drug research, selling the policing of drugs, medical hospitals, and tracking the disease effects of their drugs and junk foods. The Center for Disease Control, the Food and Drug Administration, World Health Organization, drug companies, hospitals and secondary health support industries maintain the contagious disease stupidity. If they cannot blame a disease on a virus, they blame a bacteria. They create and maintain the public's fear of an evil virus and bacteria in order to sell medicines, all types of soaps, antibiotic deodorants, toothpaste, creams, lotions and greases, all of which have not stopped an attack from contagious germs.

Bacteria are present in the body at all times. They are essential for maintaining health and food digestion. African people have the largest variety of bacterial flora in their digestive systems, which allows them to metabolize food more efficiently. Various bacteria help to eliminate waste toxins and neutralize impurities. A specific bacteria likes a specific type of food to eat. A Nutricidal African eats like Caucasians and eats 50% more wheat than can be accustomed to (should be less than 5% whole wheat). This causes specific bacteria to increase in numbers and become out of balance with the bacteria flora community. This creates a subclinical disease condition in Africans and limits melanin recycling ability. This weakens immunity, which alters the cleansing reflex, causing waste to accumulate, resulting in a "cold" (mucus congestion). Africans constantly catching colds are constantly committing the same Caucasian dietary error over and over again.

There are approximately 20 million Americans who have contagious "colds" each day. It is never explained why the contagious bacteria or virus does not kill the remainder of the population or why this contagious bacteria does not travel to the feet, brain, genitals or heart, causing "colds" of the brain, genitals or heart. If a "cold" were truly contagious it would destroy the entire body, as there is no medicine to stop it.

Caucasian medical science admits that it has no cure for the "cold." This can only mean that the common "cold" should have killed all people. Added to this, Caucasian medical science tells people they can catch sick bacteria but not strong lively healthy bacteria. Healthy bacteria could cause a person to catch more good health. The only thing a person can catch is ignorance, if they believe the contagious disease superstition of the primitive Caucasian culture.

Africans cannot compromise their health and be healthy. They cannot accept part of the Caucasian health science without getting damaged from part of that science. The contagious disease religious belief supports the Caucasian fear of germs and this fear economically supports the industries that produce chemicals to kill essential germs on and in the body with toothpaste, antibiotic soap, deodorants, feminine hygiene sprays, douches, foot spray, deodorizers, antibiotic sprays, lotions and shampoo. This supports the belief in purified (bleached white) processed foods. They do not trust nature nor do they trust Africans, because Africans are too close to nature in thought, behavior, spirit and culture. Africans and Caucasians may take herbs and eat food, but Africans metabolize herbs and food differently and express diseases differently. Do not mistake similarities to mean sameness. The physical or mental similarities between the Black and White races do not make them of like humanity or like in approach to health. For example, one can identify the many similarities or commonalties between the organizational structure, training and discipline of the United States Military and the African Liberation Armies. However, their similarities do not make them united in purpose or united as one. They are by definition and belief totally against each other.

There are also similarities between the Caucasian religions and African spirituality and African science, and Caucasian science but by definition they are directly opposite each other. The health science view of an African moves from harmony to harmony, while the Caucasian moves from conflict to conflict. For example, in a disease process some tissue of an organ may get overloaded with toxins or waste and the body's immune reflex moves to get rid of the toxins or waste. The African health scientist calls this a cleansing process. The Caucasian defines this as the body attacking itself or in conflict with itself.

A person may accidentally put another individual's bacterial fluid into an open sore or the mouth. Bacteria can be transported from one individual to another. The foreign bacteria enter the body and the body has a chemical reaction. This chemical reaction is similar to the rejection of an organ transplant. The African identifies this as a cleansing reaction while the Caucasian calls it catching another person's contagious bacteria. The Africans must honor their unique difference and know that there is no such thing as a contagious disease, or else they will remain in a disease state and move from one sickness to another sickness. There is nothing to catch but ignorance.

The Caucasian defines contagion and his sexuality as normal. However, disease is abnormal and Caucasian sexuality is abnormal. Caucasians are sexually aroused because they are sickly. Their sexual behavior and diseases are an expression of sickliness, which they blame on their myth of contagiousness. Their definition of sexually contagious diseases (VD, AIDS, herpes, etc.) overlooks that sex for them is a disease reaction. Caucasian sex operates on a bodily response to a disease condition created by food consumption, ignorance, famine and wars.

The Caucasian race prematurely begins sexual activity, puberty and reproduction at an early stage in the life span because they are holistically sickly. Africans who follow the Caucasian junk food diet, prescription and non-prescription drug use and life style also begin sexual activity at an early age. Caucasians have sexual intercourse primarily to act out mental conflicts and to satisfy feelings of control, inferiority, ownership and power as well as to perform self-hatred sexual perversions.

Early sexual activity is a symptom of a sickly race. A race with constant mild-to-severe degenerative diseases is on the verge of extinction. Normal reproductive sex begins approximately between 18 to 20 years of age or later. Ovulation and sperm production normally starts between 14 to 18 years of age. However, a sickly race will have abnormally early ovulation, low sperm counts, sexual perversions and pregnancies beginning at 9 to 12 years of age. Premature reproduction is a species survival mechanism. This species survival mechanism is triggered in sickly insects, animals and plants. This gives rise to the saying that "a plant that is sickly will reproduce quickly." Early sex among a species with degenerative diseases and excessive non-cyclic sex is harmful and causes diseases.

Disease such as arthritis, rheumatism, hardening of the arteries, varicose veins, constipation or low levels of testosterone can prevent the orgasmic contraction of the prostrate, uterus and vagina. Consequently, men and women do not feel sexually fulfilled and have excessive sex in a vain attempt to achieve psychological pleasure or orgasm. A nutrient-weak prostate can swell and contract quickly causing premature ejaculation. This can lead to infertility or excessive sex in order to feel fulfilled. A bodily disease affects the genitals along with excessive sex, which can lead to accumulation of toxins, waste and dead cells. The genital organs can become an outlet for impurities and have a cleansing reaction, which is erroneously labeled VD or AIDS. Added to this, increased sex and premature reproductive ability is a Post Ice Age and Post War species survival response to increased numbers of people.

The Ice Age and War exterminated a large number of people. During the Ice Age, Cold Age (Post Ice Age), famines, Ice Age Wars, World Wars, Race Wars (Caucasian War Against Africans), and Caucasian internal wars, an adrenaline response is required. Adrenaline is a hormone that the body releases to give extra energy and alertness for a "fight or flight" response to anger, disease, stress, frustration, depression, fear, danger or White Racism. Adrenaline basically stops the immune, digestive and reproductive systems from functioning so that the individual can concentrate on fighting for survival. The energy stimulation for the sex, digestive and immune systems is taken away and used for human survival. Therefore, prolonged adrenaline usage can inadvertently weaken the immune system. A typical Caucasian characteristic rebound reaction to famine, Post War and Post Ice Age behaviors is an increase in sex and domestic (non-military) violence.

The Caucasian diet can cause sex and violence to increase, because it is high in acidic foods such as wheat, oats, meat and dairy. Foods cause mental and physical illnesses by draining the body of nutrients, such as calcium, potassium, magnesium, manganese, vitamins A, B, C, D, E, K and amino acid. Acidity weakens the primary tissues and muscles of the eyes, heart, ears, arteries, veins and secondary muscles of the body. Muscles use carbohydrates, not protein as fuel. If alkaline carbohydrates are not available as fuel, then the energy that would go to secondary muscles (i.e.. legs, arms, back, etc.) is allocated to primary muscles. Consequently, the individual can lose weight, degenerate, lose muscle mass and immunity. The loss of muscle mass is superstitiously labeled as the body eating itself or self-cannibalism.

The acidic Caucasian meat-centered diet is contrary to the African alkaline carbohydrate-centered diet of rye, squashes, millet, corn, pumpernickel, wild rice, sprouted seeds, fruits etc. Ancient African vegetarian laborers who built the walled cities, temples, colleges, statues and pyramids, ate alkaline carbohydrates and included figs, dates, onions, lentils, barley, yams, plantain, sprouts, pollen, tropical fruits, etc, in the diet. The cabbage family provided foods which could be used to alkaline the body such as broccoli, green collards, dandelion, figs, kale, mustard greens, sesame seeds, turnip greens, watercress, etc. Ancient Roman, Greek and European athletes, laborers, peasants and gladiators copied this vegetarian diet. Later in Caucasian history the laborers and peasants started following the acidic cooked and raw animal flesh and acidic vegetable diet of the rich, victorious and barbaric clans of rulers. A vegetable shortage caused them to start making meat taste like vegetables by using herbal seasonings.

The contagious sexual diseases, along with "colds" and infections, are a superstitious myth created by Caucasians to scientifically hide their race's sickly, disease and infertility predicament. It would be cultural treason for an African to accept the superstitious belief that the Caucasian diet is not directly related to colds, AIDS, infections and death. Again, the only thing one can catch is ignorance, if they allow the Caucasian to miseducate them about health, nutrition, food and disease.

AIDS

(Collection of disease signs and symptoms)

CAUSES OF AIDS POSITIVE

Alcoholic Hepatitis
- Another Retro Virus
- Arthritis
- Cancer
- Clotting Factors
- Cold Virus

- Cross Reaction
- Drugs
- Fungus
- Hemodialysis
- Hemophiliac Blood Products

❏ Hepatitis
❏ Hepatitis B
❏ Herpes Simplex II
❏ Infection
❏ Influenza
❏ Lupus
❏ Malaria
❏ Malnutrition
❏ Microbes
❏ Myeloma
❏ Parasites

❏ Pregnancy
❏ Prior Pregnancy
❏ Semen
❏ Silicone Implant
❏ Toxins
❏ Tuberculosis
❏ Vaccinations
❏ Worms

Center for Disease Control data indicates
False Positive = 83%

Wake Up, Eat Breakfast and Die

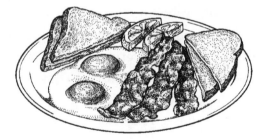

African infants, babies and children under 2 or 3 years of age cannot eat starches. Carbohydrates (starches) such as wheat, corn, rice and oat breakfast cereals cannot be digested by the child. Refined carbohydrates such as a white sugar, candy, cake, potato chips, pretzels and teething biscuits should not be given to the child. The child does not have the enzyme (ptyalin) that allows starches to be eaten. Starches eaten by children become liquid mucus manure that floats in the blood resulting in childhood diseases. Aside from this, the immune system gets weak and the kidney, liver, pineal, adrenals and spleen get exhausted from starches.

The Caucasian junk food companies and doctors want the baby to fatten up for the profit-making disease journey to death. Breakfast cereals (starches) are usually combined totally improperly, so if they could be digested it would not occur. Starches should not be combined with sugar as sugar causes the starches to spoil. Spoiled starches are absorbed in the intestine and create toxins and an acidic body. Further, fruit and cereals are another improper food combination which causes toxins and an acidic condition which weakens all cells, tissues, organs and bones. Added to this, milk should not be combined with fruits or sugar or starch. It causes toxins and an acidic condition which weakens the heart, bones, tissues and organs. Nonetheless, the Caucasian junk food industry, dieticians, medical hoodlums, milk industry and sugar industry tell the public to combine cereal, fruit, milk and sugar. These food combinations are totally against food combining laws, logic and the health of the pineal gland, brain, nerves and every cell in the body.

Africans are also indoctrinated to drink cooked orange juice and eat bread, which is a baked, constipating combination of sugar, wheat, milk, eggs and grease. They also eat bacon (grease) and eggs (chicken fetus) another concoction combined improperly. They eat this along with jelly (sugar and cooked fruit) and butter (milk grease) on toasted bread (starch) and a glass of mucus-forming cooked cow's milk. This is a breakfast that can greet you at the cemetery. Aside from this, protein is easily digested between 10 am and 2 p.m. Starch protein cereals in the morning are extremely taxing on the digestive system of the body. If cooked starches are eaten; they would naturally require fermentation to be eaten and should be digested alone or with vegetables. In the natural African breakfast diet, figs and dates were eaten or other fruits. This is Osirian Law or Cyclic Laws of nutrition. Food should ideally be eaten between the hours of 12 noon and 7 p.m., as this is the ingestion phase. The food is utilized by the body (assimilated) between the hours of 7 p.m. and 4 a.m. Digested food is ideally cleansed from the body from 4 a.m. to 12 noon. Consequently, the African breakfast was usually cleansing fruits. Until the child has developed a full set of teeth and is capable of fully chewing and mixing the food with saliva, starches should not be eaten.

The junk breakfast contributes to eating disorders. Caucasians have a diseased psychological attachment to food, which their American Psychiatric Association classifies as a mental disease. It stems from the Ice Age and superstition. Eating becomes a diseased mental craving and, emotionally, a habit with no control and is a way of letting food control the person. Food helps Caucasians to bury and stuff their true feelings of racial inferiority. Food helps hide the fear, adult delinquency, melanin albinism, dysfunctional family heritages, lack of control, anger, violence, sexism, lack of normalcy and helps bury and stuff their history of murdering over 200 million Africans and stealing every aspect of African civilization except harmony with nature and God.

Caucasians stuff their babies as if the Ice Age is still going to freeze the food supply. They force their babies to eat as often as possible or every two hours and in between meals or suck on amputated breast's rubber nipple. Sucking on a milkless amputated nipple (pacifier) is negative. The babies try to reject the overfeeding of food by drooling, vomiting, burping, having hiccups, diarrhea, stomach gas and childhood diseases. Finally, the babies that are overfed become bloated with fat. Fat babies resemble any of McDonald or Burger Kings or Wendy's or Huddle House's fat pigs or fat cows. Fat Caucasian babies like fat pigs are only fit to be led to a feeding trough and slaughtered so their fat can be used to fill a can of lard. African babies are forced to be overfed by well meaning Caucasian indoctrinated African parents.

This Caucasian mental illness with food becomes another means for the dairy, junk food, drug and medical industries to make large profits. The industries cause Nutricide and use the "break-fast" to reinforce the eating disorders. They create a stable profitable Negro consumer market. Africans are Caucasian trained food addicts that, like all Caucasian experimental laboratory animals eat garbage and beg for more. The Africans are the only experimental animal specimens that buy their own food. They are paying for their own nutritional suicide with a smile on their faces.

The African wakes up eats an undernutritious breakfast and prepares his body for the Caucasian medical sacrifice and dies with each mouth full. If breakfast cereal is not available then jelly (or syrup) cereal sandwiches in the form of bread, waffles, pancakes, or Pop Tarts are eaten. They are just as harmful. It is a hypoglycemic mucus forming breakfast designed in lower Hell. It can cause obesity and a sudden energy drop while in school. This results in the child feeling bored or disinterested in schoolwork. The sugary breakfast sets the child up to dislike school. The white sugar energy collapses in the morning hours of school resulting in low energy, fatigue, depression, inability to concentrate and learning problems. Obesity is not normal in adults or children. It is a sign of a diseased body, mind and spirit. Feeding African children like they are being fattened up for the slave auction block or an animal slaughterhouse is Nutricidal. A baby eating constantly gets fat and bloated The fat gets into the digestive system along with plaque in the cells, tissues, organs, glands and brain. A fat baby is a sick baby. Caucasian animal farms treat baby cattle nutritionally better and only feed them twice a day because it best for their growth and health. A natural foods diet and breast milk are the only defense against fat bloat and childhood diseases, though they are not used. Breast milk regulates feeding intervals and is biochemically balanced, is spiritual, cyclic and has the electromagnetic charge of melanin. Denying the African child the melaninated milk is denying the child the gift of Blackness (Africanity). African children sucking on amputated rubber nipples or bottled milk are eating their way into the Caucasians' Ice Age and caves. Aside from this, there is the negative psychological imprint on the body's subconscious of White being associate with nurturing it is given a white bottle of milk. Added to this when the baby gets ill it is taken to a hospital where all the medical supplies are wrapped in White, and the doctor wears a white laboratory jacket. Consequently, the Black baby associates being made normal and healthy with the White color. In any case, Caucasian diet habits are still connected to their cave eating customs. The custom of fattening the child and feeding them breakfast cereal concoctions along with denying the child breast milk presents a bonding problem, nutritional problem and mental illness problem.

Caucasian babies who are not breastfed begin to develop mental illness and feel that nature denied them a future and that nature cannot be trusted. This stems from the complete interruption of the breastfeeding "rights of passage." The Caucasian mother, raised on nutrient poor soil with poor nutritionally fed plants, could not continue to breastfeed, so she was forced to have her baby suck on a lower animal's breast (cow. goat, etc.). This has mentally instilled in the baby that nature/mother cannot provide (milk) security or be trusted.

Then once the Caucasian child became older, it was famines, disease, constant deaths of dysfunctional family members, hunger, violence, rape, cannibalism and eating plants that could not make him feel full. The constant episodes of starving and then overeating when food was available made life insecure and deficient of higher meaning. Life was explained by superstitions and wars between their many dysfunctional good Gods and evil Gods.

It is this mentally ill and deficient Caucasian civilization with its nutritionally deficient mind and dietary ignorance that is now trying to control the diets of Africans. Further information on diet is in White Racist studies by the Eating Disorders Program at Michigan State University and biased books such as *Managing Your Mind Through Food*, by Judith Wortman. Aside from the mental illnesses caused by denying breastfeeding, the replacement of breast milk with cow's milk is harmful. All of this causes physical diseases called childhood diseases.

Caucasian childhood diseases are normal for them. Childhood diseases are new to African children and directly related to the Caucasian diet and their dietary customs. These diseases are Nutricidal and disruptive of family harmony. They weaken the immune system. The childhood diseases are usually treated with toxic drugs that cause secondary diseases and the destruction of the "so-called" immune system.

The Caucasians combine food ignorantly. Their food combinations are anti-melanin, constipating and actually cause the diseases that are blamed on a virus or bacteria. African parents should fit the child to the food instead of fitting the food to the child. In other words, it is not proper to put sugar, fruit and milk on a cereal in order to get a child to eat it. Feed the child simple food combinations and do not combine starches with fruit, starches with meat, starches with sweets, or give cooked fruit or a sweet and acid fruit combination. These combinations cause fermentation in the stomach, gas, and manure to form in the stomach and a toxic, acidic body.

It is not correct for the African parent to let children eat (past 7 p.m.) at night, or when the child is overheated, feels bad, is tired, stressed, excited, chilled, in pain or is angry. Help the child work through negative emotions or to relax so that the food will get digested properly. The Caucasian cereals are usually not chewed but swallowed, and this ultimately causes disease. The child under 3 years of age does not have the enzyme ptyalin to metabolize the cereal foods. Stuffing the child with cereal, milk, sugar as if he is a turkey or pig can lead to flu, tonsillitis, colds, learning problems, gastritis, personality problems, mood swings, hypertension and a melanin deficiency.

The majority of childhood diseases can be tested with herbs and supplements. An enema with catnip and garlic is cleansing, also herbs (extracts are more useful) such as echinacea, gingko, chickweed, golden seal, yarrow, pau d'arco, peppermint and red clover. Supplements such as vitamins A, B, C, E, zinc, calcium, magnesium, and digestive enzymes are very beneficial.

The childhood diseases are basically the child's body trying to defend itself from adult nutritional ignorance. For example, **chicken pox** is toxins released through the skin with pimples that ooze fluid and form a crust in a 3-to-7-day cycle. The child's fingernails should be cut, as the skin is very itchy. **Measles** is a cleansing through the lungs and skin. Usually the child has bumps, a furry tongue, white spots in the mouth and throat and is sensitive to light. **Mumps** are usually swollen Lymph parotid glands in the back of the jaw between the ears. The Lymph glands get toxic from acidic, overworked food. The glands swell with toxins in an attempt to defend the child from the Caucasian diet. It can be contagious 48 hours before the swelling and up to 6 days after.

Tonsillitis is the inflammation of the tonsils caused by constipating food combinations and cereals. The tonsils get sore, swell and there may be an earache, coated tongue and bad breath. **Rheumatic Fever** is an arthritis type condition of the heart and bone joints (elbow, knee etc.), with pain and stiffness caused by crystallized waste and liquid manure mucus. Flu (influenza) is similar to mucus congestion called a "cold." It is characterized by a dry cough and dry throat. The body tries to defend itself by ejecting the mucus out of the lungs and nasal cavities by coughing. Asthma is basically a type of muscle spasm in the lungs that can be caused by waste in the body and muscles. The muscles around the lungs tighten the chest, which results in wheezing, coughing and difficulty in breathing.

All of the Caucasian caused childhood diseases are accepted as normal. However, they are not normal for African children unless they eat like Caucasians. Childhood diseases are an early start on the path of nutritional self-destruction. Breakfast is a tool used as a wake up meal for death. Caucasian caused nutritional, behavioral disorders and personality disorders are related to the cereals and the hoodlums of the junk food industry, absence of breast feeding and bonding. The social factors created and maintained by White Supremacy place the African child in jeopardy of not having a holistic Africentric future. The book titled *Kids Count Data Book: State Profiles of Child Well Being*, which is a study done by the Center of Social Policy and the Annie E. Casey Foundation, used government statistics and primarily the categories of unmarried teens, birth weight, arrest rates, violent death rate of teens, and single parent households.

This book reveals that Nutricide is preordained if the African parent does not take action to change the diet. The National Research Council (Jayne and Williams, 1989) indicates that African American poverty is 2 to 3 times higher than Caucasians at all times and the mortality and morbidity of African Americans is poor and getting worse. Caucasian created and maintained poverty and social conditions make the African child imprisoned by Nutricide.

The idea that breakfast gives immediate energy is a myth and part of Caucasian mental illness and ignorance. Africans who accept this dietary myth have a fear that if they don't eat breakfast they will get sick or very weak. Fasting at night while asleep and melatonin secretion helps to create the morning energy felt, not "breaking the fast" so-called "break-fast." The body gets accustomed to weight in the stomach, small intestines and the weight of impacted manure in the colon. An absence of the weight and sensation of impacted food and manure causes the African to feel the need to eat.

It is not true hunger but the Caucasian culturally created appetite that must be satisfied with a pasty breakfast. The food eaten will take approximately four hours to leave the stomach and six to sixteen hours to be metabolized in the small intestine with some electrolyte absorption in the large intestine. It is in the small intestine that the energy nutrients are absorbed from the food. In most cases, the drug stimulation reaction to white sugar and bleached white flour is mistaken for the nutrient energy of breakfast. The energy from the food eaten at a 9 a.m. (0900 hours) breakfast will not be nutritionally available to the body until 2100 hours (9 p.m.). At 9 p.m. the body's circadian clock is in the assimilation/melatonin phase. The pace of assimilation is slow at this hour. Consequently, the body won't use the energy from breakfast until the next day.

There is a constant slow energy flow that sustains functions but not the high-energy release that Caucasians assume the body has at the hour of breakfast. If the constipating Caucasian diet is followed, then the energy from food eaten 1 to 7 days in the past is the energy being used during the breakfast hour. In this case, the constipated African is using liquid manure, drugs and toxins for energy. An African who follows this Caucasian, stupid habit of eating an anti-melanin, constipating breakfast concoction is a human sacrifice that worships ignorance.

In general, the food eaten required energy and this energy is diverted from other organs, organ systems and immunity so that an increase of blood can go to the stomach in order to transport nutrients. Often the African feels sleepy or fatigued after eating stimulants such as sugar, dairy, caffeine, condiments, bleached white flour, etc. Condiments (spicy irritants, mustard, pepper, chocolate, nutmeg, cinnamon, etc.), and stimulants are used to overcome the energy drain of sugars, lard, grease, dairy, meat, white flour, refined carbohydrates, etc.

The Africans addicted to Caucasian junk food breakfasts are directly causing degenerative diseases such as arthritis, cardiovascular problems, varicose veins, weak eyes, fertility problems, senility, weak bones, learning disorders, mood swings, cancer, AIDS, venereal diseases, etc. They are eating breakfast to die and waking up for the rehearsal of death. Breakfast should be of cleansing fruit, whole foods, spring or distilled water and/or fruit, juice. It should be eaten in a calm unhurried state, and without talking.

Sugar And Spice, But Not Very Nice (Aspartame = Nutrasweet, Equal)

Aspartame is an artificial sweetener that is 200 times sweeter than white sugar. It is totally synthetic and is made with a toxic poison called methanol. Methanol is combined with aspartic acid and phenylalanine and called aspartame with the commercial trade name Nutrasweet or Equal. Methanol is toxic to the thymus while excessive amounts of aspartic acid and phenylalanine are toxic to the liver. It is cheap to make and yields high profits.

The U.S. Food and Drug Administration has reported that the common symptoms of too much aspartame is dizziness, nausea, vision problems, seizures, malaise and recurrent headaches. The Center for Disease Control has reported that the majority of complaints about aspartame are neurological. Canada, one of the first countries to use it, has noted that aspartame causes menstruation problems, mood swings, numbness and migraine headaches, especially among teenagers. They discontinued its consumption for 10 days and the teenagers' migraine headaches, numbness, mood swings, and other symptoms cleared up.

Children are not tested for toxic levels of aspartame, nor are the secondary effects or permanently damaging effects known. Aspartame is a sweet way to use children as laboratory test animals for the economic profits of Caucasian business. Aspartame can be found in diet foods as well as the following products: chewing gum, wine coolers, sodas, instant tea, milkshake mixes, yogurt, drugs, laxatives, cocoa mixes, cereals, candy, cake, instant breakfast, frozen deserts, gelatin deserts, breath mints, juice drinks, toppings, multivitamins, milk, instant coffee and most foods that say sugar free.

Aspartame is used in carbonated sodas in order to use the word "diet" on the label. The word "diet" on the label actually indicates that the soda is part of a diet. It is never specified on the label whether the word "diet" refers to a junk food, vegetation or weight loss diet. The consumer assumes that the word "diet" means a weight loss food. Aspartame and other synthetic sugars have never been scientifically proven to cause weight loss. In aspartame diet sodas and all sodas, the carbon dioxide used to make carbonated sodas is a poisonous gas. The body exhales toxic carbon dioxide, in order to get rid of it. The consumer ironically buys traces amounts of carbon dioxide and drinks it in carbonated sodas. This is against good health. Carbonated sodas demineralize the body and cause cirrhosis (hardening) of the liver. Harmful synthetic sugars are in "sugar free" foods. If a food taste sweet a type of sugar is in it. The Food and Drug Administration only classifies white sugar (glucose) as an official sugar. The word "sugar free" means white sugar is not in the product. "Sugar free" means a synthetic poisonous sugar such as aspartame is in the food. Synthetic chemicals such as artificial sweeteners are addicting and harmful.

The aspartame users have moved from sugar addiction to aspartame addiction. They never get treated for the sugar (sweets) addiction. Sweet addiction (aspartame, white sugar) doubles the disease-causing effects when combined with bleached white flour, white flour, polished (white) rice, salt, saturated fats, animal flesh and high cholesterol. Heart disease, diabetes, varicose veins, senility, coronary artery disease, circulatory problems, cancer and many other diseases are directly related to refined carbohydrates such as white sugar, bleached white flour, white flour, etc. It was not until they were added to the traditional saturated fat and high cholesterol diet of Caucasians did these diseases arise. When aspartame is added to the combination of saturated fats, high cholesterol, salt and hidden white sugar in junk foods, the health problems will increase. These foods are toxic (poisonous) to the pancreas, liver, pineal gland and the entire body.

Drugs such as aspartame are synergistic (enhancers) to other synthetic chemicals and synthetic junk foods. They may spice up bland food and give a sugar taste to them, but they are not very nice to the health of the body. Books that can reveal more information on the subject are *Sugar Blues*, by William Duffy, *Natural Health, Sugar and the Criminal Mind*, by J. A. Rodale, *Body, Mind and Sugar*, by E. Abrahamson and A. Pezet and *Killer Salt*, by Marietta Whittlesey.

Caucasian businesses use lies to sell white sugar to those desiring natural sugar. For example, brown sugar, is usually white sugar with caramel color sprayed on. Natural raw cane sugar sold in health food stores is white sugar with caramel color. There are other harmful sweeteners such as corn syrup, fructose, sucrose, dextrose, honey, etc. As a result of sugar consumption, over 50% of Americans are hypoglycemic and diabetic while the remainder are prediabetic.

The only truly safe sugars are those found within the raw vegetable or fruit. The herb stevia is a natural sweetener. For those who want a fairly safe sugar, grains such as malt, rice or barley syrup would be best. They are used slowly by the body and are less toxic to the pancreas.

The commercial health foods are loaded with sugars and toxins as well as combined with other foods improperly. There is a large junk health food variety of sugary sweet foods. The problem with junk health food is that deceptive misguiding words such as "natural" are used. A few wholesome ingredients are mixed with brown sugar, corn syrup, aspartame, salt, toxic, hydrogenated oils and processed foods. These foods start out being natural but are gradually converted to junk. The Caucasian health movements usually ruin themselves because they are part of the Caucasian mentality. Salad dressings are junk and another form of liquid sugar "equally" dangerous.

SWEET 'N LOW
INGREDIENTS:
Dextrose **(glucose, corn syrup)**

Causes:

❐ Diabetes
❐ Cancer
❐ Reproduction Problems
❐ Digestion Problems
❐ Genetic Alterations

❐ Mutations
❐ Hardening of Arteries
❐ Decreased Oxygen to Brain and Blood Circulation

*Note: - Contains traces of Hydrochloric Acid (Lye), Sulfuric Acid, Arsenic, Pig and Cattle Blood (Albumin)

❐ 300 Times sweeter than white sugar

❐ increases weight of food (has odorless, tasteless form)

❐ Does not have to be put on label

Calcium Saccharin **(made from Coal Tar)**

Causes:

❐ Cancer
❐ Digestive Disorders
❐ Skin Diseases

❐ Blood Clotting and
   Collagen Formation
   problems

Calcium Silicate

Causes:

❐ Respiratory Problems
❐ Headaches
❐ Diarrhea

❐ Eye Problems
❐ Hives
❐ Shock

*Note: Used to make Cement and Glass, Aspirin, Food Dye, Cosmetics, Anti-Caking Agent

Cream of Tartar

Causes:

❐ Skin Problems
❐ Edema

❐ Mineral Imbalances

*Note: - Can Contain Salt, Dyes, Emulsifiers, Waste, Etc.

ASPARTAME:

Nutra-Sweet.

Contains: Wood Alcohol, Aspartic Acid, etc. (changes into formaldehyde: Embalming Fluid)

Causes:

❐ Alteration in Brain Chemistry
❐ Birth Defects
❐ Blindness
❐ Cancer
❐ Genetic Mutations
❐ Headaches (Brain Aches)
❐ Leg Cramps

❐ Menstruation Problems
❐ Mental Confusion
❐ Mood and Thought
Disorders
❐ Nerve Damage

HONEY

Contains: 70% Fruit Sugar (Fructose)
  30% Sucrose Sugar (White Sugar)
Causes
Causes:

❐ Blood Levels of Insulin
❐ Blood Vessel Damage
❐ Contributes to Uterine Fibroids, Endometriosis, Cystic Mastitis, Breast Cancer Stomach Ulcers
❐ Gouty Arthritis
❐ Hardening of the Arteries
❐ Heart Attacks
❐ Hyperactivity
❐ Increases Blood Fats
❐ Increases Uric Acid, Cholesterol,

❐ Kidney Fatigue and Disease
❐ Liver and Adrenal glands get larger and damage
❐ Mood and Thought Disorders
❐ Pancreas shrinks and deteriorates
❐ Periodontal Disease (Teeth and Gums)
❐ Strokes
❐ Triglycerides, Cortisone,

Sugar Craving Remedy

Gymnema Sylvestre   = sugar craving
Chickweed   = craving
* Bilberry (Huckleberry)   = increases insulin used for diabetes, heals pancreas
Guggulipid   = sugar craving

Minerals

* Vanadium (Vanadyl Sulfate)   = heals pancreas
  Chromium   = increases energy, stabilizes blood sugar

* *considered most effective*

Yeast Infection Remedies

(Yeast causes desires for sugar)

Pau d'Arco   Garlic

Take A Bite Out of Crime

A diet of raw fruits and vegetables naturally brushes the teeth. In fact, the Caucasian tooth brushing ritual is only needed if you eat slimy, mucus-pasty, gummy, fiberless cooked vegetables, fruits and animal flesh. The same slimy, mucus tartar-causing cooked, concoctions put a liquid manure coating in the stomach, small and large intestines, colon, veins, arteries, muscles and joints. The small toothbrush is given the task of cleaning less than 1% of the digestive system while leaving the remainder caked with liquid manure called plaque. The only thing the toothbrush can successfully do is brush cavities and the air (breath) while the teeth rot away from every mouthful of junk food.

The cavities of the teeth actually started prenatally. African women are the worst nourished, which impacts her unborn baby. The Caucasian myth of telling African women to eat for two people is also responsible. This myth causes pregnant African women to overeat, resulting in constipation, tumors, fibroid tumors, cancer, varicose veins, stops melanin recycling, enlarges the womb, causes amniotic fluid to be mixed with liquid manure, obesity, swelling legs and feet, mood swings, personality problems, digestive disorders and weak teeth in the unborn baby. Excessive eating of the highly acidic Caucasian junk food drains the vital nutrients from the fetus' bones and teeth. This helps the Nutricide journey to the cemetery.

Salt (sodium Chloride-table salt) can cause cavities. Sea salt is 7 times saltier. If you eat salt then it will raise the salt level in your biochemical system. Therefore, you would have to raise all the minerals (calcium, magnesium, potassium, iron, etc.) in order to keep the healthy minerals, vitamin and amino acid ratio. If you don't raise all the nutrients level then you are putting yourself in an electrolyte imbalance and in disease crisis. Salt is an astringent, bleaching agent and irritant. It causes skin rashes, insomnia, hair loss, kidney disease, heart disease, obesity, tension, and irritants the roots of the teeth. Salt causes waste to stay in your body, edema, cyclic depression, anxiety, migraine headaches and it is addicting. Chemically it is a toxic poison. It is not classified as a food. Table salt has many ingredients added to it, which are not listed on the label. Salt makes you crave for sugar and compounds the addiction to salt. This increases the deterioration of your teeth.

Sugar is considered the major problem causing cavities. However, it is processed, milled, bleached white flour that causes more cavities. The Caucasians, bread that looks like whole wheat, bleached flour and enriched bleached flour are totally dangerous to the teeth. These synthetic mucus-causing flours are a gooey slime, which is devoid of vitamins, minerals and fiber (roughage). It is fiber that naturally brushes the digestive tract and teeth, not the toothbrush. In any case, processing flour decreases the teeth's life span and only serves to increase the flour's shelf life. It is strictly a moneymaking device that increases profits.

The University of California scientifically researched the deadly value of bleached white flour ("Science" magazine 93, 1941). They found that animals on a diet of enriched white flour died from malnourishment while animals on plain bleached white flour became crippled, senile and sluggish. The diseases that enriched white flour causes are far more dangerous than the diseases plain bleached white flour causes. The addition of synthetic calcium (or calcium from oyster shell animal bone, or dolomite) causes acidity which results in draining the body of calcium. This causes weak bones, bone loss and cavities. A digestive enzyme added to synthetic tricalcium phosphate and calcium carbonate is alkaline and adds phosphate and carbon to the blood, which results in biochemicals that lead to bone loss and cavities.

Ancient Africans were over 9S% cavity-free without tooth-brushes. They used the balchew sticks and raw vegetables and fruits, not toothbrushes. The Caucasian has an almost 100% cavity rate and uses the toothbrush nearly 100% of the time. This obviously means the toothbrush ritual is a failure. In fact, most of the Caucasian dentists have false teeth. They still preach the religion that says the solution to rotten teeth and a rotting away digestive tract is to brush teeth.

Tooth brushing is a fad (fashion) that is supported by no scientific research. Obviously, it was and is a business plan to increase profits for Caucasian companies that sell toothbrushes, toothpaste, toilet hygiene items, teeth braces, teeth bleach, teeth plastic enamel and gold, flossing strings, fluoride and mouthwash. Historically, Caucasian dentists were allowed into schools to examine teeth and they recommended the toothbrush. A brush salesman, not the dentist, started the ritual of brushing the teeth. Ironically, synthetic toothpaste is used and spit out. It is supposedly dirty once it is used and since it is synthetic, it is probably wise to spit it out rather than swallow, which may harm the body. Natural toothpaste is not harmful and can be swallowed after use. The toothbrush ritual includes the superstition of spitting out toothpaste. Mouthwash is an alcoholic beverage which alcoholics drink to get drunk. A mouth freshly rinsed with an alcohol mouthwash can indicate drunk driving if you are tested too soon after using it.

The Caucasian toothbrush cannot stop the deterioration of the bones or rotten teeth. It merely represents a medical ritual used to get Africans' minds conditioned for Nutricide. They have truly taken the bite (teeth) out of crime against Africans.

No Laughing Matter

Laughter and joy are a scientific part of the most scientific people—Africans. In African civilization laughter was an accepted part of events (i.e., funerals, birth, illness, etc.). Laughter is joy. Africans feel the joy of a deceased person going home to the spirit world. Africans will laugh during funeral ceremonies. Caucasians labeled this African spiritual joy as foolishness, childish and the stupidity of a backward primitive. African Americans began to adopt this White Racist oppression of funeral joy and now wear sad faces at funerals. Laughter is a fundamental part of healing and health. Without laughter, the diseased African cannot make a truly holistic recovery from an illness.

When African adults and children laugh, it is more than just joy and happiness. It is a chemical and electrical holistic activity that stimulates melanin. Laughter creates electrical impulses that turn an electrical wave into a chemical (neurotransmitters). Neurotransmitters are living cells. Laughter and thinking actually make cells. It is a spiritual process and helps strengthen the cell immunity and stimulates melanin production.

Aside from this, it is a physical exercise that increases the heart rate, exercises muscles, increases hormone action and can increase oxygen use. Laughter increases alertness by releasing catecholamines. The brain secretes endorphins (a relaxing morphine-like molecule) that relax muscles, get rid of pain, lower blood pressure, aid digestion, reduce inflammation, relieve stress and create antibacterial tears.

Laughter in the African community helps share feelings, crises, heals and bonds people. It helps to defeat depression, bad feelings, tension, inferiority, anxiety, panic and conflicts in relationships. Depression and a negative image of oneself can create cells that decrease immunity, lower melanin levels and make you easy prey for disease. Laughter can be used as a type of self-defense. In children, laughter is a common holistic language that can bridge the gap of a small vocabulary, which cannot express the child's full range of ideas and feelings.

Caucasians are slowly starting to scientifically understand and accept the holistic dimensions of laughter. The Caucasian Duke University Comprehensive Cancer Center in Durham, North Carolina uses laugh wagons. These wagons are filled with comic materials and pulled in the hallway to spread laughter. In the book *Anatomy of an Illness*, by Norman Cousins, laughter is mentioned as therapeutically important for disease recovery. Laughter truly is not a laughing matter but a scientific body language used for holistic health.

Read Labels or Comic Books

Labels are used to identify and control food and ultimately control the African American consumer. Historically, African prisoners of wars were labeled "slaves." This was a method of deception for the Caucasian slave owner and a method of using the power of words to control Africans. An African who believed himself to be a "slave" would live as a slave. The same White Supremacy mentality that labels Africans as slaves is nutritionally labeling harmful foods as valuable. The nutritional labeling of foodstuffs is not to educate or protect, but is used to biochemically control and destroy the melanin of Africans.

The federal government, along with the food industry, has decided to enter the natural foods, vitamin and mineral supplement and nutrition market. They are jointly moving to control the natural foods nutrition market. They have set recommended nutrient daily allowance standards and list the nutritional value of fruits and vegetables and other foodstuffs.

The nutritional value of plants varies according to crops, soil composition, type of seeds, type of rainfall, cycle variant, type of fertilizer and cultivation method. These factors are ignored and a standard value is set for a crop based on a "random sample" (science words for the best guess). The labels fail to list the anti-melanin, anti-nutritional values and the dangerous effects of the toxic chemicals used to grow and process the foods and the toxicity of the packaging or cans. The African American's attention is "turned off" to the harm the food does and is "turned on" to the nutritional value. It is a deadly game that the African American loses while the food industries win.

The same government that failed to protect human rights, civil rights and "ethnic medical rights" is the same government that cannot and will not stop noise, water and air pollution and toxic chemical pollution of foods. This government is now concerned about the nutritional value of foods and the same companies that pour lethal chemicals on fruits and vegetables are now concerned about nutrition. They are putting nutrition labels on foods that have synthetic disease-causing chemicals. Food labeling is a way to protect anti-nutritional, anti-melanin crimes and profits. The label tends to give an atmosphere of respectability to the crime. There are a new group of words to use to sell the same chemicalized foods. Nutrition appeals to the latest consumer health fad.

The White Supremacy government and private industries have once again completely ignored African peoples' unique biochemistry and nutrition levels and have allowed synthetic food chemicals to retard melanin (pineal gland) production. Both the government and private companies function to make profits. The only difference is one files income taxes (private) and the other does not (government). Once again they have decided what is nutritionally and medically (not allowed to use herbal medicine by health insurance companies or hospitals) best for their "darkies," "coons," "niggers," "colored people," "Negroes," blacks, Afro-Americans, African Americans and Africans. To them it is automatic to dictate what is best for their African wage slaves.

They will not and do not allow Africentric consumer scientists, health practitioners, nutritionists, disease treatments or diets to be considered or change their White Supremacist minds. Their only argument is whether to use chemical or nutritional language on food labels and ignore the nutritional slaughter of African Americans. They are concerned with the ritual and ceremonial use of words.

The ceremonial and ritual use of Greek and Latin words on food labels is more important than an African American's life. Words such as "essential," "non essential," "dispensable," and "indispensable" are used to confuse and control African American's nutritional awareness. For example, "essential" amino acids (protein building blocks) are amino acids the body needs while "non-essential" amino acids the body can make. This sounds simple, but actually it is word nonsense or Caucasian "Latin word" or "Greek word" ceremonial and ritual usage, which is word trickery. The body can make (convert) non-essential amino acids into essential amino acids and essential amino acids into non-essential amino acids. Amino acid or vitamin and mineral conversion is a melanin mediate action. Highly melaninated Africans have the ability to change one nutrient into another nutrient, if and only if they are on a natural foods diet.

A synthetic Caucasian food diet stops melanin's ability to convert. Amino acids such as tryptophane, tyrosine, methionine, Lysine and glutamine are absolutely essential for melanin usage. In the melanin albino Caucasian diet, these amino acids are not that essential. Africans have essential amino acids, which are not too essential to Caucasians. Nutrients (including amino acids) are plentiful in a natural foods diet.

Sunshine is an indispensable nutrient for Africans because it helps in food digestion, melanin regulation and also stabilizes calcium. In the Caucasian, sunshine stimulates the diseases and cancer in their bodies, which results in skin cancer, so sunshine is considered dispensable to them. The words essential or dispensable are giving a false scientific value to junk foods and chemically polluted produce. Words allow genetically and chemically polluted cow's milk, (or any animal milk for that matter) which is not nutritionally fit for humans to be sold because it meets the poor health safety standards and lists its nutrient value on the label. Words also allow chemically polluted meat (animal flesh) to be sold because it meets safety standards and lists nutrient value on the label.

The nutritional labeling of food with vitamin, mineral and amino acid content is not easily understood, in fact, it is a legal way to give scientific respectability to food that is chemically toxic. A vegetable, fruit or other foodstuffs with an excessive amount of one particular nutrient can be labeled as fortified. This gives consumers a false sense that they are getting nutrients when actually, they are being nutritionally drained. It is the ratio of nutrients in balanced proportions that increase its value. Increasing one nutrient requires all other nutrients to be increased or else the body drains its stored nutrients to make a balanced ratio.

It is best to combine natural foods to achieve balance rather than let the Caucasian food industry play God by synthetically creating stupid ratios. For example, cereal proteins are naturally high in the amino acid methionine and low in the amino acid Lysine. Legumes (beans, peas) are high in the amino acid Lysine and low in methionine. Therefore, the combination of cereal and legumes provides balanced proteins (amino acids). The ratio of synthetic herbicides and pesticides combined with food processing chemicals causes undefined lethal destruction to the human body. No indication or measured amounts of toxic chemicals are labeled on vegetables, fruits and foodstuffs, only the nutritional value is placed on the label. This accentuates the positive (nutrients) and causes the African American's mind to ignore the negative (chemical pollution). Nutrition labels have now become the newest way to cover up the health destruction (Nutricide) of African people. Nutrition labeling has now spread to the fast food industry.

The fast food industry does not use nutrition to sell its disease-producing, immune destructive, anti-melanin and constipating, synthetic junk foods. This industry has never provided educational information that could help the consumer select or combine food properly. They only meet health sanitation standards. The same government that allows food to be chemically polluted is now concerned about nutrition standards that they cannot and will not enforce. It is a case of "the blind leading the blind, one white racist capitalist telling another white racist capitalist how to protect African Americans' ethnomedical, ethnonutritional and ethnophysiological rights. Nutrition labeling in the hands of a white racist is another tool of "nutrition restraint" and Nutricide. Nutritional labeling has combined the White Racist Health food industry with the "White Racist junk food industry."

Africans failed to obtain ethnonutritional rights when Caucasian were eating health foods. Caucasians' diets were of health foods up until the 18th century. Then, African Americans failed to get ethnonutritional rights in the junk food era (19th century to the 20th century) and now they have failed to get those rights during the current Caucasian health food fad era. The Caucasian diet wheel has made a complete turn and only serves to roll over African bodies, except now they have added nutrition labels.

The current food ingredient labels actually give a vague idea of what the foodstuff contains. The food manufacturers and the Food and Drug Administration (FDA) have no idea of the true ingredients. They are just as puzzled as to what the food products contain as you are with the Greek and Latin words used to label ingredients and nutrients. The FDA does not set standards for identification or limits as to the chemicals used to make ingredients or the toxicity of chemicals used to make nutrients. They are not aware of the medical and melanin problems Africans can have from eating lethal chemicals or unbalanced nutrients. For example, carbonated sodas contain emulsifiers, artificial colors, synthetic flavoring, aromas, flavor enhancers, glycerin, anti-foaming agents, salts, caffeine, dirt, foaming agents, retardants, buffers, synthetic sweeteners, preservatives and "optional ingredients." The "optional ingredients" are synthetic chemicals that do not have to be put on the label. Added to this polluted water is used to make soda a liquid.

At best, the soda companies and other food companies' labels amount to a chemical make believe, pretend fairy tale type of ingredient story. It would be better to read a comic book than the ingredients of a soda; at least the comic book is entertaining. If you were to separately eat one of the chemical ingredients of a soda all day you would get brain damage, become physically ill, permanently damaged or die. In fact, you can eat a natural food or ingredient all day without getting sick. However, an unwholesome food eaten all day such as mustard, vinegar, salt, white sugar, mayonnaise, pickles, black pepper, cayenne, oil, grease, nutmeg, salad dressing, wine sauce, tartar sauce, etc., will cause an illness, because they are not foods.

If you were to eat the ingredients of a natural juice all-day you will not get sick, you will be healthy. Natural juices list their ingredients. For example, the ingredient label of natural apple juice would list organic apples or apples (no chemicals or water would be in it). You can read a natural foods label without the help of a dictionary or interpreter. On the other hand, if you want to confuse your mind, destroy your melanin and put nutritional restraints on your ability to be African, then the FDA and junk food companies are waiting for you at the store so they can deliver another Negro to the cemetery. Commercial grocery stores should have a label (sign) on their building that reads "Caution, the foods in this building are harmful to your health."

Talking Can Make You Sick

Conversations with supposedly nice, well-meaning Caucasians can cause destructive emotions, anger, boredom, frustration and stress in African people. Since African people are highly melaninated, it causes them to be highly emotional psychic and spiritually sensitive. Therefore, Africans can feel Caucasians are deceitfully hiding their insincerity and dependent on word order or a logical, rational conversation that makes no holistic sense. It is Caucasian abnormal thinking, which relies on word process. In other words, Caucasians feel that if something makes sense to them it must make sense to everyone. This is arrogance. This is part of their religious belief in the myth of White Supremacy. Caucasian conversation has no rhythm and relies on words (fragments) to explain their ideas.

African conversations are chemical and rely on the holistic visualization of the concept (picture) to explain holistic ideas. Caucasians typically move to prove their ideas with statistics, research, or laws of average. African people typically are in harmony with nature and themselves and use direct, honest and open ideas as proof. This is confusing to hear for the linear communication ear of Caucasians.

Words to African people are used in a ritual and ceremonial ethnic fashion and paint pictures. Words for Caucasians are not culturally based but imagined to be a pure form of logic process. They do not see how Eurocentric their words are. Caucasian words are based on superstition, self-centeredness and the collective mental illness of being a psychotic (White Supremacy is a psychosis). They tend to focus on a single idea (fragment) and ignore the total ideas as a concept of spiritual and communal rhythmic harmony.

Fundamentally, the problem with Caucasian and African communication is the mentally ill (Caucasian) talking to the sane (African). An African would have to be "out of his mind" and into the Caucasian mind in order to communicate effectively with a Caucasian. An African "out of his mind" usually has adopted Caucasian thinking processes and does not see the Caucasian as a part of a mentally ill civilization. In any case, Caucasian conversation is nutritionally draining to Africans because of the built-in psychosis of it, the arrogant insulting tone of it, and the double-talk nature of it (conflicting ideas, right and wrong mixed, important words are long words, etc.).

Caucasian conversation is a series of words being processed and is self-centered. It causes Africans to have stress, emotional torture, mental confusion and it is spiritually upsetting. Africans may not consciously be aware of the sympathetic nervous system reaction to the Caucasian verbal assaults, but they do feel a sense of vagueness and emptiness from Caucasian "word salads." Caucasians typically use cliches, socially pleasant sentences, "I am a nice white person talking to a Negro" tone in their voice; "I am not a racist, but I am white and superior" tone, and the Africans, inner self reacts to this toxic verbal energy. The melanin dominated African holistically feels the toxic energy and they must ignite the immune system to defend them from Caucasian toxic word use. It nutritionally requires extra vitamin B6, phenylalanine, yucca, suma, gingko, tryptophane, rosemary, gotu kola, L-dopa, niacinamide, methionine, tyrosine, ginseng and a natural diet consisting of raw food to cope with the subtle energy loss caused by the "word" abuse (unholistic conversation) of Caucasian White Supremacists.

Caucasian mental illness saturates their mind, mood, state of consciousness and use of conversation. Their conversation is diseased. Caucasian arrogance, hostile negative temperaments and diseased attitudes are directly and/or indirectly felt by highly electromagnetically charged Africans. Caucasian conversations are usually never identified as being as crazy as they are. It is not examined by them or taught in Africentric education or Black Studies, but it is obvious that racism has polluted their ability to honestly communicate.

Therefore, Caucasian conversation is not healthy, but part of their mental illness. If an African immediately reacts to this disease type Caucasian conversation, the Caucasian labels the African as too emotional, not intellectual and inferior. The normal Caucasian conversation is mentally oppressive to the feelings, mind and emotions of Africans. Their conversation oppression causes an energy drain. This can lead to self-imposed or Caucasian imposed chemical restraints (drugs). An African chemically restrains the depression, anger, rage and need to defend self from the craziness of a psychotic conversation. This Caucasian polluted word use can lead to nutritional restraints (junk foods). This junk food with white sugar, bleached white flour, grease, synthetic chemicals, milk and salt drain nutrients and puts the African below the problem. It helps numb the mind, spirit and body from the pain of hearing a psychotic talk psychotically. The chemical and nutritional restraints weaken the pineal, adrenal, liver, hypothalamus, thymus and gonad glands and drain the body of melanin. Ultimately the effect of talking with or listening to Caucasians talk can make you as mentally sick as they, and lead the African to Nutricide.

Safe Drugs - Ritual Superstition

Superstitions are deeply rooted in Caucasian society and science. In medical science they still practice superstitious beliefs such as using animals or African people as sacrifices to prove a toxic (poisonous) drug is economically safe for human use. Drugs used on animals are a Caucasian scientific ritual called an experiment. This ritual testing has been proven scientifically stupid by the United States government's Office of Technology Assessment that published this in publication No. 286 929, titled "Assessing the Efficacy and Safety of Medical Technologies" (September 1978).

For example, scientific drug tests are still performed on guinea pigs when it is known that guinea pigs can eat "strychnine" (a poison that kills humans) without harm. "Penicillin" is an antibiotic that kills guinea pigs while only destroying the immune system in people. "Tuberculin" vaccine causes tuberculosis in people while curing it in pigs. "Digitalis" causes high blood pressure in dogs. "Aspirin" causes birth defects in animals. A heart medicine such as "emidin" proved safe for animals while in people it kills and causes digestive and eye problems. Aside from this, a scientific method for converting lower animals, physiology so that it equals human physiology is an impossibility.

When animals are not used, Africans in ghettoes, jails or at government-supported medical facilities are used as experimental sacrifices. Sample sizes of drugs are given out which allow the drug clans of companies to use Africans as sacrifices that they call clinical experiments.

Also, the Caucasian cannibalism is still being mislabeled as science. The drug clans use human cells to pervert, freak (hybrid), and stimulate plant growth. The consequences of eating cannibalistic plants that have been raised or mated with human or animal cells is dangerous. Human cells used as plant drugs is a clear example of the psychosis of Caucasians. If the United States government cannot use the entire African body or African cells, then they use people in foreign countries. The U.S.A. pays countries to abort fetuses up to 5 months for organ harvesting or cell use. Sacrifices are used in the scientific "double blind" studies (experiments) in which physically or mentally ill people are given medicine or a sugar pill (placebo). It is called "double blind" because the doctor is not aware (blind) who is getting medicine and the sick person is not aware (blind) whether he is getting medicine or a sugar pill. However, the laboratory workers are aware. Double blind studies are a violation of the sick person's human rights and medical ethics which states that a doctor must help the sick get healthy instead of allowing a disease to kill them.

African Americans are also sacrificed for another Caucasian superstitious ritual called a clinical trial. In clinical trials, an African is paid to use a toxic, untested drug. Whether the African takes the drug or throws it away is really not researched. Nonetheless, the Africans that do take the drug are usually damaged in some way. If the drug is 20% or more effective, then it passes the clinical trial and is sold to the general public. The clinical trail with synthetic chemicals is nothing more than a ritual with no purpose other than to satisfy superstitions.

All synthetic drugs work by slowing down, speeding up or destroying Melanin. The sciences of biology and chemistry that they use to make synthetic chemicals are based upon Melanin. The science of chemistry (Keme-Black-Melanin) is based upon studying Melanin particles called electrons, protons and neutrons. The science of biology based upon the action and reaction cells Melaninated nucleus (brain) operation upon tissues, organs and systems. Drugs like chemistry and biology are Melanin based. Drugs chemically lynch, cripple and/or enslave Melanin. Caucasians call their "chemical and Biological Willie Lynch" and "Biochemical Plantation" army of antimelanin drugs science. Caucasian science is merely another translation of White Supremacy. Their White sugar synthetic chemical sweetener destroys the Melanin centers of the pancreas (Island's of Langerhaus) The Prozac synthetic drug works by stopping the melanin hormone (serotonin) from being used (reuptake inhibitor). A scientist has a culture first (cosmetology) before he can choose his profession second science is culturally confined. It cannot exist without people. People cannot exist without a culture. Caucasian science like Caucasian culture is a collection of superstitions and rituals.

The New Drug, T'is The Season To Be Healthy

Drugs are used, abused, misused and misunderstood. We are trained to rely on drugs to change our poor health to good health, to change our bad moods to good moods, and give us a false sense of life (reality). Drugs answer our immediate needs. If we need energy, we take uppers (amphetamines, speed); if we need sleep, we take downers (sedatives and depressants); if we need relief from pain; we take aspirin. To stay awake we take wake uppers like caffeine, and if we want to feel good, we take alcohol, marijuana, heroin or cocaine. We live in a drug-oriented society (European society).

In the past the drugs of choice for Africans have been depressants (downers) such as alcohol, marijuana and heroin. Oppression causes the drugs of choice to be depressants. They are downers and psychologically slow down the depression. The illegal drugs of choice for white society have been speed (e.g., cocaine and mind-altering drugs like LSD). Over 70% of Caucasians are drug addicted while less than 30% of Africans are addicted. This is related to melanin's protective ability. The Caucasians' life is considered the good life, and they want to travel the good life faster with cocaine or LSD. Africans have the bad life and want to go through it slower and use drugs to get down below and underneath the hurt and pain of oppression, so they would take "downers"—(depressants). Now Africans are trying to rush through their oppression by taking addictive accelerators like cocaine.

The slave master gave the African chattel slaves drugs to get more labor out of them. Then, after chattel slavery, Africans advanced to wage slavery (barely enough money to feed themselves, pay rent and bills). Now, Africans have advanced to mental slavery. They freely volunteer to put on their own chains and whip themselves. These are the most dangerous types of slaves because they no longer need the slave master; they have become both slave and slave master. They are the new Negroes from Negro-land. These Africans are not out of their own mind; they are out of the white man's mind. The end result of drug usage (and addiction) in African society is family destruction, death and more wealth for the white society that promotes the manufacture and sale of these addictive poisons.

Addiction of any type follows a simple step-by-step process. You can become addicted to anything by following these steps. All addictions are not bad or evil. For example, addiction to exercise, natural foods and herbs, good manners, and being truthful are good addictions. Then there are bad addictions, such as illicit sex, drugs, Whiteness, slavery, violence and junk foods.

The steps to addiction are as follows:

- **Step 1: Introduction**—to the drug (or negative activity) usually by a friend.

- **Step 2: Re-introduction**—the victim requests the drug.

- **Step 3: Craving**—the person develops a desire for the drug and associates it with pleasure.

- **Step 4: Mental dependence**—the victim must have the drug or destructive activity in order to "have a good time."

- **Step 5: Physical dependence**—drug withdrawal pains will occur if drug use is stopped.

A person can go through these addictive steps in one week, one month or one year. They can take the drug once a day or once a year and still be an addict because the drug controls their life, mind and body. A drug is really any substance that is isolated and concentrated. For example, white sugar, once you take it out of the sugar cane plant, becomes a drug because it is isolated and concentrated. Nicotine is isolated and concentrated by burning the tobacco in cigarettes. Alcohol, white sugar, salt, bleached flour and caffeine are just a few of the many drugs.

If you take the Africans out of Africa, then isolate them from culture (using slavery, oppression and exploitation), and concentrate them in the ghettos (concentration camps), put them in the social underclass (lower economic class), and educational prisons, you have created a new social drug. This is the hideous work of Europeans and European-Americans. They get high from African music, dance, entertainers (actors, athletes, politicians), and then they advance their high with African science, sex, violence and White Supremacy. Nutricidal Africans have become the white man's new drug. These Negro men and women dress up like Europeans in order to advertise European culture as Supreme. They are living commercials for the Caucasian culture and sex psychosocial high. Then, these Negroes wonder shy they marry and have sex with white folks. They have become intoxicated on the White psychotic high. They are a cloned high of White Supremacist.

ADDICTION

- Is built into the predatory European society (poverty, rape, crime, violence, self-hatred, dysfunctional family, homosexuality, etc.).
- It is symptom of White Domination (victims of White Supremacy)
- Social conditions create drug suicides (buy drugs to kill oneself)
- Associated with oppression, Slavery Trauma, Cultural Stress.

- Is part of African Co-Dependency upon European Domination and psychosis.

TREATMENT

- Must bond to African Culture (defines a Black persons' reality, self, solutions).
- Must have basic needs of spirituality, family, shelter, food, health, job or self-employment.
- Must provide personality adjustment, not personality change.
- Counseling must be at arms length, do not touch or force eye contact.
- Starts after detoxification from drug, behavior, etc.

STEPS IN TREATMENT

- Bond to Maat, culture, customs, rituals, natural foods, exercise, herbs etc.
- Solve need and act upon need to destroy White Domination.
- Heal relationship with self, family, children, and friends.
- Develop Psycho social and Historical Awareness.
- Identify Problem.
- Design method to change negatives to positives.
- Evaluate Achievements (Rewards, Punishments, etc.)
- Follow treatment schedule, goals, relapse therapy, etc.

Spit in the Face
(The Medical Symbol)

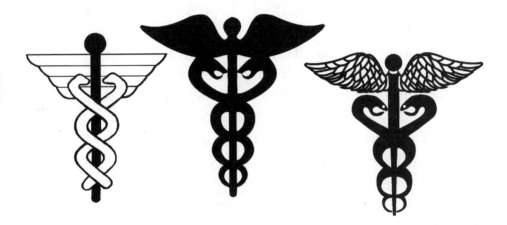

The healing arts symbol, born on the continent of Africa, reflects the origin of medical sciences, nutrition and civilization on this planet. The healing arts symbol called the caduceus, serpentine fire, tree of life or Aesculapius is used by many organizations (Taber's Medical Dictionary edited by Clayton Thomas, M.D.). It is erroneously believed to belong to European medical doctors. It is not exclusively a registered trade mark, copyrighted symbol or creation of any European organization. This symbol predates all European civilizations and its earliest usage was part of ancient Africa's religious (spiritual) based orders (schools).

The ancient Africans were the first to use the medical symbol. Greeks and Romans called this mythological symbol Aesculapius. Aesculapius is the European name for an African man named Imhotep. He was an Egyptian doctor. Hippocrates was a student of Imhotep and was called an Aesculapian.

In the Aesculapian symbol, or tree of life symbol, the two snakes (serpents) intertwined indicate the connection of the cycles (laws) and the unity of the two great truths (i.e., day/night, female/male, life/death, health/sickness, right/wrong). The crossing snakes are intertwined around a divine Rod (Scepter) which was carried by Hermes Trimegistus (Greek/Roman word) who was originally called Thoth by Africans. Thoth was the healing attribute of God, inventor of calculus; geometry and the "word." Thoth wrote the name of King Seti I on the tree of life in the Temple of Karnak. "Seb," the ruler of snakes, (order, cycles) joined the snakes together to show the harmony of the two truths (female/male principles of life). The circle at the top of the scepter represents the cosmic circle of the whole that contains all creation or the astral (stellar) that has the solar and lunar inside it. This is a sign that the Greater contains the Lesser.

The triangle or symbolic pyramid of the tree of life represents the sun being born in the east. The three points (corners) on the triangle indicate God, humans and nature or the pineal gland, pituitary gland, and hypothalamus gland or the heaven, earth and nether world which was also called the Orion Star of Horu. The bird's wings represent the Vulture or Eagle's wings which symbolize the Atel (judgment) or the twin truths (day/night, female/male etc.). The two wings also indicate the double Horus (order, law, structure, cycles) which are separated and united by the Urem or Rem or Nile River. These two truths are symbolized by the City of Coming Forth by Day (City of the living) on the East Bank of the Nile River and the city of Coming Forth by Night (city of the dead) on the West Bank of the Nile. Aside from this, the tree of life symbolizes the solstices, equinox and solar opening of the earth (Harris Papyrus).

The snakes, wand, wings and cosmic circle combine to form the tree of life. Trees in ancient Egypt were called Teru and indicate order, structure, academics, rites of passage, cycles, the generative principle and woman. The tree of life symbolizes holistics (body, mind, spirit). The crossing of the snakes represents the crossing of the nervous system and primary energy force fields (acupuncture meridians). One snake represents the mind while the other snake represents the body intertwined and united around God's divine rod (scepter)

The symbol is also called the Caduceus and the word "cadaver (body)" is derived from it and is a Latinized African word. The tree of life is symbolic of reincarnation as the snake sheds its skin and is born again. In African mythology one snake died (body) and was reborn when the other snake gave it a healing herb (spirit). The serpents (snakes) were given the names of Imhotep's children such as Panakia (pancreas) and Hakia (hygiene).

If the tongue, fangs and deadly sting of the snake are exposed, it represents allopathic medicine. European MD's use this type of suppressive medicine to treat disease. When the serpents shed their skin, it represents homeopathic medicine. This medicine treats symptoms in order to purify the body. When the serpent has its tail in its mouth, this represents naturopathic medicine. Naturopathy nourishes the life force in the body and allows the body to cure itself.

Imhotep's Greek/Roman name, Aesculapius, reveals further the African origin of medicine. "Ashe" means human, "scul (school)" means instruct, and "aphe" means snake and the combined words mean "to instruct about the snakes." The Greeks/Romans/Europeans learned from stolen knowledge of the world's oldest books on medicine, the African books called the *Hearst Papyrus of The 7ᵗʰ Egyptian Dynasty (2000 BC)* with 250 remedies, *Kahun Papyrus of 12ᵗʰ and 13ᵗʰ Dynasty (2133 7 T0 1766)* with gynecology treatments and in the 18th Dynasty (1500 BC), there are the *London Medical Papyrus, Ebers Papyrus, Edwin Smith Papyrus, in the 19th Dynasty (1000 B.C.), Chester-Beatty Papyrus and Berlin Papyrus.*

Aside from these medical books, there are other African books, which are still secretly held or were destroyed. For example, Clement of Alexandria A.D. 200 and Iamlichus A.D. 363 reported that 42 books on Human Knowledge called *Hermetic (Thoth) Books*, were destroyed or stolen. Book number 37 on Anatomy, book 38 on Disease, book 39 on Surgery, book 40 on Remedies, book 41 on Eye Disease and book 42 on Female Disease are missing.

Aside from these books on medicine, there are many more African books by countless African authors that Europeans destroyed such as the 40 books written by Ahmad Babo, who was the first Black President of the University of Sankore in Timbuctu.

Ancient European historians such as Dioscorides, Galen and Theophratus wrote and quoted the medical prescriptions that they learned from the books in the library of the Temple (University) of Imhotep at Memphis, Egypt. Hippocrates (who Europeans say invented medicine) quotes the African textbook called the *Carlsburg Papyrus* #4. Many of the symbols of Latinized letters and Latinized African words were passed to the Europeans in 1600 BC when Thutmose II colonized Cyprus, Crete, Syria, Babylonia, Kadesh and other Mediterranean and Asian countries.

Thutmose Stela at Karnak contains the "Hymn of Triumph" which states that 110 European colonies paid taxes to Africa. In fact, the European colonies would protest to Africa for not providing enough African soldiers to protect Europeans from other European barbaric raiding hordes of thieves, rapists, cannibals and dysfunctional families. Historically, this contact with African civilization allowed the European to learn of medical science and its African symbol, "The Tree of Life."

In contemporary times, Africans brought to America and en-slaved demonstrated that they learned medical science and nutri-tion in Africa. The enslaved African women and men (doctors) knew the exact medical healing principles of herbs. African doctors were sold as slaves because they were expert medical scientists. These African doctors were used by European physicians and pharmacists until laws were passed that made it illegal (1749 Gen-eral Assembly of South Carolina).

The African healing art and symbol have been stolen by Euro-peans. However, the medical symbol, whenever it is seen an-nounces to the world that Africa and Africans are the originators and creators of medical science. Despite the Europeans' stealing the science and symbol and destroying valuable books that belonged to African people, they remain the most diseased race. Caucasians are constantly seeking cures, drugs, surgery, and technology to slow down their bodily diseases and disguise their disease of mental ill-ness (White Racism is a psychosis). The Caucasian White Suprem-acy mental illness causes them to use any and every means to con-trol and destroy African people. They use peace, nutrition, educational religion, computers, movies, sexism, government, drugs, jail, food, science and medicine to control or destroy African people. The medical symbol represents not only Afiica's knowledge, but is also another means by which Caucasians spit in the face of all African peoples.

Guide for Classification of Energy Chart

Energy that enters the body or acts upon the body can be placed into two general categories. Energy can be in the form of herbs, foods, vitamins, minerals, disease or it can be emotional, mental as well as spiritual. Energy can either add or take away from health. This chart is designed to help you to classify herbs, food, nutrients, disease, etc., so that you can be aware of the treatment needed. For example, if one properly of an herb or disease is known, it can be classified. Once classified, the organs or organ system that is weakened can be strengthened or cleansed by the correct herbal remedy. For example, an herb such as Yohimbe speeds up the bodily nervous system Therefore, it would be classified as a sympathetic nervous system activator and it would have all the other characteristics that are under Male Principle. This herb's continued use would drain or weaken the male principle. An herb classified as a Female principle such as alfalfa or chamomile would help to balance the energy drain of yohimbe.

Another example would be valerian. This herb is a sedative to the nerves. Since it relaxes the nerves it would be classified as Female principle and would decrease (slow down) breathing (respiration), slow down (decrease) circulation and at the same time increase the digestive process, and increase secretion from sex glands. Further, a disease reaction such as constipation indicates that it is Male principle so the bodily state would be acidic. Consequently, an herb such as catnip or senna could be used because they are alkaline and would promote the excretion of waste (bowel movement).

Additionally, drugs such as refined sugar, salt (sodium chloride) as well as meat are contractive. The biochemistry of the body reacts to the eating of drugs and meat by trying to expand (dilute) them in order to neutralize their harmful effect. The rush of neutralizing biochemicals of the body results in speeding up the body, which gives a stimulating effect. The body's reactions feel stimulating; the drugs and meats are not. The drugs and meat are not stimulants but destructive depressive immune retardants.

Too much speeding up of reactions in defense against drugs, meat, dairy and junk foods causes an energy, drain resulting in a drop of energy that is exhaustion and mislabeled relaxation. For example, white sugar increases the blood sugar and overstimulates the liver and pancreas, which in turn causes an oversecretion of insulin. An excessive amount of insulin causes sugar diabetes or turns sugar into fat. Excessive insulin (hyperinsulin) results in weight gain (obesity) or weight loss. Too much blood sugar results in low blood sugar (hypoglycemia) causing mental sluggishness and fatigue. There is also a biochemical reaction to overstimulation of the Male principle resulting in Female Principle rebound. There are other holistic relationships. This energy classification system is related to all energy available to humans be it cosmic, spiritual, intelligence or unseen. The human is part of all and all is part of the human body. The human body is similar to a tree. The Ankh holistically represents that tree's aspect.

The Tree of life (Ankh) is also symbolic of the physiology of the human body. The body's physical, mental and spiritual functions are plainly explained in the *Book of Coming Forth by Day and by Night*. In the Bible and Koran the Caucasian priest cults and power elite distorted these books with myths and superstitions in order to control people.

This chart divides the Tree of Life into two parts (branches) called the Female and Male Principle. These two branches grow from the tree's trunk (backbone and spinal cord). Nerves receive and carry all types of information (sound, sight, psychic, electrical, chemical, etheric) and broadcast all types.

The Ra factors or law of balance cause the Isis principle and Osiris principle to be drawn together (united). The Ra factor is the liquid cerebral spinal fluid in the backbone and the brain that transports nerve information to and from the brain and the pineal gland's auric forces (chakras). The pineal's galaxy-shaped aura gives the African to the universal creator.

The body is part of and related to the universe, colors, sun, music, Ankh force, stars (zodiac), vitamins, moon, minerals, planets and all things seen and unseen. For example, the pineal gland is solar (sun), pituitary is air, uterus/prostate is water, and ovaries/testicles are earth.

The Seven Halls of Osirius, the seven colors of the pineal gland and the seven seals refer to the solar, pharyngeal, cardia, cavernous, conarium, uterus/prostate and sacral plexuses. The body's five senses, five ventricles, (solaristic chambers), five points of the Pyramid and five endocrine glands (thyroid, parathyroid, pancreas, adrenal and ovary/testes) are interrelated. The symbolic Seven Halls of Osirius refers to the plexuses and the five points of the pyramid refer to the endocrine glands.

The chart is a guide to understanding the complexity and simplicity of the human body. The body can be diagnosed for disease by finding the aspect it most identifies with or it can be treated for a disease by identifying its opposing principle compliment. The chart is a tool that can be used to help you to use your body as an instrument for healing.

Classification of Energy Chart

(Chart of the Two Great Truths & Four Principles of Life So-Called Mystery System)

Male Principle	Female Principle
Science	Art
Square	Circle
Pyramid	Pyramid
Electricity	Magnetism
Serotonin Increase	Melatonin Increase
Speeds Up Action	Slows Down Action
Contracts Energy	Expands Energy
Sympathetic Nervous System	Parasympathetic Nervous System

Male Principle	Female Principle
Acidic Bodily Condition	Alkaline Bodily Condition
Uses energy	Gathers energy
Adrenergic	Cholenergic
Thoracolumbar	Cranialsacral
Involuntary Motor Muscles	Voluntarily Motor Muscles
Blood Flow to Brain:	**Blood Flow to Brain:**
Decrease	Increase
Contracts Vessels	Expands Vessels
Blood flow to Muscle:	**Blood flow to Muscle:**
Increase	Decrease
Nervous System Action:	**Nervous System Action:**
Increase	Decrease
Excretory System:	**Excretory System:**
Decrease	Increase
Digestive System:	**Digestive System:**
Decrease	Increase
Respiratory System:	**Respiratory System:**
Increase	Decrease
Circulatory System:	**Circulatory System:**
Increase	Decrease
Reproductive System:	**Reproductive System:**
Decrease	Increase
Spiritual System:	**Spiritual System:**
Decrease	Increase
Kingdom of Gods:	**Kingdom of Gods:**
Decrease	Increase
Pingala Nerve	Ida Nerve
Back	Front
Anus	Mouth

Male Principle	Female Principle
Flaccid Penis	Erect Penis
Active Vaginal Muscles	Passive Vaginal Muscles
Melanin:	**Melanin:**
Solid Crystals	Gas & Liquid Crystals
Pineal	Pancreas
Kidney	Heart
Thyroid	Spleen
Lungs	Liver
Large Intestine	Small Intestine
Thymus	Pituitary
Upper Jaw	Lower law
Negative Energy Enters Left Foot and Exits Right Hand	Positive Energy Enters Right Foot and Exits Left Hand
Cosmic Energy Enters Right Foot and Exits Left Hand	Cosmic Energy Enters Left Foot and Exits Right Hand
Positive Anger, Fear	Love Bonding
Sun, Mars, Mercury	Venus, Moon (Sun's Reflection)
Elements:	**Elements:**
Fire, Air	Water, Earth
Electrical	Magnetic
Vertical	Horizontal
Initiative	Receptive
Visible	Visible
Temperal	Eternal
Exoteric	Esoteric
East, West	North, South
Electromagnetic	Electromagnetic

Male Principle	Female Principle
Negative	Positive
Osiris (North Pole)	Ra (South Pole)
Nephthis (East Pole)	Isis (West Pole)
Cayenne, Mandrake	Garlic, Ginger
Licorice, Comfrey	Mints, Blue Water Lily
Phoenix	Hippopotamus
Ape	Crocodile
Gold	Silver
Pungent	Sour
Salty Taste in Foods	Sweet Taste in Foods
Orange	Green
Red	Violet
Blue	Indigo
Frankincense	Jasmine, Calamus
Lavender	Pine
Oak, Cedar	Rose, Sandalwood
Beans, Roots, Vegetables.	Fruit, Sprouts, Sweet, Celery
Fecundity	Aridity
Fall	Rise
Contractive	Expansive
Clairvoyance	Audiovoyance
(Seeing Divinely)	(Hearing Divinely)
Nitrogen	Carbon
Oxygen	Hydrogen
Phosphorus	Sodium
Copper	Iron
Tin	Nickel

Male Principle	Female Principle
Lead	Titanium
Zinc	Cobalt
Bismuth	Potassium
Sulfur	Magnesium
Heru	Hathor
Ra	Nu
Pyramid	Circle
Cup	Magic Wand (Caduceus)
Scepter	Pentacle
Vitamin K	Vitamin E
Vitamin C	Vitamin B
Vitamin A	Vitamin D
Protein	Carbohydrate
Epinephrine	Acetylcholine
Snake	Vulture
To Know	To Will
To Dare	To Keep Silent
Action	Completion
Resistance	Result
Study	Will
Intrepidy	Discretion
Gemini	Cancer
Libra	Scorpio
Aquarius	Pisces
Aries	Taurus
Sagittarius	Virgo
Leo	Capricorn

Chapter Three
Children

"Let us not forget that it is our duty to remedy any wrong that has already been done and not ourselves perpetuate the evil of race destruction."

Marcus Garvey

Born into Diseases

The Caucasian has waged full-scale war against the health of African babies. African children are highly melaninated, highly biochemically responsive, highly spiritual and electromagnetically united to the galaxy, sun, moon, cycles, planets, parents, water, plants, and the earth. Each African child has the specific prenatal rhythm of its zodiac sign. The prenatal movements of a Capricorn child are distinctively different from the prenatal movements of a Libra child. Consequently, the zodiac sign and ancestral aura of the child requires that the mother alter her diet to meet the specific nutritional needs of the unborn child.

The Caucasian medicine, nutrition, disease and remedy systems ignore rhythm, melanin and White Racism. Their health practitioners have no rhythm and holistically do not understand rhythm. They ignore the zodiac specific movements of the prenatal babies' growth and development as well as zodiac specific nutrition requirements.

Sound, which is melanin driven, is very important for the African child. A child's pineal gland and ears (the first mature physical senses) are very important. The ear drum is fully developed before birth and translates sounds (light energy) just as the highly melaninated skin can convert light energy into images that are interpreted by the brain as that of sound, smell, touch, sight, psychic energy and extrasensory information. African people have the highest melanin content in their ears. The prenatal child's ears act as part of the brain. The correct cultural music and drumming should be a definite part of the parent's surroundings and in the prenatal child's environment. This would help to stimulate melanin properly and prevent predisposing the prenatal infant to melanin deficiency.

Cancer

The Caucasian doctors, nurses, drugs, hospitals, diet, test standards and birthing techniques are an unnecessary interruption in the prenatal child's rhythm, nutrition and brain function. The child is subject to cancer-causing ultrasounds. The needles used for taking the amniocentesis fluid (determines whether baby is a girl or boy) is guided by ultrasound. Fetal monitors that are strapped on the mother's abdomen use ultrasound. The internal metallic devices that are screwed into the unborn baby's head cause inflammations with pus-filled abscesses. X-rays given to the mother cause a 50% increase in various types of cancer. Aside from this, the increase in electronic and computer machines has caused an increase in Cae-sarean Sections (C-Section). C-Section babies have an increase in learning problems. Their biochemical "rites of passage" and bonding have been Nutricidally interrupted.

Sound

Rhythm (cycle laws) is melanin dependent in African babies. For example, pendulum operated clocks can all be started at different time intervals. However, they all will synchronize to one rhythm. This has been found true even if a house where several women live, each having a different menstruation period cycle. They will eventually have synchronized periods and menstruate at the same time. An African baby and mother will have synchronized heart-beats. Sounds become human cells in the baby's body. Since the ear matures first, sound is important because it produces s waves that are absorbed by melanin and translate into thoughts, feelings, emotions, spirit and ideas. Babies should not be exposed to sounds of arguments, hostility, fighting, violence, White Racism (cultural insults), and disharmony. Consequently, Caucasian medical principles ignore the melanin rhythmic importance to the baby and mother causing a conflict within the body and towards the mother. Rhythm controls the growth of organs and bones. A baby can grow up to l inch in height in 24 hours. Growth cycles (rhythm) are controlled by melanin. When melanin is imbalanced, or not nutritionally fed, a sudden growth spurt can occur internally and/or externally. This can result in sudden irritation in a baby (*Growth Research*, University of Pennsylvania by M. Lampl, M.D., Ph. D.)

Brain-Assault and Battery

Bonding is further interrupted by birth techniques of Caucasians. Labor is induced by synthetic drugs causing the contractions to be out of rhythm and violently forceful. This results in too much pressure on the child's head. This increased pressure decreases the air, blood and nutrient supply to the African child's brain. The skull is squeezed together too hard causing the bones to collide resulting in a fluid-filled bruise on the top of the head. Drugs in any form (including synthetic food) cause the bones to collide together resulting in dimples in the chin or improper growth such as cleft tongues and lips or dimples in the ear.

Further, Caucasians use a pair of pliers (forceps) to clamp and squeeze the head so they can pull the baby out of the womb. This further decreases the air, blood and nutrient supply to the brain. They also use a vacuum pump, which they clamp on the head to forcefully pull the baby out the womb. This drains rhythmaticity, electromagnetic energy and nutrients out of the brain and can stop nutrients from getting to the brain. Aside from being unnatural, it is a shock to the baby, beyond any criminal assault and battery. It could be classified according to the United Nations Human Rights Charter as an assault and battery with the intent to maim, mutilate and harm for life.

Furthermore, Caucasians interrupt the proper rhythmic bio-chemical rites of passage of the child by cutting the umbilical cord before it stops pulsating. This further deprives the baby of air, nu-trients and blood and shocks the baby's entire system. Additionally, the Caucasians will turn the baby upside down and slap the baby's behind for no other reason than to follow a primitive Caucasian ritual based on some weird cave man superstition.

Aside from this, the unborn baby lives in a diseased amniotic liquid slime that is full of mucus and liquid manure instead of healthy amniotic fluid which is a light weight clear liquid which occurs on a natural African diet. The diseased amniotic fluid of to-day's mother is thick, fowl, sticky and is mostly caused by synthetic foods, drugs and constipation. This unhealthy slime is what Afri-can babies live in while in the womb instead of the natural elec-tromagnetic melaninated amniotic fluid.

Furthermore, the newborn baby may have a white crusty sticky slime over the face caused by the man ejaculating on it during the woman's pregnancy. Sex is erroneously promoted by Caucasian medical science as being ideal for couples and the baby. The total of poor prenatal nutrition, ignorant superstitious medical techniques, violence, and money driven medical activities work to push the baby to a nutritionally self-destructive path. Then the bonding does not occur between mother and child. The baby should be placed on the mother's breast after being born in order to stimulate bonding and placenta release. Bonding for the African baby starts before con-ception and prenatal growth. The placing of the baby on the mother's stomach near the breast is an extension of bonding.

Drugs

Caucasian medicine treats a child's birth as if it is a disease process. They interrupt birthing by giving the parents' junk food that retards growth. They give the mother drugs that go directly into the baby's body. Drugs and Caucasian nutritional standards cause the African baby to try to breathe before being born. In this case, the baby may have a bowel movement and attempt to breathe causing it to swallow amniotic fluid that can have its bowel movement (manure) in it. The baby has a bowel movement before birth due to shock and overstimulation in response to junk food and drugs. Drugs retard growth, slow down learning and interrupt the baby's ability to bond with its mother. Drugs cause the baby's immune system to get exhausted and junk foods deplete the immunity as they overstimulate the sympathetic nervous system. They activate serotonin out of its natural cyclic pattern and depress melatonin.

Caucasian—Lowest Humanoid

African people are the highest on the human development chain. Caucasians are the lowest developed humans of all the races of man. The Chinese, Japanese, Indians, Native Indians are in between Africans and Caucasians on the chain.   The   Caucasians using a lower, four-legged animal for milk to feed them are closer to that lower animal (cow) than an African. However, Africans giving their babies cow's milk or synthetic formula milk are interrupting bonding. Cow's milk helps cows to bond and may influence a child to bond with animalistic characteristic behaviors or the Caucasian race, but not the African race. African breast milk provides scientifically balanced milk that nourishes the baby, stimulates melanin, and stimulates and builds immunity. While cow's milk and formula are only good for breeding humans and building a physical body that can work for the benefit of White Power.

The races of man are classified according to the concentration of melanin, and melanin density. This scientifically measures human mental, physical, spiritual superiority and inferiority capabilities. There are basically six types of human beings. Black people (Africans) are rated the highest with a number "6." Eumelanin, Pheumelanin, Pseudo-melanin grades of pigmentation cause the highest-grade rating. The Brown people such as Mexicans, Malaysians and Puerto Ricans are rated "5." The Chinese, Japanese and Indians are at "4" along with Vietnamese, Koreans etc. Then mixed whites are at "2" to "3" and finally, white people with blue, green and gray eyes are rated the lowest at " 1."

Playground or Deathground

The Caucasian culture's playgrounds are made with equipment, which makes the play area a death ground. They usually have a ground of concrete, chemically polluted sand, asphalt, outdoor carpet, din or wood chips, which aside from being pollutants, may include broken glass, urine, fecal matter, fungus, etc. The playground toys and exercise devices can be made of steel pipes with assortments of plastic, jagged or razor-edged devices that are hazardous to health. The exercise devices are usually made for monkeys and do not allow all muscle groups to exercise. The toys are unholistic and based on the Caucasian culture's idea of toys.

African toys were spiritual and geared to help the child towards higher growth. The African play activities were communal or a sharing activity rather than individualistic or competitive Caucasian play. There were the African games such as Kea (similar to tic-tac-toe) which was played with stones. In contemporary African American history, the Kea type play board was drawn on the ground and a shoe heel was used. A game such as "Hop Scotch" has patterns drawn with chalk on the pavement or in the street, which were patterned after Kea. It had a large chalk drawn play board which incorporated the symbol of the Sun (Ra) at the apex, pyramid shape inside a square, and symbols of the female and male principle as connecting boxes. This was played with a shoe heel as a moving peg.

Belenin (similar to marbles), Beleta (similar to jacks), Wali (count and capture) and action games such as Kele (chicken fighting) were played. Kele is an action form of Duck Duck Goose with participants jumping in a frog position and trying to push each other over. These games were played by African children until the early 1960's.

On the other hand, Caucasian toys and playgrounds are made so that the child becomes accustomed to violence and can isolate and divorce himself from others. Additionally, the Caucasian playground toy devices are not organized by gender nor do they reflect spirituality, cosmic reality or have any relationship to family life. Most playground accidents are influenced by the violence and sex abuse caused by adults forcing children to watch R-rated movies and videos. This causes children to violently damage themselves in playground activities.

The Caucasian playground is usually a fenced-in cage of steel pipes and wires. Falls and miscalculated play activities can cause permanent harm. No professional athlete would consider training or exercising on the devices or under the conditions that children are forced to play under. In 1990, almost 80 percent of the children taken to hospital emergency rooms were between 5 and 14 years of age and the other 20 percent of the children were below 5 years of age. The climbing toys and monkey bars caused over 70,000 children to be taken to the hospital. The number of children treated by parents, teachers, school nurses, self-treated, treated by other children

or that go untreated would increase the total of playground injuries. Aside from this, the number of injuries children inflict upon
each other on playgrounds has not been determined. The injuries
adults inflict upon children that they are helping to play at playgrounds would also increase the total injuries of children. As far as
monkey bars are concerned, a safe way to decrease a child's risk of
injury is to measure the distance between the bar rings. If the child's
leg is shorter than the distance between rungs, then he will have a
higher chance of his foot slipping and inflicting an injury to his
body.

The playground lacks instructions for proper use of the devices.
The playgrounds do not have warnings for the appropriate distance
to be away from the swings nor is any child's exercise safety moni-
tored by another child or adult. Play at the playground using the
Caucasian devices is usually designed for individual and not for
group or family orientated play. The playgrounds do not have first
aid kits available. Children can be scarred, maimed, mutilated or
injured for life at the caged playground that should be called a death
ground. Some are on legal drugs and can be in withdrawal or high.

The playground and Nutricide form a doubly destructive combination against the African child. The child presents its body at the
playground and the condition of that body is nutritional depriva-
tion caused by the Caucasian junk food diet. The child is nutritionally crippled. The neurohormonal and neurophysiological response
are degenerates. In other words, the mind and body reflexes are
near zero, muscle reflexes are slower or inaccurate, nerves are irritated, mood swings burst sporadically, near-arthritic and rheuma-
toid conditions and heart failure conditions are present.

Added to this, the muscles, nerves and brain are floating in liquid manure and lactic acid waste. The child is carrying around approximately 3 pounds of caked-up toxic manure in the rectum
(adults usually have 7 to 15 pounds) which Caucasians calculate as

normal body weight. The internal organs, tissues, nerves and cells are clogged and activity-impaired with liquid, slimy manure called mucus or plaque. Additionally, a low energy hypoglycemic level can strike at any moment caused by the sugary breakfast or dessert or snack or soda or candy. This can instantaneously cause loss of muscle, brain and nerve control. This is directly related to the bleached white flour, grease, salt and white sugar, hypoglycemic Caucasian junk foods.

The obstacle courses called playground toys require 100% physical efficiency that the Caucasian diet cannot and will not provide. The African child is escorted to the deathground nutritionally crippled and asked to perform 100% on a nutritionless diet. It is a prelude to an accident prepared for them by Caucasian Nutricide. To make matters worse, the parents, teachers, school nurses, doctors or extended family members are drugged on the tasty Nutricidal diet and do not see the obvious dangers of the situation.

Computer Trained Dogs =African Children

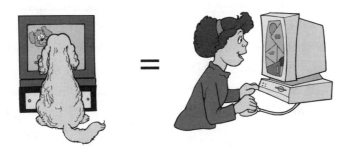

The African child watches television and plays video games for entertainment. However, the mental and emotional effect of these activities are subtle and yet dangerous. It may be that the video games are playing the child instead of the child playing the games.

The video game synthetic sounds and synthetic music sounds are associated with violence, sex, food and the Caucasian thinking processes. It has been proven by Caucasian physiologist, Ivan Petrovich Pavlov (1849-1936) that by repeated associations with a bell and dog a desired reflex action can occur. He used sounds to produce desired mental and physical behaviors. In later experiments he used people. In other words, the synthetic sounds of the computer games can cause thoughts, feelings, emotions and physical behaviors, violence, sex, desire for junk food, and Caucasian linear logic.

Linear logic video inducement means that the African child is trained to think like a Caucasian. Eventually, the African child will see computers, computer games, and hear the synthetic sounds of music instruments, synthetic action sounds, see computer generated people and associate it with violence, sex, people and food. The child will apply Caucasian thinking and behaviors to African people. The collective Caucasian psychosis (mental illness) is a part of video games (music videos and television) as well as Caucasian rituals, superstitions, group sex, ceremonies and social customs.

The Caucasian diseased logic indoctrinates the African child and adult to view life in terms of inferior versus superior, rule or ruin, win/lose, cowboys and Indians (Native American), sane/insane, crime/police, war/peace, African, poor, powerless/White, rich, powerful, kill or be killed, live/die, violence wins/lesser violence loses, food/famine, master/slave, bad guy/good guy, White beauty/Black ugly, or smart/dumb. In this one-dimensional psychotic (craziness) process, a person's feelings get mixed-up inappropriately. The craziness (psychosis) of Caucasian thought mixes feelings together, inappropriately as a feeling sensation. For example, sex, violence, junk food, conflict, love or harmony are mixed together as one feeling. In other words, the normal feeling of love may cause a violent reaction or a feeling of love can result in conflict. This is the primary reason why Africans who act lovingly or non-violently towards Caucasians get a reaction of conflict and violence.

This same diseased psychosis is programmed in computers, put in video games, and in synthetic video action sounds. Ironically, the Africans use synthetic sounds in their music. Synthetic sounds do not resemble the natural sound of a musical instrument. A computerized synthetic sound that imitates the authentic sound of natural instrument (drum, piano etc.) is not to be confused with an alien synthetic sound. Synthetic sounds train the ear to make an association with Caucasian culture, violence, junk food, sex, thinking and reflex behaviors. The sounds and music of African culture are no longer heard by the child who plays computer games.

The computer games, synthetic action sounds and synthetic music sounds are attached to Caucasian civilization's psychosis. Computer games, like all Caucasian cultural aspects, serve the needs and wants of White Supremacy. The former Caucasian slave master's cultural "gifts" to the African are used to keep the psychosis of White Supremacy and Black Inferiority alive. The slave master's government gives Africans the right to vote. Then the Africans' political vote is used for their own destruction. The slave master gives the former economic slave (prisoner of war) an education. Then, the miseducation is used to destroy Africans. The slave master gives Africans money. Then money is used to destroy Africans.

It should be noted that 99% of Africans monies goes to maintain and support white businesses. The slave masters give Africans guns and train them to be police or soldiers. The African then uses these guns to destroy other Africans. These Black police and soldiers kill Africans in order to defend Caucasian law and order. The slave master gives Africans junk foods and allopathic medicine which he uses to destroy Africans. Now the slave master has given Africans computer games. These games are used to destroy Africans or at least ruin Africans.

Computer games, videos, movies, cartoons and television programs are used to entertain, to escape financial, mental or physical problems. However, they cause the African to escape African culture and get polluted in Caucasian culture. Videos and computer games cause difficulty in relating to others, boredom, irritability, mood swings, and personality problems. They drain energy from the African American community. The energy spent on computer games could be used to do positive things for the African family, community and individuals. Instead, the energy is spent to become more Caucasian.

Clinically depressed children view more television, eat more junk food and are the most undernourished. They usually have a melanin deficiency. African children usually watch 25 hours more television than white children and spend more time with computer games. The computer games and television programs are used to escape oppression and side effects of racism. Unfortunately, they cause the same problems. This makes being an African child twice as painful, more prone to disease, and more nutritionally drained than being a white child. The National Institute of Mental Health conducted a 13-year study using 1,200 people which validated the many mental and behavioral problems viewing television causes. It was found that viewing television causes reduced social ability, poor ability to interact and negative moods. This has been revealed in the book *Television and the Quality of Life: How Viewing Shapes Everyday Experiences*, by Lawrence Earlbaum Associates.

Video games are basically structured similar to the arcade games of the 18th century. African children become addicted to these games and the Caucasian psychosis in the games. Their melaninated Black skin identifies them as Africans while their mind, moods, personality, self-centeredness, behavior and thinking process identify them as Caucasians. These games can help in problem solving of space and movement, sequence in Caucasian logic, but are carriers of Caucasian, diseased thinking. The child becomes devoted to fantasy, solo-play and develops an unreal idea of his competence based upon unholistically winning against a computer opponent.

The African child develops competitive behavior instead of the African communal, family-centered thinking and cooperative sharing of knowledge and resources. Selfishness is rewarded by a selfish-competitive way of life. In the real world, the African child loses the holistic Africentric ability to interact with real African people, African cultural artifacts and objects. The child gains a low tolerance of human failure, socialization, rejection and compromise. Added to this, the African child (and video games-addicted adult) has increased aggressive behavior. He/she also associates synthetic action sounds and music with real life.

The child uses mindless amusement as fun and increases the potential for doing anything for excitement, along with fully developing the Caucasian mental illness that mixes violence with sex or love and cultivates a need to ruin or destroy others. In books such as *Playing with Power in Movies, Television and Video*, by Marsha Kinder, it is estimated that well over 1 out of 3 African American children own computerized Caucasian mental illness (computer games).

The child begins to lose the responsiveness to Maat and the natural cycles of nature, subtle weather changes, natural sunlight variations, slight changes in the taste of natural foods as well as changes in cold, hot, others, parents, music, moods and thoughts. African children begin to react only to mindless synthetic sounds. The sound of rivers, the wind, digestive organs, African music, African drum rhythm (language), trees, and wild life become meaningless.

The result is that the child is not attached to his African body and mind and becomes attached to the Caucasian mind. The Caucasian behaviors of violence, sex and destruction are copied by the child. African children in actuality are not playing the games but the computer games are playing them—playing them into a tool of destruction of Africa, African family centeredness, African natural diets, Africentric thinking and themselves. African children are rapidly becoming the new Pavlov's dog that associates sounds with mental and physical reflexes which support White Supremacy and make them easy prey for Nutricide. They are becoming computer-trained dogs that behave like humanoids (Caucasians can be considered a primitive collection of genetic leftover waste).

Bonding—The Betrayal

Bonding between parent and child connects the child to the parent, world, culture and spirituality. It defines life and empowers the child. It is a function of White Racist institutions (education, health, nutrition, psychology, sociology, etc.), to destroy or damage the African human right to bond. Bonding is a political issue and is used to sustain White Supremacy. An African that has bonding damage is easy to control, economically exploit, and manipulate. A woman who has bond damage is prone to abuse children, has inadequate mothering skills, and lacks mental and emotional stability. A bond-damaged man is prone to be self-destructive, has poor social skills and has emotional problems.

Bond damage causes men and women to be violent, suicidal, sickly and have a short life span. This human tragedy also causes the man to hide his feelings, to be easily agitated and have conflicts understanding and using his cycles. The bond-damaged woman waits for unbalanced mental and emotional cycles to complete before altering behavior, distributes feelings to others or traumatizes herself.

A damaged bond does not allow the child to complete the defining of personality. Personality relates to the spirit. Marriage helps in bonding mind, body and culture. If the personality is bond-damaged, then concrete thinking and the physical world are used to fulfill the missing ingredients of an ill bond. This is typical of Caucasian personalities. In any case, White Racist institutions continue to damage Africans by dislocating the bond. They transfer the bond to White Culture and this causes spiritual, physical, mental and emotional illnesses.

For example, the original idea of Carter G. Woodson of a Negro History Day is now a White institution (Black History Month) with role models picked by Caucasians. These role models, heroes, sheroes and great African Americans qualify as Caucasian African American heroes because they worked for White organizations, served White institutions or organizations or entertained Whites such as Joe Louis, Marian Anderson, Thurgood Marshall, Jackie Robinson, W.E.B. DuBois, A. Phillip Randolph, Madame C. J. Walker, General Colin Powell, Hank Aaron, Jesse Jackson, etc. African importance is defined only if it relates to Whites and helps to transfer the bond to White culture. The extreme ugliness of Caucasian bond destruction is that Caucasians have become Africans' surrogate mother, reality, culture and world. This results in Negroes becoming nutritional imbeciles.

Bonding is a necessary rite of passage and is the foundation of an African's growth, development and contact with the holistic world of seen and unseen energies. Bonding is a rhythmic (cyclic) process of the body, mind and spirit. Without bonding, the child is isolated from Africentric holism. A natural foods diet and breastfeeding are essential for bonding. A bonded African child discovers why they are on earth and what their purpose is in life. An unbonded child struggles to discover whether they are safe enough to survive. The unbonded child tends to be violent. There is much conflicting information about bonding caused by White Supremacy which forces Africans to adopt white standards for growth and development, nutrition, spirituality, and psychology.

Caucasians are sickly, and for Africans to adopt sick Caucasian standards of health is cultural treason and sheer ignorance. For example, the U.S. Public Health Service indicates that over 250,000,000 junk food-eating Americans are in some state of disease while 1,000,000 can be vaguely classified as healthy. In other words, sickness is generally classified as health and this has an effect on bonding. Bonding is a unique rite of passage for Africans. White Racism has destroyed or totally impaired healthy bonding.

The African parent and adults have to re-evaluate parenting, bonding, breastfeeding, nutrition and the Male and Female Principles based upon the rapid holistic growth and development of the African child. Bonding destruction occurs when the African child and parent use Caucasian superstitious health, bonding, growth and development standards. For example, the African child uses words rhythmically, synchronizes the words with facial expression, voice tone, mood, and body movements. Thinking is a spiritual and physical activity for the African child. If the child is not rhythmically moving the body and using facial expressions, then the African child is not thinking.

Historically, movement and the drum were used for instructing and educating the child in school. The Caucasians outlawed the drum, and continued to keep it out of the African child's education, which caused damaging effects on the child. An education without rhythm is a Caucasian education. The drum, dance and music are a natural part of learning all school subjects and not a separate, isolated, scheduled school activity.

In Egyptian mythology Osirus taught mathematics with the use of the drum and harp. Learning is a melaninated process. Melanin is a cyclic rhythmic substance that is dominant in Africans. Words are rhythmic sounds (phonic). Children associate sounds with body rhythm and senses. Consequently, words used by parents when speaking to children should be sense orientated with words associated with smell, sight, hearing and touch. The adult should perform the child's instructions. Modeling and learning by doing is instructive.

The child views activities as cyclic—each movement has a beginning and an end. For example, the adult tells the child to put on his shoes. The child reacts by putting the shoes on. The child will sometimes put the shoes on the wrong foot. Putting the shoes on is one complete cyclic task while putting the shoes on the correct foot is a separate cyclic task. Consequently, the adult should wait until the child has completely put the shoes on the wrong feet before telling the child to remove the shoes and start over—another cyclic task. In order to avoid this side effect of racism, the adult should demonstrate the activity with the use of shoe/sock identifiers such as a color, number, floor print, letter or symbol codes etc. The adult should perform the task in a play learning-fashion. "Putting on the shoes" is understood by the child to be a name or label which is a property of the cyclic task. This is similar to taste, smell and touch being a property of a mango.

One of the side effects of White Racism is that the African adult assumes that the child has the same thought process as an adult. Consequently, the adult uses adult logic to communicate to a child. This causes a conflict and impairs parent/child bonding. The child thinks from the outside inward while an adult thinks inside outward. In other words, the adult puts together words without associating action or body movement.

The child up to 2 years of age is merely collecting data, such as, properties of events activities, words, spirits, drumming, music, food, breast milk and adults. The acceptance of this can help to avoid the signs and symptoms of Caucasian-caused bonding impairments. For example, the parent's failure at bonding causes them to give adult instructions to a child. The child does not understand the instructions and acts according to its own ability to comprehend. Consequently, this can result in parents saying to the child "I told you," when there is a failure to communicate. This statement merely pacifies the adults failure to bond. Other statements often used by parents with bonding impairments are "Next time you will know better," "If you listened to me it would not have happened," "why is your head so hard? "When I tell you to do something, you do as you want," "You play too much instead of doing as you are told," etc.

It has to be understood by the adult that the child is processing an abundance of information while doing a task. The child sees colors around objects or senses auras (spirits) and does the task in time (in cyclic rhythm) as opposed to on time (Caucasian abstract). Instructions mixed with play are helpful for the child. For example, Twa (Pygmies) children play at adult reality and the adults play with the child and enjoy the play. The play leads to adult work. The child's play merges with the adult world The child's thinking is one cyclic movement from spiritual to concrete to abstract then enlightenment.

A child's thinking may give meaning to events or activities based on the aura-light or sensation that the child feels. The adult *must* answer the child within the child's reality thinking. For example, the child my ask "Why does night fall and don't break?" The adult answer could be that the night fell into the ocean. The child may ask, "Who is God's father?" The response could be Ra. The child requires answers that will match its level of understanding. Therefore, the adult answer to questions should not be abstract, scientific or theoretical but more aligned to concrete and action orientation. The acceptance of the child as going through to and with a melaninated rhythmic bonding process is essential. The child will give holistic meaning to events or activities based on what is felt electromagnetically, cyclically, spiritually or melaninately.

The child may say it saw a lion in the kitchen. The adult true or false judgment of the lion's presence in the kitchen is not the issue. The meaning of the child's statement is the issue. The child does not need adult correction or to be called a liar. The child is working through, to and with the rites of passage of idea nurturing and maturity. The child perceives the lion and the maturity of perception is the development of concepts. Concepts change and mature.

Children act upon energy (i.e., lion) and that energy (lion) acts upon them. The child's verbal explanation of psychic, spiritual, emotional, electromagnetic, or sensed energy (lion) is not a hallucination, illusion or fantasy, but concrete in the child's logic system. The adult reality has the ability to deal with abstract concepts. Therefore, an adult calling another adult Leo (Zodiac) the Lion or a football team a Lion presents no logic problem while in the child's mind this is confusing. In this lion fantasy or child's warning that a lion is in the kitchen, the adult could go to the kitchen with the child and talk to the lion and ask it to leave or offer it food or chase it away or ask it to protect the house. This would address the child within its logic system, much more realistically than calling the child a liar. The child seeing the lion is an issue of idea maturation and is a necessary step in the experiential learning, practice of idea formation, and the ability of the child to understand understanding.

The child sees the world through the mind, diet, body and behavior of the adult. Therefore, it is still within the bonding cycles. The child is considered to be connected biochemically with the mother for a year after birth. Incidentally, this mother bond is still apparent in adulthood as music with the same rhythm of the mother's heart beat (usually a walking pace) is the most soothing, best for learning, increases endurance, reduces stress and helps food metabolism. The child's consciousness is an extension of the parent's consciousness in a blended feedback and feedforward system.

Mentalistically the child's consciousness is a function of the melaninated mid-brain (corpus callosum) which unites the right brain (hemisphere) to the left brain. This harmonious mixture of the hemispheres causes fantasy and reality (concrete) to be united in the child's logic system. The African's mid-brain is larger and has more melanin centers than the Caucasian mid-brain. In ratios of proportion, the midbrain has nearly completed its development and is large. It unites and exchanges electrical and chemical information so that hemispheres are not very distinct in function. Consequently, language is a function of both hemispheres instead of being primarily a left brain activity.

Impairment of bonding by poor nutrition and bottle milk also impairs the electrical, chemical, melanin unity and exchange between the brain's hemispheres. There is conflict and confusion in fantasy because there are unbalanced mixtures of reality, rhythm, spirituality and play. A child with a White Racist-caused impaired or weak bond, can fear monsters, animals, objects, and can have nightmares that continue into the day. The child is lost, unfocused, nutritionally restrained without completed holistic bond cycles. Children may verbalize their damaged bond by projecting their loss of empowerment, control, anxiety, isolation, and fears upon objects or animals such as lions. In other words, the child uses its logic system to express the damaged bond.

Children are capable of understanding adult body language, voice tone, mood shifts, facial expressions and not abstract adult logic. An African adult diseased by White Racism may not be able to understand the child's logic or be aware that the child understands them because children have a different logic system. The child lives in the "here and now (present)." Consequently, children believe a dead person is in a different living state. They think that the dead may wake up at night or cannot physically move because they are punished or that death is a result of bad behavior (Karma).

A game such as "Peek a Boo" is a "here and now" game which allows the adult to become conditioned to the child's logic and allows the child to accept the adults "here and now" unity with them. When the adult "peeks" they are here (present) and when they hide they are an unseen presence (spirit) and when they return to say "boo" they verify that life is seen and unseen. "Peek a Boo" is a logic game that demonstrates that life is cyclic and a continuous flow between the living and dead. It also introduces the child to rhythm in speech and the three phonic sounds (peek-a-boo) which develops into number usage and games of numbers.

This and other African games are subjected to White Racism values and become fragmented and lose their connection to life as a continuum. If games are not extended into mathematics, music, drum rhythms, spirituality or logic they become lost and valueless. A White Racist education defines African games as unholistic and worthless play of primitive peoples.

Caucasian education emphasizes abstract nonspiritual thought without body movement or rhythm (cyclic) or the drum. This type of education damages the bond to African culture and is combined with junk food, junk medicine, junk history, junk religion and junk culture. The Caucasian school education divorces the African child from the African community, family, spiritualized games and play. Caucasian abstract play results in depression, self-hatred, Caucasian cultural addiction, confusion, and/or Caucasian logic and anxiety which holistically cripples the African child's learning rites of passage.

In African culture, games, toys, tools, music and dance allow the child to explore the world. These games, toys and tools gradually develop into adult games, toys and tools (hobbies such as collecting real or toy cars, dolls, jewelry, etc). Caucasians, in order to avoid the shock and damage of their education founded on survival of the strong over the weak, smart over the dumb, rich/poor, have/have not's, white is right/Black is wrong, either/or and fight/flight logic, believe that starting school early (preschool) solves the anxiety conflict that education causes. It actually amplifies the damage done to the child's nutritional, spiritual, cultural, and parent bonding. In African culture the storytellers used in educational and cultural activities keep the parent/child bond intact. It is a living continuum of the importance of fantasy between adult and child. Aside from this, parents who read to and with children help the child to use story telling and to see the world through adult eyes. This increases the child's reading skills and desire to read. African children historically are naturally literary. They read words and symbols on tools, toys, and games. African children naturally become adults who read literature on statues, walls, ceilings, floors, coffins and in books.

The Caucasian lesser evolved use of the mid-brain and the conflict or split they have between the right brain and the left brain causes them to define the right mind (brain) as creative, spiritual, feminine and evil. Consequently, the right mind that controls the left hand causes the left hand to be classified as evil and is associated with death. The right hand is controlled by the rational, intellectual, conflict-oriented, male or good left brain. Consequently, the right hand is associated with "life" instead of death. This gives rise to such statements as "if your right hand (life) betrays you, cut it off." White Male Supremacy superstitions, late development of bio-feedback, melanin deficiencies, the generally sickly condition of the

White race and the overabundance of damage bonding cause their education to be miseducation.

The absence of bonding and the anxiety, mistrust and fear that it causes result in the child being powerless. The child learns to not trust the parent as a source of nurturing and power and as a medium between themselves and the holistic worlds. The bond-damaged child grows to be an adult who fears the holistic healing powers of the body. The child firmly believes that drugs, natural supplements and herbs heal the body and mistrusts African science that states that food is medicine and medicine is food.

Food naturally excites the holistic healing forces in the body. Natural or synthetic supplements and herbs can only act as mediums between the individual and food as medicine. The bond-damaged child watches the parent give up control over her own body to a Caucasian superstitious medical system that is firmly based upon the standard that the sickly Caucasian is healthy. A bond-damaged adult reacts to situations instead of acting upon a situation. The child learns that she/he has no personal power over his life, no spirit power, and cannot act upon reality.

Bonding "rites of passage" emphasize the utilization of holistic powers to act on reality and clairvoyance reality. The trance "rites of passage" teaches the child when first awake in the morning to go into a trance state and perceive the day and act upon it (change it for the better or avoid negative events). The Trance State before sleep is used to see the spirit world and act upon it and/or with it. Holistic bonding teaches the child to see dis-ease as an alarm that a healing crisis is in progress. No cure, remedy, herb or supplement should be used to stop the body from having a healing crisis. Drugs are typically used to disconnect the dis-ease alarm while the cause of the dis-ease remains unchanged. Ironically, Caucasian thinking causes Africans to continuously look for a cure for the body's self-curing process erroneously called a disease. Caucasians, looking for a cure for a cure is based on superstitions and stems from their bond damage. Bonding for the child has a cyclic, task-like motion. An example of a bonding activity could be as follows:

1. Be calm, hold (embrace) the child or look the child in the eyes and smile.
2. Ask the child to listen.
3. Give the child instructions in action words. ("Put on your shoes, please," or "Lets go see the lion")
4. Then ask the child to repeat instructions with you. Saying instructions together assists bonding.
5. Model the task or perform the task with the child until they master it unsupervised.
6. Thank the child for his/her good actions.

In the bonding process, the child's logic sees words as properties of a behavior, words as living actuality and words as truth. They understand that word and action are combined as one cyclic task and one motion. This helps the child to conceptualize and bond. The child conceptualizes that creating with creation and form with function are one motion (cyclic). In other words, learning and doing are one cyclic task.

The child's logic is the standard for communicating with and understanding the child. Their body goes through obvious changes. In some cases the legs, arms, torso, hands, feet, toes, fingers, nose, ears, eyes and bone structure as well as internal organs may grow out of proportion or sporadically or in synchronized harmony. Growth is physically obvious while mental and spiritual development may not be apparent. However, physical growth influences the parent/child bond.

Mental, emotional and spiritual Africentric growth is not given importance by parents suffering from White Racism. Bonding is distorted by a Caucasian diet. The Caucasian main food groups of dairy, protein (meat), starch and vegetable is forced on the African child. A child's primary dietary focus should be centered around starches with raw fruit, raw vegetables, sprouts, beans, raw nuts, raw seeds and supplemented with breast milk. The bond restraining Caucasian diet dis-eases African growth and development. It alters, slows down or stops melanin cyclic utilization. It causes subclinical malnutrition and reduces the brain's ability to function. This makes the child easy prey for White manipulation and control. Thus, true Bonding is betrayed and Nutricidal.

Bonding Repair Remedies

Bond Damage is a dis-ease and, as such, it can be treated. The accumulation of damaged thoughts, words, behaviors, moods, spirituality, or cohesive relationships, that compromise ability, is imprinted in the holistic personality. This accumulation can be released from the system by healing. A bonding-healing crisis will show signs and symptoms of what appears to be a dis-ease. Dis-ease is merely the body, mind and spirit's attempt to rid itself of harmful toxins, such as a Bonding Disease. The healing crisis may manifest itself by the child (or adult) showing anger towards parents or parenting, rejection of Africentric activities, withdrawal from relationships, confusion, emotional instability, acting lost or being disturbed during nurturing.

This is merely the re-orientation phase of healing. The individual must go through a definition of self, parents, culture, and spirit and get accustomed to new feelings and concepts. The bonding-healing crisis will soon give rise to acceptance by the Bond-damaged parent, adult, family and/or child. Added to this, the Bond-Damaged individual must learn to defend themselves from the constant reinforcement of Bond Damage built into the White Racist institutions, social lifestyle, entertainment media and male/female relationships. It is important nurturing is applied while the parent and child or affected individuals go through healing.

Remedy List

- Carry naked infant in a sling close to the naked breast whenever possible. Use a sling to carry the child. Do not use strollers
- Do not bottle feed; Breast Feeding is a must.
- Do not use Caucasian dolls, toys or Eurocentric games.
- Do not use cages such as playpens or cribs. (The African child is made a prisoner by cribs and playpens. She psychologically can then easily accept cage schools with metal detectors, iron bars at windows and police patrols in the building.)
- Do not use leashes or body harness to walk the child. (This is how animals or trained dogs are treated.)
- Use natural foods, vegetarian milk substitutes and a vegetarian diet.
- Avoid nursery school, preschool, day care and other baby-sitting services until Bonding has been established. Use African culturally oriented services and people.
- Avoid hospital delivery. Use natural home birth.
- Do not play sexual and/or violent music, television programs or movies in child's presence.
- Engage in storytelling. (read Africentric stories)
- Play cultural music, put African (includes African American) Artwork and pictures in the home.
- No acts of physical, verbal or spiritual violence or cursing in the child's presence.
- Do not call child's behavior or action bad or disrespectful.; do not call the child bad, stupid, dumb, hardheaded, or a liar.
- Sing African songs to the child.

• Allow the family to bond with family activities. In some African
cultures, the bonding mother and child are alone for up to two
weeks and the mother is the only one allowed to handle the
child. If the child is handled, it is by a family member. Usually a
female family member will assist the mother of a newborn. A
family member, as well as the family, are essentials of the bonding remedy process.

Obviously, the remedies chosen from the list vary according to
whether the person is a single adult, parent. Child, prisoner, recov-
ering addict, teenager or whether it will be a group healing process
or family healing process. It should be noted that burial of the dead
according to African cultural ceremony and ritual helps the person
see and feel the bonding imperative in their life. A Bond-Damaged
African is one of the most potent weapons a Caucasian can use to
rule, destroy and Nutricide the race.

Bonding Disease Stages

There are major and minor signs and symptoms of Bonding Disease. Below are a few generalized symptoms that can help identify
the need for Bonding Remedies.

Bonding Disease Stage Symptoms

Acute:
• mistakes ancestral spirits for dangerous ghosts
• easily agitated
• lacks social skills
• mood swings
• failure to complete cyclic task in time

Subacute:
- opposite sex relationship problems
- underreactive to culture or Africentricity.
- underreactive to White Racism
- all of Acute symptoms

Chronic:
- mixes African culture with Caucasian
- confuses spirituality with religion
- speaks excessively logical and concrete and does not use spiritual terms.
- lacks improvisational skills
- straightens hair and men cut their hair very short so kinks won't be apparent and calls it neat
- all of Acute and Subacute symptoms
- believes all races think alike
- believes all races are the same

Degenerative
- believes self is one with all races; excuses the Caucasian race's behavior.
- lacks rhythm
- angers or prefers to protest truthful statements about White Folks psychosis
- dates White Folks and socializes with them in preference to own race
- all of Acute, Subacute, and Chronic symptoms

Growth and Development of Infants

The African baby natural development of the mind, spirit, and body is suppressed. It is forcefully retarded, twisted, distorted and perverted by subjection the child to the very slow Caucasian growth and development standards. African babies who have parents that follow Africentric standards, ethno medicine and a natural African diet have children who develop and grow quickly. This is also related to melanin's effect on the body. The African baby at birth can make eye contact, sit up, smile, and can intellectually participate in life. Its neurohormonal development is complete at 12 years of age (becomes an adult). Caucasians' retarded adult growth (melanin-deficient) is not complete until ages 18 to 21. Consequently, the African is forced to depress its naturally accelerated holistic growth. This causes subclinical physical and mental illness, emotional reactions to suppression, intellectually antagonistic reactions, which result in, decreased nutrient metabolism, ill bonding with parents, family and ancestors and a weak immune system.

Forcing the baby and child to follow Caucasian health standards and a junk food diet is ethnomedical racism. This results in development and growth constipation. The amount of damage done to African children and adults by this type of White Racism is beyond estimate. It is reflected in school drop-out, juvenile jails, crimes, drug addiction, violence, broken homes, learning problems, diseases, psychosocial genocide and nutricide (nutritional destruction of Africans).

The African baby at birth is able to consciously make social contact with its parents. African babies can sit erect, respond to and know least three to six years behind in growth and development. In other words, they raise an eagle bird (African) to believe that it is a chicken (Caucasian). This constipates the African child's growth and development and makes them easier servants to White Supremacy. Also, it helps Caucasian to destroy the family and relationships. Consequently, any threat to unify and mobilize is directly defeated by White Racism.

Works by the following authors can be a resource for growth and development, melanin, nutrition and Bonding: *Melanin (Protective Intoxicant Capabilities in the Black Human and its Influence on Human Behavior)* by Carol Barnes, is a three-volume work; all volumes are recommended. *Magical Child: Rediscovering Nature's Plan for Our Children*, by J. C. Pearce, *Magical Dilemma of Victor Neuburg*, by J. Overton-Fuller, Diet *Crime and Delinquency*, by A. Schauss, *Infancy in Uganda*, by Mary Ainsworth, *Ethnological Studies of Child Behavior*, by Burton Jones, Biological Rhythms in Human and Animal Physiology, by Gay Gaer Luce, *Specific Health Standards for Pre-Adolescent Children of Three Races*, by Wingerd, Solomon and Schaea, *Problems in the Nutritional Assessment of Black Individuals*, by S. Garn and D. Clark.

Functional Ability

The functional ability of the African child develops faster than in other races. If the child's parents and the child itself are on a natural foods diet, herbal medicine and the child is breastfed, then the holistic effect of bonding will accelerate its biological chemical functions. Generally, the functions of the African child start decreasing in the absence of bonding and from the impact of Caucasian junk food. The longer the duration of nutricide, the more retarded the functions of the body become.

African child	Caucasian child
18 minutes after birth or sooner: • can make eye contact • can stop head from falling back • recognizes parents	**6 weeks:**
2 days: • can hold head steady	**2 months:**

African child	Caucasian child
7 weeks: • can support self while sitting • looks at self in mirror	**5 months:**
2 months: • can hold self erect	**6 months:**
2 months: • standing ability	9 months:
2 months: • can play board games and re-move pegs	**1 year:**
5 months: • climbs steps	**13 months:**

Growth and Development
(Stages For The African Child)

The Caucasian studies of African children scientifically validate that the African child is superior to all children of other races. African children who come from a somewhat natural foods diet without junk food-addicted parents and are allowed to Africentrically bond with their mother have a faster growth and development rate than Caucasians. This is dietary and melanin related. African children grow and develop faster than children of other races because of their high bodily melanin content and neurohormonal superiority. In other words, the melanin saturation of the nervous system (neuro) and superior control and responsiveness of the glands that secrete fluids (hormones) causes superior and faster growth and development. Further, the melanin-saturated muscular structure responds fast and reacts to growth faster. The African child has the largest amount of "Fast Twitch" muscles than a child of any other race.

The child's brain has the most melanin saturation and has 12 melanin centers. This allows the brain to transmit, receive and interpret more mental information. These melanin clusters or melanin centers are sometimes called chakras. The African child's intellectual, spiritual and extrasensory abilities are highly developed. The parent bond, especially the mother and child bond, is accomplished faster. It starts prenatally and birth is a continuation of the spiritual, psychic, mental, electromagnetic and biochemical bond Therefore, the African baby who has parents who eat natural foods and is breastfed will mature faster.

However, an African child will be Africentrically retarded when the parents eat anti-melanin Caucasian junk food, cooked foods and meat. This junk diet holistically (body, mind and spirit) forces the child to follow the retarded growth and development of Caucasians. This nutritional restraint causes the child to follow a path of nutricide and menticide. The Caucasian synthetic diet stops melanin from being recycled and constipates the child. This results in the brain, organs, nerves, pineal gland and muscles constantly floating in liquid manure called mucus. The African child's reactions to this Caucasian nutritional poisoning is usually misinterpreted as behavioral problems, genetic violence learning problems, attention span deficit, disease or hyperactivity. The child's natural self-defense responses are erroneously called physical or mental disease. The physiological fact of the matter is the child's entire body is trying to fight against the Nutricide.

Stages of Growth and Development

Birth through 2 years of age
- at birth is holistically aware of itself, parents and fully in contact with environment
- synchronizes mouth and body to mother at a slower, usually un-noticeable pace
- sensory and motor coordination
- uses reasoning, logic and memory
- has ability to respond to slightest variation in environment.
- places esthetic values on objects.
- can be toilet-trained before 6 months of age.
- enjoys rhythm games and activities.
- feels safe when on a schedule/routine/rhythmic lifestyle.

2 years old
- responds to verbal instructions
- enjoys intellectual games; will laugh at logic substitute jokes
- likes to challenge environment, improvise and create different variables
- forgets task or ideas not in the "here and now (present)"
- politically manipulates and controls environment and others

3 to 4 years old
- social skills become complicated
- extrasensory and psychic abilities increase
- has increased vocabulary to apply to child's logic
- does not have vocabulary with adult logic and usage
- corpus collostrum completes growth; can mix Right Mind into verbal and listening vocabulary
- focuses on the concrete and not the abstract

5 to 7 years old

- enjoys cultural learning with tools, numbers, Trance, spiritualism and dance
- likes to apply learning to activity immediately
- samples intellectual ideas and acts or reacts to them in play or fantasy
- development of worldview
- sees adult world as play of adults and plays at adult work, customs, behavior, rituals and logic
- likes to disassemble adult ideas, artifacts, gadgets or toys made by adults (child thinks by doing)
- transitional Bond from Parent to include culture
- concrete thinking decreases in utilization and imaginative thinking increases
- thinking becomes action
- able to reverse reality (i.e., walk on fire without getting burnt)

7 to 9 years old

- natural cycles of mental, physical, spiritual, emotional and psychic energies acquires cultural meanings of adult
- spirit world increase in awareness and may have visits by deceased ancestors, strangers, animals and objects
- seeks clarity about White Racism
- challenges reality within self

9 to 11 years old

- selective about types of fantasy, Trance topics and play reality
- separates word from word meaning
- uses mind powers more; if the child can mentally balance a table (concept) with two legs missing then the power to enter a different reality is possible
- experiences other experiences

Development Quotient

African Child	Caucasian Child
Supplemental Eating:	
bananas, yams, squash, papaw (with Breast Milk)	meat, cereal
(*alkaline foods*)	(*acid foods*)
Greets Parents:	
musical voice, sounds, claps hands, lifting arms, smile	similar to mock play of wolves, tigers embraces, hugs (kill's prey) kissing imitates eating prey, lapping blood (tongue kissing)
Toys:	
musical, radionic, fruits, berries, plants, stuffed animals	hunting type spiritual devices, guns, hammers, mathematical
Faces:	
family and environment	face-to-face while sitting with parent
Beating:	
none–Is too young to understand purpose, 14 months or older	slapping of infants
Food:	
Raw grape or orange juice powder herb at 3 months	meat (cooked or raw) cereal pastry, cow's milk
No digestive problems	Indigestion, causing burping, drooling, nose dripping mucus; requires patting on back after feeding to relieve indigestion.
Sensormotor and Psychomotor Skills:	
12 months or less	2-3 years or more
Indicates hunger with sound:	
cooing and whimper	cries

Growth and Development
Through a Child's Eyes

The African child's growth and development of spirit, body and mind have noticeable changes at different ages. However, these changes at different ages are interpreted and defined by adult logic. This is a mistake that causes a negative effect upon truly helping to Bond with the child. The child has to be accepted on its own terms, in its own language and by its own holistic feelings. Children do not conceptualize or feel abrupt changes at each stage of holistic growth and development because nature has had over a billion years to smoothly perfect the continuous transitions of growth. Abrupt growth spurts in anatomy, spirit or mind are usually caused by junk food diets, physical traumas, disease, drugs and/or damaged Bonding between Parent and Child.

The child comes from a spirit world where energy is energy and can freely transform into different forms. For example, the chromosome of the male is Y and is carried to the uterus upon ejaculating sperm, which fertilizes the egg in the fallopian tube. The chromosome of the woman is X. The XY chromosomes unite causing fertilization and conception of a boy. If the XX chromosomes unite, a girl is conceived. However, these chromosomes are simply energy and do not possess a gender or sexuality of their own.

In about 6 to 8 weeks during fetal life, the XY chromosome can change to an XX pair. In other words, the slow moving, long living Y chromosome with a missing leg grows another leg and becomes an X chromosome. The Y energy is simply spirit energy that is free to change. Incidentally, a change of this sort causes the girl to be born with emotional and mental imbalances and to have sexual confusion.

Energy is energy and free to transform. The child comes from an undifferentiated energy state called spirit. Consequently, the child's spirit must adjust to a differentiated world, a world where energy is concrete and fixed in a state of existence. For example, an apple (energy) is an apple and different from a grape. The child tends to touch, hear, smell, taste and see objects, events and people in a concrete (unchangeable) manner. The child understands that the doctor's bill is simply a doctor whose name is Bill. This is concrete thinking. An adult understands the doctor bill to mean a financial charge for services. This is abstract thinking. Once the child has fixed or associates a concrete property to an object, event or person it then can abstract (change) it. Then after the child makes changes and variations (improvises), it can see the spirit content (Ra Factor) of the object, event or person once again. This completes the cycle of an object, event, activity, task, or concept that a child subjects all things to that enter its mind. A complete cycle allows the child to see activities, tasks or an event in time (rhythm) rather than on time (non-rhythmic melanin albino characteristic). The African child performs tasks in time while the adult may come to social events in time (rhythm). This is negatively called "Colored Peoples" (C.P.) time.

The African child's mind is spiritual, physical and mental. The brain is a physical structure that operates with chemical and electrical energy. It has electromagnetic melanin centers (clusters) and is melanin saturated within all its cells. The brain's ventricles (open spaces) are filled with continuously moving electromagnetic cerebral spinal fluid (holy waters).

The brain has a force field that physically resembles a galaxy (sometimes called the Third Eye = Horu). This galaxy looks like a cloud and hovers (floats) above the pineal gland and hypothalamus in the third ventricle. Historically, the ancient Africans called the fluid-filled ventricles "holy waters" to denote their spirituality.

The 12 melanin centers have properties similar to the 12 signs of the zodiac. Information, ideas, data and energy are processed through the brain and translated by the mind. The mind is partially in the body (biochemically limited) and partially outside the brain and body (not limited by time and space). When the mind needs past, present or future information, it gets it from melanin and processes it through the chemical and electrical reactions of brain cells and calls it intelligence. Melanin allows the mind to be a part of all things and in all places. Melanin bonds all Africans in the seen and unseen worlds. They are genetically Bonded to ancestors and unborn children, and aware of the slightest changes in the present and future of the galaxy, plants, waters, earth, animals, weather and climates, are spiritualized and are united with the Earth's intelligence (Mother Nature).

Melanin allows the child's spirit, body and mind to be in unity and harmoniously synchronized. However, the African child should have parents who are spiritualized, on a natural foods diet (vegetarian) and had been breastfed and Bonded with their parents. If this is not possible, then the child must have parents who have taken Bonding Remedies. Bonding would help to eliminate confusion on how and why the mind functions.

Melanin makes the brain one functioning unit. There is no split in the brain, only areas that may have specialized functions. For example, the human eyes have a specialized function (sight), but are not split or separate from the body. Without the body the eyes have no purpose. The mind sees, while the eyes merely absorb stimulation.

The Caucasians view life, nature and the mind as in conflict. This is superstitiously how the linear Caucasian's brain primitively attempts to understand the concept of the Right and Left Mind. (Caucasians see the Right Mind against or opposite the Left Mind, Predator against Prey, Man against Woman (Battle of the Sexes), Good against Evil and Rich against the Poor. This is a symptom of the Mother and Child Bonding damage.

The mind is one. There is only consciousness. Caucasians have divided the mind into fragmented parts called subconscious, pre-conscious, super-conscious and unconscious. The African mind is melaninated, cyclic and rhythmic. It takes rhythm to understand and operate the mind. Melanin albinos (Caucasians) do not have enough rhythm to understand or attempt to perform a few simple dance steps. It is a total mistake to refer to or rely upon Caucasian psychology to do anything other than reflect the dis-ease state of their White Supremacy psychosis (craziness). They are Bond damaged and nutritionally delinquent.

The African child's spiritualized thinking does not depend on memory or the content of ideas. The mind reflects its own unique growth and development as well as its harmonious, synchronized growth unity with the emotions, spirit, and body. A Bonded African child's growth has been overlooked, and the Caucasian child's growth and development have been racistly forced upon the African child. This has caused Bonding damage and the perpetuation of White Supremacy.

Africans following the growth and development unique to the African child further Africanity and create a child who is a change agent. This child will not compromise freedom or Africentric learning. Learning is a cyclic process. There are basically three "progressions to learning." *The first stage*: a new idea is introduced to the child. The child translates the idea from adult logic to children's logic. During *the second stage*: the new idea is experimentally learned. In *the third stage* the child transposes an idea and treats the idea as if it were a toy and uses variations on the new idea either in play or in fantasy. The child uses its own language to coordinate, define and redefine a new idea similar to the use of sight to coordinate the senses.

The child sees all of life as a symbolic property of energy. All of the child's early symbolic use is merged with self, spirit, the concrete word, fantasy, play and the Parents' Bond. It is important to remember that words are symbols, just as letters, music, dance, fantasy, play and Bonding are symbols of energy that the senses detect. The holistic mind interprets energy for the child.

However, an adult or child with a disease caused by a damaged Bond can be in the acute, subacute, chronic or degenerative stages of Bonding disease. The essential way to understand Bonding and Bonding disease is through a child's eyes. It is the child's world as seen by them that leads to the adult world that can be seen. The child's holistic "vision" advances to "supervision" and they must be respected as little "people" not little "children." For example, a child given the freedom to eat any type of natural food will nutritionally balance the diet within a week. The adult needs to read books and take nutrition courses in order to eat a nutritionally balanced diet. A child forced to see the world with adult abstracts would eat himself into poor health and disease. The African child has the all-seeing and all-knowing Eye of Horu within, and the adult has to use the child's eyes in order to complete the Adult Bonding.

Mentors

The Mentor is the key agent for nutritional wisdom and the development of the African child. Mentors are commonly called a "hero," a "shero," a famous ancestor, educator, athlete, social activist, freedom fighter, scientist, relative or any significant person. Mentors not only serve as role models, but also have three primary functions. First, the Mentor is a "coach" that encourages the child's highest [ability] good. Secondly, the mentor is a " Tutor" that instructs in the use of rules or theories as they apply to their ability. Finally, a mentor is a "Counselor" mat gives guidance on the quality of life needed for that ability. Ability has a broad meaning and includes talent, career, aspiration, family life, community life, business development, leadership and the child's individual concerns. An education is the primary expression of mat ability. The origin of the Mentor demonstrates its significance in "family-centered" African life.

Mentors have a long history in African American heritage and culture. Mentor in Greek means Divine Teacher. In African civilizations such as the Kush, Ethiopia, Nubia and Egypt, it is explained in mythology. The mythological God named Osiris (his name means guide of the Soul) was a great ruler. Before Osiris was born, the world had no order; there were no buildings and life was crude. Osiris left his country to travel all over the world to teach the laws of cycles, order, proper worship and technology. In his absence from his children, a highly developed person was chosen to teach his son Horus the laws of man, God, universe, science, ethics, nutrition, agriculture and holistic health. The person chosen was named Thoth. Thoth was a God in charge of the written laws of Maat. Thoth taught Maat to Horus. Maat is morals, righteousness, ethics, truth and justice which includes the divine image of humans, perfection, teachability, free will of humans and also moral practice in human development. Maat Thoth (Mentor) is also represented by the Kabala, Caduceus, Mancala or Ankh, which means "Tree of Life." The "Tree of Life" is symbolic of the utilization of 12 Melanin centers of the brain, the 12 cranial nerves, the 12 steps of Jacob's Ladder, the 12 steps on the God Shun's stairs, the 12 principals of Metutu, or the 12 cyclic degrees of the Zodiac (attributes of God). These 12 steps plus the Sun God equal number 13.

The "Rites of Passage" of growth and development are degrees, which are called the mystery system and are taught by Mentors. The mentor is basically responsible for the fruit (child) of the "Tree of Life" and is part of the African American extended family. Sometimes, the principles or steps are combined such as the 7 principles of Kwanzaa or the 7 Halls of Osiris or they can be reduced to 3 steps or levels. For example, the mystery steps could be (1) "Mortal." In this step there is no "inner-vision" and the person learns how to holistically care for his family-centered life, (2) "Intelligence" –in this step the person receives mind or consciousness and attains "inner-vision" and (3) "Creator" or "Suns of Light" or "Enlightenment or Endarkenment." In this step the person becomes united with the light of God (RA) and receives "super-vision." Mentors and Maat can be used to combat Nutricide.

Male and Female Communication for Family Maat

Energy is processed differently by the Female and Male.

When the Female is in the Feeling Stage, the Male is in the Thinking Stage.

When the Male is the Thinking Stage, the Female is in the Feeling stage.

In order to avoid conflicts, arguments, or confusion in talking, translation is needed between the different stages

The purpose of communication is to create more harmony, balance, justice, peace (Maat). If the conversation is not serving Maat stop talking

Female Principle (Cycle Stages)			
Stage	1	2	3	4
Energy	Senses	Feel	Think	Maat (Balance, Adapt)
Element	Earth	Water	Air	Fire

Male Principle			
Stage	1	2	3	4
Energy	Senses	Feel	Think	Maat (Balance, Adapt)
Element	Earth	Water	Air	Fire

Grease

The oils, lotions, cremes, moisturizers, softeners, powders, bleaching cremes, rejuvenators, sheep fat (lanolin), and other assorted concoctions do not allow the skin to breath and clog the pores. It is basically harmful for babies, children and adults. It eventually is absorbed into the blood. Cosmetic chemical companies, solely interested in profit, ignorantly advise the greasing and oiling of the baby's skin. It is the same greased baby that grows to adulthood and greases its body for whatever reason the synthetic chemical companies advertisement says. The grease concoctions feel smooth when touched because the hand slides over the oiled skin. The skin remains unchanged because skin is nourished and made smooth because of what is eaten not what is put on skin. Oddly enough, the upper layer of skin is dead and cannot utilize the grease concoction. The chemicals can be fabric-like softeners, bleach, hydrogenated fat, which destroy bodily nutrients and weaken the body.

The Caucasian custom of greasing their skin has nothing to do with health. In fact, it is mostly steeped in superstition. During the many plagues in Europe, it was believed that open skin pores allowed diseases to enter the body. Consequently, they stopped bathing with water and started using animal grease to bathe their skin. They used cooked sheep fat, which was believed to be good for the skin because sheep have curly fur. Today, Caucasians use lanolin (sheep grease) in many of their skin care products based on this ignorant superstition.

In the 1600's Europeans used protective alcohol spirit water (cologne) to bathe babies and protect them from evil diseases, this resulted in inflamed eyes and skin and severe pain in babies. Many concoctions were used; even blood (human, menstrual and or animal) combined with superstitious ceremonies. Today, remnants of the rituals still exist, as a grease cleansing is followed by a spirit mask (clay is used as the mask), then followed with a holy water (skin cologne) rinse or a skin peel (facemask removal), then another greasing. The ancient Greeks used salt, the biblical Hebrews used salt, and Soranus of Ephesus used salt and honey. The Ice Age Caucasian mentality led the Britons, Scythians, Germans, Russians, and Greenlanders to use ice or snow to bathe newborn babies. This damaged the baby's skin and was an emotionally and mentally abusive act.

In ancient Africa, warm water was used to bath babies. In fact, most races of color use warm (not cold) water, such as the Natives of Pitcairn's Island or the Araucanian Natives of South America. Today, the Caucasians add synthetic chemicals, antiseptics and dyes to baby grease. When grease is mixed with water, it is called a lotion. Basically, lotions are emulsified grease floating in water. The antiseptic lotions kill germs and also irritate the sensitive skin of the baby. Fossil oils (mineral oil) destroy oil-soluble nutrients such as vitamins A, D, E and K in the skin and dry it. They cause the skin to peel and chafe and rob it of nutrients. Aside from this, the oil and grease concoctions are absorbed into the blood and find their way to the brain. The hospitals grease babies because they do not have time to change their diapers. It is an economic convenience. A gentle massage of the baby's body would help the skin to release its own natural oils. Aside from this, massage is beneficial for the baby's intelligence (increases it) and emotional well being. Good hygiene is all the baby or an adult needs for skin—keep it clean. In the case of fat-bloated babies, the layers of fat and folded fat should be kept clean. Greasing baby like an automobile or metal motor is a way to avoid keeping the baby clean. It is a chemical solution to break the Parental Bond.

In African Bonding, the mother can sense when the child has to urinate. When the child needs to urinate, the mother lowers the child to a squatted position and the child urinates. Soon, the child learns to signal and attempts to get to a squatting position so it can urinate. The Africans do not need diapers or to grease the baby. A child on a raw food diet would not have slimy-paste gooey-manure (bowel movements), so toilet paper would not be needed. Greasing, toilet paper and diapers are symptoms of a sick Caucasian race. They denote psychotic fear and have destroyed the mother and child bond. This causes a dysfunctional family and mental illness. They try to cover up this mental illness with cow's milk, toilet paper, diapers and grease. In fact, the Caucasian's abnormal fear and behavior is forced upon Africans as normal along with Nutricide.

Caucasians superstitiously have a fear of the weather. This is understandable considering their Ice Age heritage with earthquakes, loud thunder, floods, landslides, huge boulders moving, animals constantly running, food shortages, starvation, diseases, cannibalism, rape, dysfunctional families, no education and no water supply, all of which the Caucasians associate with the weather. They fear the weather, fear God, fear nature, and fear each other.

In fear of the weather, they overdress babies. Babies should be dressed for the type of weather. In the summer, lightweight and light colored clothes. In the winter, the home's temperature should be between 75 and 80 degrees. Summer clothes should be put on the baby while indoors. If going outside in the winter cold, then winter clothes should be worn. Skin rashes are usually caused by putting on too much clothing, which results in sweating. The wearing of synthetic clothes can stop air circulation resulting in sweating and rashes.

Tight underwear worn by men and women (especially synthetic instead of cotton) can cause sweating and fungus growth. It must be noted that the long gowns and full-length clothing of African women and men may appear hot. However, when walking, the clothing creates a type of air conditioning and causes cool air to circulate over the body. The fully clothed African garments are actually cooling. They help to prevent dehydration.

If keeping the baby clean and dry is done, then there is no need for antiseptic soap, medicated concoctions, boric acid, starch powder, talcum powder, vinegar, oatmeal or bran baths, greasy, oily, lubricated wipes and other Caucasian superstitious substitutes for good hygiene.

Using Babies As Toys

The African adult can abuse babies by over-handling them. This can occur because babies are abused by being used for entertainment. A baby should not be used to get a laugh or physically manipulated to get reactions. Adults laugh at babies' reactions to stimuli such as sounds, light, touch or muscle manipulations. Adults assume these human responses are cute, as they make the baby perform circus tricks like a clown or a pet dog. Babies placed in the center of an adult's attention are being abused. Babies put on display like a store window mannequin (plastic dummy) while adults' stare at them, commenting on their physical features and personality, is holistically harmful.

Then added to this, many toys, plastic gadgets, stuffed animals plastic nipples, bottled milk and noise-making devices are put in their face or hands. The baby is treated like it is a toy and talked to in Caucasian mumbled, no-syllable words while it is being passed back, forward and around the room like a remote control device or a computer game (Nintendo). Aside from this, the baby is forced to endure loud talking, bright anti-melanin artificial light (should be full color spectrum), loud music, loud laughter, and disturbed rest/sleep periods. African babies, with their immature immune systems, are subjected to the adults, synthetic and/or non-synthetic germs and bacteria.

Usually the African family members are the only ones allowed to hold the baby. During the first few days after birth only the mother handles the baby as bonding is taking place. A child subjected to weird vibrations and unholistic emotions of strangers is actually being abused. A baby is a gift from God who deserves the highest good and cleansed spirits in its presence. The continuous display of babies as the center of attention can cause them to be self-centered and egotistic. They become conditioned to think that other people or gadgets (toys) must entertain them. They also begin to develop the idea that the absence of entertainment brings boredom. The baby gets accustomed to thinking that amputated animal parts and stuffed beasts or people are fun and normal. They are given an amputated Mr. Potato head or a rubber amputated breast's nipple pacifier or a deformed animal face (Miss Piggy), etc. Eventually, they grow up and accept amputated mannequin body parts in store windows or in store displays. In stores on display there will be an amputated-human head, amputated breast (modeling a brassiere) or a body with only the hips and thighs (modeling underwear).

The baby is conditioned to accept the mutilation of the human as part of normal life. Mutilated human mannequins (dummies) and toys are associated with fun that gives the self, or ego, pleasure. It is a crazy mixture of human and animal mutilations and amputations and fun that the child gets conditioned to. The destruction of other (mannequin amputations) is viewed as part of getting attention and pleasure. This, along with sexual abuse from watching R-rated movies, music videos, Nutricide and violent films is damaging. Toys, especially Caucasian toys, present a mixture of something to love, destroy and to have fun with.

Silent Guilt—Caucasian Woman

The Caucasian woman is a powerful force in Nutricide. The Caucasian media does not openly show the Caucasian woman's participation in Nutricide, so it is silent. She is as guilty of White Supremacy as the Caucasian man. She inherits the wealth exploited from Africans from her family or deceased male. She controls the major stocks in the junk food, medicine and drug companies (usually by inheritance). Caucasian women dominate Caucasian civilization, as there are over 600 million women per 300 million men.

The Caucasian woman is the controlling and dominating labor force in the public schools teaching profession, nurses, cookbook and fairy-tale writers. In these positions she pushes junk foods, cooked foods and toxic, poisonous medicine to African children. Historically, the Caucasian woman made prisoners of war (slaves) breastfeed her babies. She raped and helped her Caucasian men to rape African women, children and men. She used African women as homosexual toys and African men as sex toys aside from preparing slaves' flesh in culinary dishes for Caucasian cannibalistic meals and rituals.

Further, the Caucasian woman educated or indoctrinated Caucasian boys and girls to be White Supremacists. Additionally, she controlled and acted as manager of slave plantations while her husband was away on trips. She also worked in machine factories during the World Wars. Her labor helped to exploit, destroy and/or kill African Americans. Additionally, the Caucasian woman still works in junk food factories that make synthetic foods for Nutricide. She directly and indirectly promotes herself as the symbol of beauty and culture by inferiorizing Africans.

The White woman as a symbol of the highest form of beauty and sexuality for the Black woman and man is a mixture of deeply embedded homosexuality. She wears clothes that have sexual connotations. The high heel shoes she wears are symbols of perverted sex. The heel on the Caucasian high heel shoe is symbolically a long erect penis. Historically, the long pointed toe on the Caucasian shoe represents an erect penis. The pointed leather toe was stuck into the vagina and/or anus (man or woman) for sexual masturbation. They were erotic decorations and jewelry for the penis like toe of the shoe. She basically dresses in the clothing of ancient Caucasian men (dress, skirt, stockings, lace, bikini, high heel and pointed shoe)

The White woman is physically created by her father and mother. Therefore, she is half man and half woman with a dominant physical expression of a female. However, she carries within her the subdominant traces of the mental, emotional, sexual and physical characteristics of a white man.

In the Black man's act of sexual intercourse with a white woman a subtle form of mental illness and dysfunctionality exist. The Black man may be consciously having sex with the white woman but he is also subconsciously (subliminally) having sex with the White man. The Black man can be having sex with the White woman in order to satisfy his need to be loved, nurtured, raped, sodomized, protected and/or possessed by the white man. If the Black man is having sex with the white woman what is he doing emotionally with the White man within the white woman? He is in a homosexual relationship with the white man thru the sex act with the white woman. He psychologically becomes the white man's homosexual 'nigga' boy.

The Black man in the act of sex with the White woman or homosexual act with man is a boy. The White persons in this White Supremacy dominated world controls all rewards and punishments via their military, money, schools, media, capitals, resources and stolen African lands. Therefore, they are the adults and all Black men and women are their children (subjected to Caucasian adult system of rewards and punishments). Consequently, in the Black/White sexual act Whites are adults and Blacks are the child (boy, girl).

A Black person that has sexual intercourse with a White woman (or man) is satisfying a psychotic dysfunctional desire to be loved by the white man. It is a cowardly act. Instead of picking up a gun and destroying his White enemy the Black man picks up his penis and mentally destroys himself. His sexual intercourse with the White woman is a form of self-hatred. This type of sex shows that he hates the image of the Black woman, which means he hates the female part of himself (mother), thus he hates himself.

The Black man that has sex with a Black woman is practicing Maat and spiritually uniting himself with God. Sex is a political, social and spiritual language of a culture. It is not simply a physical reproductive or regenerative activity. African sexuality is a holistic (spirit/mind/body) cultural language that Africans use to serve Maat.

A Black person having sex with a White person is emotionally masturbating a dysfunctional ingredient in the mind. A dysfunctional African is one that is not free to practice African culture at all times and in all situations. You, your family, your culture and the continent of Africa has to be free of White domination and able to defend itself and attack its enemies in order to be holistically healthy, functional and free. Therefore, any sex with a White woman merely represents another form of African dysfunctionality.

The crazy sick part of the Black man and White woman sexual intercourse is that the White woman enjoys the dysfunctional social situation. She enjoys and gets a sexual thrill from the Black man's sexual hatred, denial of Black female love and subliminal hatred of his own man hood and race. She gets animalistic exotic erotic sexual arousal from his symbolic sacrifice of himself on her symbolic vagina cross. He symbolically imprisons himself in the cave jail of her White vagina where he is safe from his Blackness and lost in her Whiteness. In many ways this same sexual dysfunction occurs with the Black Woman that has sex with the White man. Added to the Black woman's dysfunctions is the Mother Principle. The Black woman destroys her Mother Principle, which means she is also destroying Mother Africa. In any case, this White/Black sex is a way of committing spiritual suicide and African cultural castration.

It is often said, "The hand that rocks the cradle controls the civilization. In other words, the Caucasian woman is the foundation for White Supremacy and Nutricide all over the world. The majority of the Sunday school (religious school) teachers are Caucasian women, so she is the primary teacher of racism to her children at church and in public and private schools and colleges.

The Caucasian woman may meekly or silently hide her guilt. However, she enjoys the benefits of White skin and lets the White man take the total blame for her crimes against Africans. The Caucasian woman creates the fantasy image that the mentally and physically weakest man on this planet is the most powerful man the Caucasian. The Caucasian woman is a companion and co-dependent partner in the maintenance of Nutricide and will do anything that is required, by any means required, in order to be the Supreme Caucasian Woman even if it means destroying the Caucasian man in the process.

The mental illness, which defends her spiritual, mental and physical inferiority, works as a paranoia. Paranoia acts on the assumptions that the mind creates. Added to this, the Caucasian woman has a phobic (fantasy fear) reaction to her own phobias (exaggerated, illogical fear) combined with a melanin albinism brain that lacks enough electromagnetic charge to regenerate itself and think holistically. She is by no means half-guilty of White Supremacy, but fully guilty of the crimes she has inflicted against African peoples.

Historically, it was the Caucasian woman who castrated the African man after and while they were being hung. It was the Caucasian woman who made African babies drink cow's milk so that her Caucasian babies could drink the African woman's breast milk. It was/is the Caucasian woman who does not allow African children to bond. It is the Caucasian woman who teaches White Supremacy and African Inferiority to African children. The Caucasian woman lacks the mother instinct and does not and will not allow the African woman to use hers.

The Caucasian woman in American democratic elections has the majority of votes that can control the government. Her inherited stock controls the major wealth (power elite) of the country. She displays her lack of respect for Africans by putting her sexual immorality and spiritual perversion in television dramas called soap operas. Caucasian women have perverted nature, perverted bonding and perverted the Mother instinct in order to hold claim to White Female Supremacy mental illness. It is a characteristic of the Caucasian woman's mental illness to avoid being responsible for her behavior and life. Rather than cope with her own fantasy/joy of being the supreme woman on earth she puts her feelings on her man and tries to tell Africans that she is not as angry, violent, sexually perverted, phobic, paranoid, devious, self-centered, inferior and as racist as her mate.

The Caucasian woman has a dependent and competitive dependent relationship with her Caucasian man. The Caucasians' collective (racial) mental illness teaches them to be dependent in order to be intimate. They are intimate only because neither one of them can operate White Racism or Nutricide without the other. One of them may feel dependent upon and exploited, while the other feels taken advantage of. The solution to this dependency is another form of dependency, called control. It is similar to the left brain and right brain bonding together by the mid-brain. In this case, the Caucasian woman and man are bonded together by their mental illness, which controls the relationship. Control is one of the paranoid phobic aspects of their mental disease.

Caucasians need to control Africans with diet, medicine, democracy, socialism, jails, religion, schools, jobs, drugs, food, sex and violence. In this way, the Caucasian feels that they won't be dependent on African civilizations, science, social systems, resources and land. In reality, Caucasians are dependent on African people's culture, God, science, resources and land. This is an obvious contradiction, because control and dependency in the mind of the mentally ill is a mixed feeling (mixed with sex and violence) and is confusing. Within the Caucasian mental disease, it is taught that intimidation helps to confuse (double talk, word trickery) Africans. This is a way to be superior. Intimidation could have been learned from the Ice Age in which the weather, animals, cannibalism, food and violence intimidated their very existence.

The Caucasian woman continues to enjoy the benefits of her mental illness while she pretends to be innocent of Nutricide. She uses her sexuality to sell junk food, cooked food and medicine to Africans and at the same time creates the fantasy image that she is superior in mind and beauty. Her guilty behavior claims her while her White Racist words indict her. She is guilty and has committed a sin against mother instinct—the instinct that says nurtures, nourish and protect all children. Instead, she commits Nutricide upon African children.

Birth Marks (Maternal Impressions)

The Caucasian myths and superstitions that surround birthmarks cloud their true meaning. In health matters, it is best to leave African health concerns to Africans and leave Caucasian concerns to Caucasians. We must learn to differentiate and separate Caucasian health from African highly melaninated health imperatives.

Maternal Impressions are the impact of the spirit, environment, people or events upon an unborn child. The ancient Greeks believed that a mother could make her baby a genius, artist or warrior by looking at mathematics, art or pictures of military battles. If Maternal Impressions are solely mental, then the impression of chattel slavery upon Africans would have produced more Africans wanting to be slavers or total warriors against slavery.

The White slave master used Maternal Impressions to his advantage. Often, the mythological reason that was given for an African woman giving birth to a white baby was that it was caused by her looking at too many white clouds in the sky. Caucasian myth and superstitions are guarded by religious books, such as *The Bible and Koran*, which were rewritten by political, Caucasian racists. For example, in the book of Genesis, in Chapter 30 verses 29 to 43 it says that placing different colors of rods in front of Jacob's cattle caused them to have stripes of various colors.

There are Maternal Impressions that can be made by highly melaninated Africans. The electromagnetic aura of mother and child has a harmonious charge. This facilitates Bonding along with breastfeeding. The melanin is the bonding substance that passes through the placenta's protective barrier and communicates biochemically through the ancestral genetic pool. The baby and the mother develop a holistic language of vibrations. The parents become a vehicle of melanin-to-melanin intelligence. However, if the Caucasian junk food diet, drugs, cow's milk, cooked food, animal flesh consumption and the absence of bonding are a part of the parent's life, no Africentric Maternal Impression can be made. The electromagnetic biochemical impression can be made with melanin as the vehicle. If the parent's diet is anti-melanin junk food and poisonous drugs, then the child will have a biochemical predisposition for the Caucasian diet. In other words, the child will have the maternal impression passed to it to eat like Caucasians and be prone to Caucasian diseases.

Maternal instinct is basic for mother and father. A holistic maternal instinct is necessary for a maternal impression to be made. The Ice Age Caucasians have historically lacked this maternal bonding. The brutal molesting, cannibalism and murdering of African children during colonialism and slavery are a testimonial to the lack of Caucasian maternal instinct. In ancient European Sparta, all diseased and weak babies were drowned. In the European cannibalistic history, babies and children were captured with human traps and special roasting recipes were used. In the 17th Century, Caucasian babies were given molasses, castor oil, spirit water, herbs and combinations of drugs for medical, poisonous treatments of disease. The treatment for such diseases as diphtheria resulted in a death rate of close to 100%.

Caucasians stay heavily invested in their myths and superstitions and not facts because of their mental illness. It is obvious that the teachings of Hippocrates regarding giving natural foods and herbal remedies to children have not been obeyed in 2,000 years of Caucasian history. This is partially related to the fact that his teachings are African and are considered a religious belief rather than a hygienic fact.

During the massive European famines, wars and pestilence, medical practitioners killed more babies than the atrocities. Any semblance of a Maternal Instinct and maternal impressions were ignored. European parents continue to give toxic drugs and poisonous inoculations and vaccinations to their babies and children. While the babies were asleep in bed with their parents, they were suffocated by parents rolling on them. There were at least 20 deaths per week related to suffocation, 1 in 7 died within the first year due to disease or starvation, 2 in 5 died before age 5, and the remaining 50% died of diseases before reaching 25 years of age. These deaths do not reflect deaths caused by famine, violence, cannibalism or wars. For example, at the end of World War I in France, America and Belgium, 77 out of 1,000 babies died due to disease and nutritional slaughter. The death rate for children was higher than for soldiers, as 10 out of 1,000 American soldiers died in battle or from battle wounds.

It must be noted that wild animals' babies do not die from disease, but from violence. African people cannot rely on Caucasians to understand or utilize the melaninated Maternal Instinct or the value of Maternal Impressions, as Caucasian history is a violation of nature. (Information on babies' death rates are in such books as, *Notes on Nursing*, by Florence Nightingale, *Shut Your Mouth*, by George Catlin, *Infant Mortality*, by E. Ballard).

Birthmarks are usually highly melaninated, darkened skin areas. Generally, the Birthmark can be a spiritual signature of an ancestor, sign of a gift (or calling), or a chakra (melanin cluster), denote a weak force or organ, enhance the vibration of a chakra, indicate a cyclic force specific to a Zodiac sign, indicate an uncut attachment to a Maternal force, indicate a caution or a mind set or a nutritional weakness and/or a developmental emphasis for the child's rite of passage.

Birthmarks on children are not necessarily from the parents. Generations of ancestors' genes are carried by parents. The father's sperm and mother's egg (ova) are not solely created by them. The sperm and ova are entirely separate, living, melaninated forms. Nature does not leave the highly biochemical and electromagnetic ancestral organisms' creation up to the parents. In order to understand this God force, the birthmarks have to be viewed as God's signature. The understanding of the scientific fact that Melanin does not die will help the African to accept that African parents can leave an impression on the child's melanin. This is Maternal Impression. The correct holistic diet, lifestyle, Bonding and Breast Feeding nutritional customs must be followed in order to uplift the race. The Maternal Impression can be our guide again for the Greatness that is all Africans' destiny.

Birthmarks can act as a Divine instrument for the baby's future. However, the current Nutricide locks away the holistic meaning of an African's life. The Caucasians' mental illness can cause many of the Trees of Life (Ankh) such as birthmarks to be considered the stupid or silly thinking of a primitive African people. Once the negative effects of the Caucasians' White Supremacy mental illness is in the African's mind, the African mind becomes like concrete. It is thoroughly mixed up and cemented in ignorance. A concrete Caucasian block replaces the African brain.

Trances / Meditation / Daydreams

The trance state of consciousness can be considered a type of self-hypnosis. It has always been used in African civilization. Among African Americans, trance is used in Church. African people in church go into a trance and get possessed with the Holy Spirit (or Holy Ghost). African children use trance when they go into a daydream state. Trance, Meditation or Daydreams are a similar type of consciousness. Trance increases learning ability. It can be considered a combination of organic spirit, ancestral spirit, mind spirit and body spirit holistic awareness. Trance, vision, possession states or conjure have been used by Jesus the Christ, George Washington Carver, Nat Turner, Denmark Vesey, Malcolm X, Harriet Tubman, Martin Luther King, Sojourner Truth, Marcus Garvey, etc. Trances take on the characteristics of the culture from which they are derived. For example, African culture would have a ritual or ceremony to prepare the African person for the trance and a closure ritual/ceremony to acknowledge the blessings received from the trance. There are basically two types of trances—the isolation (self-centered) and the full awareness (communal-relationship with all energy).

The isolation type meditation requires that you lose contact with the environment and people around you. In this separation or disconnection with life around you, you become only aware of yourself. This is a popular meditation approach because of people pollution, high tech/low touch or over-saturation of people. This approach creates a meditative space that allows you to reconnect with self. This trance allows an inner journey into the silence of the body, mind, and spirit. It is believed that all life started in silence or in the non-senses or blackness or melanin. This type of trance allows the regeneration of the power of silence or non-senses or blackness. This can be a "self-centered" trance if used from a Caucasian perspective. However, Africentrically, it places the being in the blackness or melanin center of life.

The full contact, or being aware of the total environment around you and within you, is the other major approach to trance. You do not isolate self but, allow self to be communal with all energy, such as air, sun, moisture, trees, birds, insects, other people, water, breathing, the blinking of eyes, the sound of hearing sounds, the pineal gland's vibrations, heart beats, energy centers (melanin clusters called Chakras), which is holistic attention to internal and external forces. In this approach, you meditate within the world and do not isolate yourself outside the world's energy. This gives energy to the world that gives energy back to you.

African children as well as adults naturally use trance. Children easily drift into a trance which is called daydreaming. Daydreaming is a mild state of trance. It is not a structured or educated use of trance. It should be taught within the "Rites of Passage." The child should be instructed that during the trance (daydream) they are not mentally or spiritually in their body and can experience travel in the past, present and future. In the spirit travel, they solve problems, communicate with other spirits and with ancestors living as well as dead. They should be instructed that there are appropriate times for trance. Further, the African child should be told that trance is essential for African people and that their great ancestors used it before studying or doing any activity. All African children's so-called toys have spiritual meaning and many of the musical or spiritually shaped toys contacted the trance energy of the child. Play activity also included trance activity.

Trances can be done while sitting on the floor, standing, drumming, singing, jogging, walking, lying down, or dancing; they are a functional part of life. They can be done by isolating yourself from activities. It can be a melanin regenerative, and self-uplifting activity. Deep breathing and slow exhaling are essential to trances. Breathing through the nose very slowly is necessary. If standing or sitting in a chair, the legs should be at least shoulder width apart. Further, the arms should be relaxed at the sides, if standing, or hands should be placed in the lap if sitting. Erect posture, back upright, not slumped over and eyes either closed or open and focused straightforward. You can visualize an Ankh or crystal or color or use African music or incense to focus attention or use silence. The object is to go beyond the mind's limitations.

The trance state may need nutritional support. There are herbs such as Gotu Kola, Catnip, Iboga, Gingko and Yucca, which can be used. Also supplements such as Glutamine, B_6, L-Dopa, Tyrosine, Tryptophane, Melatonin, or Niacinamide can be used. Trance helps the African to utilize melanin energy, to create force fields and healthy cells in the body. The deliberate inferiorization of African trances by Caucasians has taken away a vital nutrient for health. Without the use of trance, the African is nutritionally deprived and Nutricided. The beginner in trance-learning should go slowly. Perhaps, a two-minute trance and then gradually increasing according to the child's or adult's ability.

A Divine Mess

The African Divine nutritional level (Ankh Force) is vital to holistic health. Caucasian science divorces Africans from this spiritualized ability. Spirit is merely a response to Divineness. Divineness causes consciousness, intelligence, life force, light, magnetism, air, levity, gravity, sight, sound, water or electricity to be in a form that we can physically recognize. Ankh Force (Melanin Electromagnetic Vibratory Energy) is receptive, transmitted, stored and converted more readily in Africans than in any other race. Ankh Force is a level of life's existence that is in nutrients which allows Africans to transmute.

Transmutation is the ability to excite trace elemental energies in nutrients, which causes them to be adaptive or convened. For example, sodium can be adapted (changed) to magnesium, magnesium to calcium, electrical waves to chemicals, chemicals to magnetic energy, sound to light, light to vitamins, vitamins to hormones, hormones to enzymes, etc. These Ankh force mediate activities are called transmutation because the Caucasian scientists do not like to use the word spirituality.

Spirituality leads to melanin and melanin leads to Ankh Force and Ankh Force leads to Africans' racial superiority. Caucasian science and religions use myths and superstitions to focus attention away from Ankh Force. These media (religion and science) are destructive to the harmony of Africans. For example, Caucasian science pits Good Bacteria (vaccine) against Bad Bacteria (contagion) and religions use Good Social Behavior (socially approved homosexuality) against Bad Behavior (constitutional duty to destroy U.S.

government) instead of science. The only true science is the study of Ankh Force melanin, conjuring, Divining, Maat and spirituality.

Caucasian science is not the study of Ankh Force but superstitions. It is superstition to believe that bacteria cause dis-ease. Disease is merely the accumulation of toxins and waste in the body caused by incorrect food combinations, junk food, drugs, alcohol, dairy products, animal flesh cooked concoctions and a disregard for the spiritual nature of vegetables and fruits. Africans become physically, spiritually and mentally ill when they do not use Ankh nutritional force. Ankh has to be used to maintain health. Nutricide is caused when Caucasian media (sciences, religion, school textbooks etc.), classifies Divining as unscientific or non-religious. Divineness becomes engulfed in negative taboos and confused with folk tales, which distorts its value in the science of living. Divining and Maat is part of the nutritional reality for an African life.

The Nutricidal Divining destruction is caused when Africans worship scientific or cultural ceremonies, rituals, customs, etiquette, manners, a specific culture's morality, discipline, laws and social order. Another culture's science (biology, chemistry) or religious rewritten books (*Bible, Koran*) create a Divine Mess with the African. Alien culture's religious books demonstrate how another culture accepted or rejected a religion (not to be confused with spirituality). In those religious books prophets lectured to the people of their culture and stated rules of behaviors within their culture for the people of their culture. In 99% of cases, the prophet is never a woman, which is directly opposed to African spirituality and wisdom.

Incidentally, African spirituality teaches that sin is punishment for bad behavior while blessings are rewards for good behavior. In other religions, it is believed that you are punished by your sins not for your sins. It is considered sinful not to follow the male prophet, which means follow the prophet's culture. This teaching of positive cultural customs is erroneously called spirituality. The prophet and culture become more important than spirituality. Religious preachers teach culture and social science. Teaching spirituality would demand the teaching of the subject of nutrition, melanin and taking physical action to get freedom.

Africentric spirituality requires the use of Divining ability to know who you are, what your purpose in life is and taking holistic action to achieve that purpose. In others words, the use of Divining Ankh, Crystals, Trance, Draughts, Pendulums, Egyptian Tarot cards, Zodiac, Divining Dice, Shells, etc., are an essential part of being African. Divining helps to sensitize the body and nutrients in foods for the Africans who seek spiritual Endarkenment (erroneously called enlightenment) from preachers of various Caucasian cultural-type religions. Unfortunately, Africans are taught to ignore a vital part of their spiritualization—Divining. The Caucasian preachers (Christian, Moslem, Jews etc.), do not speak directly about the Africentric rules of spirituality or Divining abilities because this would make the follower free of the preacher and religion.

The media (preacher/religion) vaguely correlates spirituality to social myths, superstitions, animal sacrifices, fables, scripture gossip, wars and battles between Gods, Prophets and tribes, murder, rapes or politics. Furthermore, the preachers give Caucasian cultural significance to Bible/Koran gossip (scriptures), and do not directly teach the rules of Africentric spirituality or Divining (Rites of Passage). This causes the believers (followers) to have knowledge about social life and none about spiritual "willing," regeneration, cyclic laws, or nutritional transmutation (Melanin-based science). African nutrition, biology, anatomy and chemistry are spiritual science that requires using Divine abilities (so-called psychic, clairvoyance, audiovoyance, etc.).

Preachers and religions omit the Divine abilities. To them, Divining abilities are erroneously interpreted as witchcraft. Religious institutions are designed to promote, create, recruit, propagandize and economically feed religion to humans. Followers (Believers) of religions worship the religion or prophet while God becomes a secondary issue. If the prophet or preacher eats junk food, animal flesh, uses Caucasian science, then the followers (Believers) do the same.

It is ungodly to harm or destroy the living Temple of God (human body) with junk food, junk culture, junk religions and junk science. It is easy for Africans to follow Caucasian junk science, nutrition and medicine because they are forms of religion. They use superstition, scientific or scriptural gossip, violence, sex and Good against Evil ideas. Disease is considered evil and Divine ability is considered evil, while in reality they are both healthy for the African. Dis-eases are a cleansing process of the body. Divining is a spiritualizing process for nutrients, melanin and the Ankh Force.

The nutritional upliftment of Africans has to be free of superstitions, myths, and Caucasian culture media, (nutrition, biology, chemistry etc.) and worship. There is a difference between respecting prophets (i.e., Akhenaton, Nzinga, Imhotep, Hatshepsut, Garvey, Muhammad, Jesus, Elijah Mohammed, Moses, Buddha, Martin Luther King Jr., Malcolm X, etc.) and worshipping prophets. The worshipper believes in a prophet/religion and gathers scientific or scriptural gossip to support that belief

The African who uses Divining, is led to respect a prophet and worship God. An Endarkened (melanin enlightened) African understands that nutrients (vitamins, minerals, amino acids) are spirits and science is a spirit language used to help understand nutrients. Nutrients merely react to a common force in harmony with the body. In other words, if you eat an apple your body does not become half apple and half-human, it reacts to nutrients in the apple. The spiritual nutrients, mental nutrients and physical nutrients are parts of all vitamins, minerals and amino acids. For example, a nutrient such as Glutamic Acid (Glutamine) is good for cellular repair (physical), improving memory (mental) and directing Ankh (spiritual). In other words, Glutamic Acid is holistic. However, Caucasian science, myth and superstition (gossip) limits and enslaves nutrients and stops their spiritual use. This Caucasian science belief can stop the Africans' ability to Divine and holistically use Maat.

Caucasian science gossip (media) limits vitamin A's nutritional use. It is believed that vitamin A is primarily good for infection and the eyes. This is true, but it is not the full scope of vitamin A's holistic capacity. This belief held in an African's mind and spirit harms vitamin A and diseases the African. Vitamin A is not found isolated in a plant. It is part of a nutrient family. Vitamin A is in a communal relationship (family) with other vitamins, minerals and amino acids. It does not function alone. It is part of a holistic team of body, mind and spirit nutrients.

However, Caucasian self-centered (individualistic) behavior projects this behavior on chemicals, vitamins, minerals, etc. It is believed that nutrients behave like White people. Vitamin A is believed to come from nothing (chaos) and return to nothing. It comes from destruction and will destroy itself. Vitamin A is considered a nutrient slave designed to serve the White Race. Africans who nutricidally follow this science gossip psychologically stop Vitamin A from being holistic. Vitamin A can be good for infections (physically), help memory storage (mental) and harmonize spirit, to, spirit energies (spiritual). Vitamin A has abilities beyond Caucasian science gossip and is in harmony when it is spiritually free to act communally within the body.

The communal nutrients from a natural foods diet cure the body of disease. Ironically, the healing (curing) of a scratch (minor skin cut) on the arm is the same biological process as the curing of cancers, fibroid tumors, VD, ulcers, colds or dandruff. A natural food diet, is assurance of a cure, not health insurance. Health insurance is a junk-food-eating Africans only protection against disease instead of the Divineness of nature. Health insurance businesses charge everyone for the illness of a few. They force Africans to use drugs and surgery and to eat junk food while in hospitals. This causes more disease and increases insurance company profits and damages the health spirit of Africans.

The Caucasians deliberately teach African children and scientists to ignore Ankh Force. This is destructive nutritionally, mentally and spiritually. Ankh is commonly labeled Life Force, Prana, Chakra, Electromagnetic Energy, Radionics, Acupuncture Meridians, Consciousness, Conjure, Extrasensory Perception, Divine, The Seventh Sense, Audiovoyance, Clairvoyance etc. All seen and unseen matter has intelligence within it that is Ankh. All matter such as thoughts, emotions, vitamins, minerals, amino acids, plants, cells, atmosphere, galaxy and planets absorb, store and transmit Ankh force. The great African American alchemist George Washington Carver referred to it as listening to the intelligence of nature (audiovoyance). He often said the peanut told him what to do. Some Africans need a medium such as Tarot cards, pendulums, crystals, shells, the zodiac, auras, Ancestors, or a Trance to help them communicate with the Ankh Force, while others communicate directly. This communication is called Divining. An African who does not use Divining and adopts Caucasian culture in the form of sciences is in a Divine Mess that is nutricidal.

Caucasian science media is simply used to enslave African's Ankh Force. This childish, Caucasian, superstitious science propaganda is called pure science while African spiritualized (Ankh Force) science is called primitive, unscientific, evil, ignorance or witchcraft. An African who does not use his Ankh force also dislocates (degenerates) his ability to be healthy. Health can only be obtained by Divine use of Ankh Force. Ankh Force is the language of vitamins, minerals, amino acids, vegetable proteins and carbohydrates. They vibrate to their highest nutrient level in a body that is spiritualized with Ankh force. Without Ankh force the African is an unhealthy imitation Caucasian and a diseased African.

Africans naturally rely upon Ankh force to feed and nourish their lives. The Divining ability (Ankh Force) was used in a Trance by all ancient African professionals such as scientist, herbalist, nutritionist, doctor, engineer, teacher, musician, athlete, agriculturist, architect, administrator as well as children and adults in their everyday life. Divining (Ankh Force) and Trance (focusing of energy) is a tradition in African culture.

Caucasians have "Whitewashed" (brainwashed) Africans to accept a cartoon fantasy science and a White religious Divine Mess. The power of the mind to cause Divining and psychosomatic diseases cannot be denied. There are those who have spiritual and mental depression. They express their depression by exaggerated and imaginary fears of physical diseases. In the case of Africans, hypochondriac diseases can be caused by White Racism, suppressed feelings about slavery and/or a melanin deficiency.

The mind reacts first to any disease and may be nutritionally, culturally and spiritually deprived which can cause a physical disease. It is suggested that Tryptophane, Melatonin Supplement, herbal combinations of Gingko/Gotu Kola, Echinacea, Saw Palmetto or fresh tropical fruits and vegetables be eaten in order to increase the melanin supply needed to protect the African mind, body and spirit. A "Whitewashed" (brainwashed) African mind can physically handicap the body. A mind-created physical disease can cripple an individual and limit the use of Maat.

For example, the miracle cures of people by Faith Healers were verified to be true. The invalids, crippled, blind, deaf and handicapped were given complete physical examinations before going to the Faith Healer. The examinations indicated that the handicapped people did not have anatomical, biochemical or organic causes for being handicapped. An organic cause for being handicapped could be a permanently destroyed bone, muscle or organ caused by injury, birth defect or spiritual damage. In other words, the physical diseases were in the mind. The handicapped persons told themselves they were handicapped and made their bodies become fixed in a diseased posture or state. In many cases, the superstitious medical community told the person they were handicapped and used science gossip, drugs and social science to attach the mind to a psychosomatic illness.

The handicapped are often the Caucasians' psychosomatic zombies created by them in order to sustain the drug companies and help create and perpetuate fear of bacteria phobias. The handicapped generate profits for research institutions. The handicapped are psychosomatic sacrifices for medical business profits.

A handicapped individual, after a physical examination, attended a Faith Healing or Divining session held at a church, in a tent or sports arena and was cured in front of witnesses. The Faith Healer told the handicapped they could walk or see and the handicapped accepted this truth, reprogrammed their minds and used belief to cure themselves. This positive suggestion cured the mind that in turn cured the body of the handicap. A changed mind changed their physical impairment.

Oddly enough, Africans have not only Caucasian psychosomatic illness but Ethnomedical illness, which causes them to be handicapped. Africans who tell themselves they are healthy can be handicapped. If African use Caucasian health standards to determine health, they are diseased. They tell their body and mind that the nutritional deficiencies caused by a healthy Caucasian standard are normal. The African believes the constant, physically weakened health condition and nutrient-deficient brain is normal and will not seek African medical advice or natural foods. The Caucasian junk medicine, junk culture and junk religions cement the African's psychosomatic disease.

Any African who is not perpetually attempting to destroy White Culture is psychosomatically ill, handicapped. This nutritionally handicapped African mind is fixed in the Caucasian propaganda that says that Africans who employ Divining are practicing Witchcraft, Black magic or some evil. The handicapped African in partnership with Caucasians helps to create the Divine Mess by separating the Africans spirit from the Divining abilities.

The obstruction of Divining, African culture, ethnomedicine and Africentric thought is at the speed of Caucasian computers. The 12 years of White Racist miseducation in Eurocentric schools slows the African's pace. Today, the computerized fast pace of brainwashing is escalated and destroys Africans' Divining ability with Caucasoid linear thought in computer programs, games and Freak Foods. The only defense an African has is natural foods, herbal medicine and Divining. Africans who eat anything on a dinner plate that looks like food, smells like food and does not talk back, move, attempt to attack him, call him a nigger or kill him immediately upon putting it in his mouth are sacrificing their Divine Kinship to Africa and ancestors.

The Caucasian cloned vegetables and fruits have been created with human cells, pig cells, insect cells, rat cells, drugs, pus, nuclear mutated cells, bacteria, diseased cells and electromagnetically perverted cells that are usually grown on petroleum waste without soil. These freak vegetables and fruits are causing new mutated spliced genetic diseases of the body, mind, and spirit.

The genes from diseased animals, insects or humans are combined with separate species or within each other's gene pool to create transgenetic eatable plant freaks. These freaks are technically classified as food additives because they are added to a plant. However, the dysfunctional Caucasians avoid their own laws by considering these freaks as natural plants because they grow similarly to plants. Actually, these freak plants are cloned animals trapped in a plant's body. They are lowest in nutritional value, pollute the soil, water and air and alter the human body, mind and spirit. They make Divining a nutritional impossibility for those Africans who eat the freaks.

Genetic altering of vegetables, fruits, beef, pork, milk poultry and seafood is estimated to be the largest increase in the food industry's profits since frozen foods in 1930. The tobacco industry is now massively invested in biotech (freaks). For example, tobacco plus tomato gene splicing has created frost-resistant tomato plants. The same cancer-causing potential exists in the combination of "tobacco-tomato" plant as the toxic, cooked oil from the tobacco plant. Some other freaks available to consumers are "chicken/potato" animals, which increases potato immunity. "Insect (Wax Moth)/Potato" plant resists bruises in processing. Human/Pig (swine) cell animals. This swine has leaner meat. The market is unlimited, as human sperm and egg cell splicing plus human brain and animal brain splicing with other plants and humans has generated another market for the pharmaceutical business. Some businesses already involved in the transgenetic (freak foods) are the National Institutes of Mental Health, U.S. Military, (The Military has cloned plants and animals as weapons or cloned people as programmed weapons and uses biochemical cellular weapons), Campbell Soup, Upjohn, Pepsi Cola, Calgene, Heinz, Frito-Lay, Dole, Dupont, Hunt-Wesson, Shell Oil, Garden and Household Plants, Pets, Animal Feed Industries, and the Cosmetic Industry. These businesses do not have any legal obligation to label their animal/plants as freaks. Therefore, an African who is eating freaks will sooner or later become a freak with no Divining, conjuring abilities or spiritual energy. It is now or never. Either Africans eat natural foods and start Divining and use Maat or become a Divine Mess.

Chapter Four
Craziness

"Not only must we teach Black people how to use food nutritionally, but we must teach them to do it within the context of their own culture."

Dr. Alvenia Fulton

Gang Warfare

The Caucasian race has a deep sense of inferiority. This is mixed with superstitions, phobic reactions to phobias, self-hatred and fear that cripple their brains. It causes them to distort the thoughts that come to and leave their brains. Their moods, feelings, logic, behavior and socialization with other races is an acting-out of that phobic mind set. Caucasian civilization is built on a foundation of dysfunctional (abnormal) families that form loosely united gangs. They have massive gangs (European countries) that attack the ecology of the earth with pollution. Their gangs attack African people with Nutricide and genocide.

Once they have made a conquest, then they begin to fight each other. A deep sense of insecurity about safety, victories, sex, nature, God and themselves causes them to attack each other in a gang-like manner. They call their gangs governments, ethnic groups, alliances, religions, the United Nations, public schools, hospitals, drug companies, the Food and Drug Administration, Congress, the military, the criminal justice system, the Department of Health Education and Welfare, banks, corporations, the Stock Market, social clubs, police, food companies, entertainment media, computers companies, etc. Their gangs attack African countries or African peoples and through pretend information (propaganda) make the world and themselves believe that the attacks are for money or power. The attacks gain security from their own minds and the disease of the inner self.

The largest Caucasian gangs are a collection of clans which they choose to call a civilization. They are a neurotic, diseased group from an Ice Age climate filled with aggression, war, violence, and the disease of melanin albinism. Their collective behavior is a reflection or mirror of melanin deficit diseased minds. The Caucasian mind that controls the junk food and medical companies (hospitals) is a mind that is aggressive, violent and at war with itself. In order to remedy the problems of the health field, the problems of the Caucasian mind have to be solved. White Supremacy and White Racism are merely a psychological shield that protects a deeply infested psychological disease.

The Caucasian civilizations and melanin albinism that shaped their inner psychosis (craziness) is different from White Racism. Once the White Racism/White Supremacy was established, it functioned as a separate disease state with its own set of psychotic (crazy) structures. Teaching Caucasians that they are White supremacists has no curative psychological effect on them. It is the same as teaching a drunk person about being sober—they are too drunk to understand. So it follows that teaching Caucasians that their junk food and junk medicine is destructive to Africans will not help the Caucasians become less racist.

It is obvious that their degenerative food causes degenerative diseases. For example, the mucus forming bleached white flour, white sugar, cow's milk, grease (lard and oil), synthetic chemical additives and salt create a liquid slime called plaque.

This constantly accumulates and collects in the veins, muscles, nerves, brain and arteries. This eventually blocks the functioning or stops the function of any organ that has veins, arteries, nerves, muscles or melanin. The effect of the liquid manure (plaque) in the body is called disease.

If the Caucasian junk foods, chemicals and medicines cause the heart to be injured or stop, it is called heart disease. If it constipates the brain, it is called senility, learning disorders, mood swings or depression. If the gooey, pus-like slime collects in the eyes, it is called cataracts or glaucoma. If it is in the reproductive system, it is called fibroid tumors, prostate cancer or sterility. However, the disease began in the diseased mind of the Caucasian and is reflected in the diseased foods, cooked foods, synthetic chemicals and poisonous medicines that they force upon Africans. Treating or trying to change the White Supremacy that mask (protects) their inner disease has no effect upon their obsessive-compulsive craziness.

The obsessive neurosis of a normal person is quite different from the obsessive-compulsive craziness of a crazy person (Caucasian). The Caucasian obsessive-compulsive mind tells them to think the way they think, because they must think the way they think in order to think. If this sounds crazy, it is crazy. The Caucasian mind gets pleasure from thinking the way it thinks, and the pleasure it gets is also a craziness which is called narcissistic. Caucasians get pleasure from thinking they are superior and pain from knowing they are not superior. Theirs is a mind in conflict and at violent war with itself. It is their nature.

Caucasians live within the contradiction (conflict) of their minds. White Supremacy is merely a reflection (mirror) of that conflict. It is the mind that lives within Caucasian people that must fantasize reality. There are approximately 5 billion people in the world, 4 billion are colored and 900,000 million are Caucasians (600,000 Caucasian women and 300,000 Caucasian men) and the majority of the colored people are African or mixed Africans. In less than 2,000 years Caucasians have murdered at least 200 million Africans and at least 50 million Natives in India, in the Americas, Australia, Caribbean, Alaska, etc.).

The Caucasian collective mind has not faced the reality of their mass murders or subhuman barbaric behavior. Their mind is constantly on trial and declares itself guilty and innocent at the same time. The Caucasian food thugs have murdered millions (Nutricide) of Africans with diabetes, heart attacks, hypertension, high blood pressure, cancer, tuberculosis, etc. Added to this Nutricide is the murder of Africans with syphilis, AIDS, sickle cell anemia, prescription and illegal drugs (23% of the people that take Valium die, at least 25% on illegal drugs die).

Further, there is the Caucasian mutilation of Africans with surgery, drugs, vaccinations and inoculations. For example, the German Measles/Rubella causes arthritis. Flu Shots cause paralysis. Measles causes the nerves to be damaged and burn the brain (encephalitis). Whooping Cough Vaccine causes convulsions, fevers and brain problems. Insulin use leads to blindness. Tetracycline use causes bone problems. Antibiotics weaken the immune system and birth control pills cause cancer and other maladies. It is quite obvious that Caucasian food gangs, medical gangs and drug gangs are killing themselves and killing Africans. The deaths are blamed on the "obsession" with money. Money is supposed to bring security. However, the Caucasian mind is insecure and "compulsively" wants more security (money). Thus, they are obsessive-compulsive, crazy people. A mind in conflict with itself never finds security. Security craves security to satisfy the need for security in order to be secure from a mind that is insecure.

Each gang is in conflict within itself which means it is mentally and morally corrupt. For example, the Food and Drug Administration allows unsafe drugs to be used and is asked to police (morally control) the Drug companies. Drug companies test drugs which are unscientific, questionable, the use wrong dosage, and forge test results. The Center for Disease Control's research indicated that 80% of laboratory test results are questionable or wrong and 20% could be loosely considered correct. The American hospital-certifying agency approved hospitals as safe for the sick while the Department of Health Education and Welfare declared that 66% of hospitals are unsafe for sick people. They demanded that the dangerous Hospitals be closed. However, the certifying agency let them remain open.

The United States Surgeon General's Nutrition and Health research declared that junk food causes disease. The Food and Drug Administration allows junk food companies to continue to manufacture and sell harmful junk foods. It is obvious if one corrupt gang is used to correct another corrupt gang. Problems are not corrected. Each gang merely mirrors the mental disease of the Caucasians.

Cell Out- Genetic Racism

The Caucasian biological and chemical rituals and ceremonies that they call science are diseased with White Racism. Their scientifically normal standards for all human races are based on Caucasian biochemistry. What little science they do use is stolen from Africa and called a Caucasian discovery. Hippocrates, the "father" of Caucasian medicine, stole from the African textbook called *The Carlsburg Papyrus*. Other thieves, such as Galen, Theophrastus and Dioscorides wrote and quoted the medical prescriptions from the Temple of Imhotep and the African textbook, *Papyrus of Moscow*. Their Caucasian founder of nursing, Florence Nightingale, did not contribute to the nursing field. Actually, an African lady born in Jamaica named Mary Seacole is the founder of that field.

In 1852 Mary Seacole was instrumental in saving residents of Central America (including Panama) from a cholera outbreak. Mary Seacole helped stop the 1853 yellow fever outbreak in Jamaica. In 1854, during the Crimean War that England, France and Turkey fought against Russia, the War Department of England used Mary Seacole's healing ability to save soldiers' lives on the battlefield. Florence Nightingale was present at the battle but too sick to work. Nightingale was of some help to Caucasian soldiers; at the same time she was infecting soldiers with syphilis. She eventually died of syphilis. The Caucasian so-called scientists have recorded the behavior of thieves, liars, acts of unprovoked violence, murder and disease warfare against Africans. This is historical criminal behavior combined with their contemporary behavior of stealing wealth and knowledge from Africa, stealing human beings (slavery), global war against Africans, rape of African women, boys and girls, destruction of Africa's libraries, art, buildings and culture compounded by their mental illness of White Racism. Their mental and physical behaviors indicate that they have a hereditary genetic disease.

The Caucasians have available to them the information that they can obtain from the African's human cells. In fact, they now have patents on the cells in the human body. Their copyrights have to be honored and money paid to scientists with human cell patents before a scientific laboratory can use the individual cells to help diagnose illness. Genetic discrimination based upon disease history is available with no way to keep it private. An individual African parent may not have the criminal mental or physical trait or characteristic, but since it is in an African's genetic cell pool it allows Caucasians to use that information to genetically identify criminals and racistly discriminate against Africans. This is genetic racism. In other words, Caucasians can hate the very cells in an Africans body because the cells are melaninated.

Africans can be labeled genetically violent and discriminated against. Genetic engineers can change African cells by using deactivated viruses as carriers of Caucasian characteristics that they want in the African mind, spirit and body. In this way, Africans will become the types of person the Caucasians want them to be. Aside from this, the mental, emotional, spiritual and behavioral reaction of genetically altered African children is chemical cannibalism. Genetic drugs are the new weapons available to White supremacists to use in their attempts to continuously dominate Africans. Dr. Leroy Hood, a geneticist at the California Institute of Technology, claims that the genetic revolution will change Caucasian medicine. In fact, it was reported in *Reader's Digest*. Volume 139, Number 833, September 1991, that the National Institutes of Health has already done genetic transfusions at their clinical center. It is obvious from the Caucasian's behavior that they do not see themselves as mentally ill and that they are going to always see Africans as inferior and servants for White Supremacy.

Caucasians, through the use of genetics, can take your genetic cells out of yow body and place their programmed cells into your body. Your Africentric, melaninated genetic cells will be replaced by Eurocentric cells. Africans will be Caucasians inside their bodies with Black skin. The African world community will eventually be a programmed community of cloned servants in search of a White master. It will be a cell out of Africentric civilization.

Mental Illness is Entertaining

Mental illness is when the mind can no longer move from one thought to another freely. The mind gets stuck in a thought process or on a thought. A mind holding onto a thought when it is against the health and well being of self or of others is sick. In Caucasian civilization, a mentally ill person is anyone who is against his or her way of life. While in African civilization, an individual who is imbalanced in thinking or uses the left side of the brain too much is considered mentally ill. Consequently, an African person too "left minded" (logical individualistic analytical =Caucasoid) would be told that they were not in their "right mind." Africentrically, we have to be aware of the subtle mental illness within the Caucasian society. In this way, Africans will not be infected by it.

It is Caucasian mental illness that leads a child to think that violence can be solved by violence. It is Caucasian mental illness that seeks the solution to immunity system failures with immunity depressants. Any disease is a failure of the immune system to protect health. In any case, Caucasians believe that immune failures can be corrected by immune suppressive drugs (antibiotics, aspirin, anti-histamines, cold depressants. etc.). For example, the Food and Drug Administration in 1991 approved the use of treating bladder cancer by giving the sick person an infection. The germ mycobacterium bovis (BCG), which is found in abundance in tuberculosis disease, is given to people with bladder tumors (cancer). This does not get rid of the cause of the disease nor does it change the disease-producing diet. This may seem like an unrelated point or it may appear unre-lated to mental illness as a form of entertainment, but it is part of the same mental illness. This type of distortion that treats an illness with an illness is part of the foundation of their mental illness. The acceptance of this concept allows the mind to be conditioned to ac-cept mentally ill ideas as "pure science" when it is the disease of mental illness. If mental illness is accepted as science, then it be-comes easy to accept mental illness as entertainment.

Caucasian cliches help to support mental illness as entertain-ment or science. For example, a cliche such as "money is the root of evil" is a mentally ill concept. African money, Chinese money, Na-tive American money, etc., was never the root of evil nor did it cause evil among them. It is Caucasians who are evil (mentally ill), and they use money to support their mental illness (evil). Money is not a living thing that can cause or create good or evil. However, the Caucasian diseased mind believes that they are not evil (men-tally ill) but their money is evil (mentally ill). This is thinking psy-chotically and further supports mental illness as entertainment.

Caucasians block out, hide, shut off and cover up feelings about true reality. The Caucasians feel that they are inferior to the su-premacy of African civilization, and this hidden emotion causes feelings of anger, violence, paranoia, murder, fear, love, pleasure, anxiety, sex, and excitement. Within this mental illness is the in-ability to separate feelings. All feelings are the same or may not be felt at all. Consequently, feelings of love are mixed with violence in their minds and in their movies, children's fairy tales, videos, computer games and religions.

The inferiority reflex causes Caucasians to block out feelings without understanding why. Caucasians feel a need to be in control that is the same as the cravings felt by drug addicts, food addicts, sex or violence addicts. However, these feelings are not understood or labeled correctly. These feelings can result in crisis behavior which is a need to create events or an issue or war or violence in order to stay in control. It is an outgrowth of "self-centeredness" instead of African "family centeredness." In Caucasian "self-centeredness" everything (events, African behaviors) is either for or against them. There is a lack of understanding of where their rights end and African rights begin. African human rights cannot be understood by Caucasians. Caucasians use linear communication ("double talk," "talk with a forked tongue," confusion between truth and lies) and act on their paranoia. Paranoids act on their assumptions while sane people check out assumptions before acting. Direct communication would require honesty and an acceptance of their crimes (massive murders. slavery, colonialism) against Africa and African people.

Caucasians believe their civilization to be highly developed, so there is no need for them to consider the rights of other civilizations or African people. Anything outside of Caucasian superiority does not exist. Since Caucasians are the only scientists (dieticians, doctors. healers) who know and understand everything, there is no need to remember that Africans founded and perfected all sciences. If it were true that the Caucasians are the supreme race, then other cultures (African) are irrelevant because Caucasian collective mental illness and mythology verify that they are the most evolved, powerful and developed race. They think that gadgets, such as machines or computers, indicate superiority in a civilization. However, it is the ability to get along with self, others, nature and God (human relationship) that determines superiority.

If Caucasians are responsible for what has happened in their civilization and what they have done to Africa and Africans, then they must be blamed for their destructive mentality, and everything that has kept them inferior is totally their fault. They are inferior because of the murderous and destructive actions that they have committed and continue to commit against Africans, natives of North and South America and of Australia, the Caribbean, etc. Despite this, they believe that their superiority has happened because they made it happen without massive murders, rape, slavery and stealing of information and land. Caucasians believe their superiority requires them to be in control; it is also believed that they have always been in control. Therefore, everything is "just and honorable" that they have done to be in control. At one time in history, they called the slaughter of Africans a part of Caucasian "Manifest Destiny." Manifest Destiny is merely a pleasant term for mental illness. "Manifest Destiny," a slogan, when translated means Caucasian control.

There is doubt that communication can harmonize or unite the African and Caucasian races because White supremacists do not see other races or cultures, and especially African, as equal or superior. There is no line that marks a separation between Caucasian inferiority and Caucasian imagined superiority. This is caused because Caucasians do not perceive African (or other races) human rights as God-given. They see African rights as something that is granted by violence (war). The Caucasian linear-communicates (confused inner conversation) within themselves and to themselves. It must be noted that Caucasians speak to themselves with "double talk" or a "forked tongue." Caucasians lack respect for African cultural boundaries. In other words, they see everything superior about African culture as Caucasian, and within their mental illness everything and everyone becomes a possession. They imagine themselves to be the center of the world. They constantly describe social activities, and even entertainment in terms of their mental illness and value structure (cosmology).

The center of Caucasian entertainment is violence, murder, sex and mental illness. The absence of this type of entertainment is called boredom. This definition of entertainment starts with the African baby and is nurtured and taught from childhood to adulthood. Consequently, the African spends his life escaping boredom by using drugs, sex, food, sex dancing, changing jobs, divorces, watching movies, television viewing, physical exercise to build muscles (not to clean up neighborhoods or to improve the community) gossip talking or listening to gossip talk shows, going to parties, dropping out of school, shopping, spending money or taking trips. It is Caucasian boredom and Caucasian entertainment that consumes African children and adults' lives.

Entertainment in the Caucasian world is mixed with violence, murder, mental illness, sex and self-centeredness. Africentrically, the purpose of "entering" the "inner-attainment" (entertainment) is designed to uplift the body, mind and spirit. The purpose of "bore (hole or holy) dom (place)" or the "holy place" is to reach the spiritual Kingdom. Boredom is not negative. Boredom occurs when an activity or thought has fulfilled itself and causes you to pass through the human limits to the spiritual unlimited. Boredom is a quiet or silent part of yourself in which the melanin speaks to you and through you.

In melanin-deficient Caucasians there is not enough ancestral or spiritual or electromagnetic energy to vibrate their brains, so "boredom" is something they must avoid or replace with violence, sex or mental illness. Mental illness is mixed with violence, sex and fantasy. Caucasians and the Africans who follow them participate in more fantasy than their children's fantasy world of cartoons, videos, computer games, movies and television. Adult Caucasians consume more-make-believe fantasy stories (i.e., movies, television programs, songs, books), use more games (good-is-White, evil-is-black themes), use more recreational legal and illegal drugs to help make mental fantasy, have recreational sex which is 90% fantasy and live a life where they fantasize Caucasian civilization as superior and Africa and African people as inferior.

Fantasy is entertainment and entertainment is a mixture of mental illness and fantasy. The fantasy is so concrete in the Caucasian mind that it is real and no longer considered a mental illness. Like concrete, it is thoroughly mixed and cemented in craziness. It is mental illness to eat a diet that causes disease, than eat the same diet while in the hospital in order to cure the disease.

The central focus of the fantasy is the good-guy-versus-the-bad-guy themes. The bad guy is any one who opposes or is fighting against the good Caucasian or good Caucasian civilization. The person fighting against the good Caucasian is labeled in some way mentally ill, a sex pervert, a savage, bloodthirsty, insane, seeking revenge; is power hungry, lives in an imaginary world, has unreal fears, wants to destroy the world and is never a person who has a legitimate right to oppose the good Caucasian. Usually, the fantasy type movie, videos, book, cartoon, television show, or dramatic play devotes the major part of the time to justify why the Caucasian "good guy" should exterminate the person who opposes him. This helps to reinforce the Caucasian myth about themselves and to sustain the entertainment fantasy that is mental illness.

The African parents' choice for their children is to teach the child to be spiritual, to use trances (daydreams), to sense the spirit presence of ancestors and to find joy in the spirit world of God. African people who choose the Caucasian entertainment of toys (gadgets), violence, sex and mental disease will affirm in the African child that you would have to be mentally ill if you think about or are about opposing (fighting) Caucasian White Supremacy. The issue remains that either African people are being entertained or are being made mentally ill. It is a subtle type of mental disease when you find mental illness entertaining.

The mentally ill person is used to entertain the audience's attention during news programs. A mentally ill person who may have committed a crime is viewed as evil, but never mentally ill. News programs constantly pick a crime such as murder, rape, brutality, illegal businessmen (drug pushers) robbery, assault and battery as evil when in actuality they are activities of the mentally ill. Consequently, mental illness is viewed as evil and a crime. Caucasians believe all crimes must be punished, not psychologically treated. The African child never sees the massive mental illness of Caucasian civilization because mental illness is not clearly stated as mental illness, but as a crime. A criminal is anyone fighting against the Caucasian will. An African child raised on this Caucasian logic in fantasy or news programs will be programmed to think criminals are sane and perverted instead of mentally ill. They will not see the so-called normal thinking Caucasian as a specimen of craziness. An African child will grow up to be an adult who mixes and confuses entertainment and mental illness as the same. The African child will not conceive or believe that it is normal for Africans to fight the mentally ill Caucasian race unless they themselves are crazy.

Epidemics, Lies, And Diseases For Money

Epidemics are the sudden spread of diseases that affect many people at the same time in a particular area. These diseases are usually considered contagious. However, the vast majority of these epidemics are usually created by the Caucasian diet or vaccinations inoculations. The vaccination/inoculation business combined with the medical business makes profits from the diseases that the food business causes. And of course, the food business makes profits selling the junk food to Africans. Vaccinations, inoculations, synthetic medicine and junk foods cause the disease epidemics. None of these Caucasian businesses will take the responsibility for the epidemics, mutilation and human sacrifices that they have caused. The African consumer is led to believe that diseases are a natural way of life. It is a natural way of life for Caucasians, but Nutricidal for Africans.

Epidemiology is another myth and fable of Caucasian science that does not have repeatable scientific proofs to document its findings. In other words, it is quackery. John Gravant founded the entire science of epidemiology in 1662. He had an herb and spirits (alcohol) business and published the Europeans' first book on the subject, *Natural and Political Observations Made Upon the Bills of Morality*. He wrote that more White men died than White women and that one-third of the White children died before they reached the age of five. This field has been called unscientific and fictitious by Caucasian authorities in the field. It has been criticized by epidemiologists such as Alvin R. Feinstine, Professor of Medicine and Epidemiology at Yale University School of Medicine in 1901 and in the 1980 Presidential Address to the American Heart Association's (AHA) 53rd Scientific Session by the Ex-President of the AHA and Thomas N. James M. D. Kurt A. Oster M. D. in November 1975 wrote an article. *"The Decline of Common Sense and the Ascent of Computerized Nonsense in Medicine."* This article scientifically pointed out the stupidity of the science and its vast errors.

Epidemiology uses insurance companies' myth of disease, "risk factors." Currently a Caucasian "risk factor" has many meanings. The "risk factor" idea has not caused an improvement in heart disease care. Aside from this, a "risk factor" differs from one report to another. Further, insurance companies use mathematical statistical reports that cannot be applied to human life. This statistical data cannot be applied to observations on African people's natural diet without a measure of melanin levels and spiritual science.

Epidemiology uses data from public records which they put through complex mathematical manipulation. For example, from the advice of insurance companies, epidemiology concluded that "risk factors" such as smoking, heavy alcohol drinking, obesity, disease history of parents with a diet high in saturated fat and cholesterol caused heart disease. This advice was given to the public without scientific proof. It was never reported to the public that this advice was merely a mathematical deduction and that this Caucasian advice may or may not be of any help or could actually cause disease or that a change of diet (lower in fat and cholesterol) would be of little help or no help. Further, it was not advised that within six months of a lowered cholesterol diet the body rebounds to its high cholesterol level. Additionally, it was not advised that people with type A blood usually have a higher cholesterol level. It was not advised that African people tend to have low cholesterol levels.

Ironically, the use of Caucasian standards to judge disease in Africans can result in Africans being considered as having a normal cholesterol level when in actuality they are sick. The African undiagnosed sickness progresses further before the Caucasian standard recognizes a disease. African people have to be on "mental alert" and must be constantly aware of the source of advice. If the advice is given by a doctor, scientist, an actor, athlete, medical organization, insurance company or the food business, it is still advice. Advice is simply a non-scientific opinion. Aside from this, medical groups change their advice from year to year.

In 1950, the normal serum cholesterol was arbitrarily set at 150 mg. Then, it was changed to 300 mg. Then in 1980 the American Heart Association gave advice that the cholesterol level should be 220 mg. Caucasian science does not take into account the cyclic laws of nutrients, hormones, organs or the human body. In African science, the daily cyclic nature of cholesterol's monthly, and yearly cycles would be a factor. The specific cyclic levels are different for men and women. In the African Rites of Passage each dietary cyclic change was taught to the individual. Highly melaninated Africans have sensitive and responsive rhythms (cycles). Caucasians with melanin albinism are not cyclic oriented and their science ignores these factors. Caucasian epidemiology relies on advice, mathematical opinions, and scientific quackery. Thus, this field is another tool used in the Nutricide of African people.

Facts about Health

Africans can see the lies and misconception about Caucasian health and medicine by looking at the facts:

Fact 1:   America's worst drug takers are probably physicians. According to a series of articles appearing in the New York Times in mid-1975, the percentage of physicians on hard drugs (heroin, opium, cocaine) was about 19 times greater than the number of people among the general population addicted to the same drugs.

Fact 2:   Numerous surveys, tests, and health evaluation programs have consistently revealed that America's "medical professionals" are no healthier than the average American is.

Fact 3:   Compared to the general population, 23% more American physicians (including heart specialist!) die of heart and cardiovascular problems. Cancer deaths among physicians are 12% higher than among the general population.

Fact 4:   "Whenever doctors strike, throughout the world, the same result occurs: The morality rate drops. The first strike was in Saskatchewan, Canada, in the late sixties. The second was in Los Angeles, where, according to Professor Milton

Roemer of UCLA's School of Public Health, the mortality rate during that strike dropped by 17 percent. The third strike was in Columbia, South America, where the morality rate dropped by 37 percent. The fourth, and my favorite, strike was in Israel when, during an 85-day strike, the morality rate dropped by 50 percent. This greatly concerned the morticians, who did a study of their own. They discovered the last time the morality rate dropped that low was 20 years previously at the time of the last doctor's strike."

Fact 5: Annual physical examinations procedures and test are a health risk.

Fact 6: Hospitals are dangerous places for the sick (because of extreme exposure to other diseases).

Fact 7: Most operations do little good and many do harm.

Fact 8: Medical testing labs are reports and scientifically inaccurate.

Fact 9: Many drugs cause more problems that they cure. (Doctors prescribe drugs "sold" to them by salesmen who use questionable research data.)

Fact 10: The X-ray machine is the most pervasive and the most dangerous tool in the doctor's office.

Fact 11: Over 900 billion dollars was spent on so-called "health care" in America in 1992. (If Americans would stop doing #5 and #6, health care expenditure would almost certainly drop to less than $100 billion per year.)

Fact 12: Over 125 million Americans have one or more chronic disease condition.

Fact 13: Only one-and-half percent (12) of Americans are regarded as healthy by the US Public Health Service-less than four million out of a population of over 250 million. This means that 982 % have some type of illnesses.

Fact 14: About one-and-a-half billion visits are made by patients to physicians, clinics, and emergency rooms every year in the USA. That is about six visits per Americans.

Fact 15: Over 5 million Americans suffer such side effects or adverse reactions from drugs and medicines administered by physicians each year, that they need to be hospitalized.

Fact 16: One in five Americans spends some time in hospital for treatment every year.

Fact 17: Over 50 million Americans suffer from high blood pressure.

Fact 18: Chances are better than 95% that your arteries are partially blocked by plaque. Almost every American child over 4-years old has arterial plaque formation. Nearly 45% of Americans die from heart disease or cardiovascular problems.

Fact 19: Three out of every ten Americans get cancer. Eighty percent of these people suffer death attributed to cancer. Over 500,000 Americans will die of cancer this year.

Fact 20: Cancer is the number one cause of death among our children.

Fact 21: Over one in three Americans suffer from some form of allergy.

Fact 22: About a third of Americans are obese. Yet nearly all Americans are malnourished in some way, despite overeating.

Fact 23: Over 50% of Americans suffer from chronic digestive disorders.

Fact 24: Some 16 million Americans suffer from ulcers.

Fact 25: Over 41 million Americans suffer from hemorrhoids.

Fact 26: Nine out of ten Americans suffer from more or less clogged colons. Constipation is a wide spread disease.

Fact 27: Over 10 million Americans suffer from asthma.

Fact 28: Over 30 million Americans suffer from chronic sinus infections.

Fact 29: There are about 15 million diabetics or near-diabetics in America.

Fact 30: Over ten million Americans have psoriasis (a skin disease) diseases: rheumatism, gout, and bursitis.

Fact 31: Over 36 million Americans suffer from arthritis and related diseases: rheumatism, gout, and bursitis.

Fact 32: One of five births in America is defective, about half being brain defects.

Fact 33: Almost every baby born in America has been polluted before birth by poisons and drugs in mother's bloodstream.

Fact 34: Over eight million American children are mentally retarded or handicapped because of brain problems-possibly caused by poisons and drugs from the mother's bloodstream, and the effect of radiation and the polluted air, water, soil and vaccinations upon their system.

Fact 35: The 4th leading cause of death is misdiagnosis, prescription and medical errors.

Fact 36: The average age of death of doctors is 58. *Dissent in Medicine Nine Doctor's Speak Out* by Robert S. Mendelsohn M.D. *Confession of A Medical Heretic* by Robert S. Mendelsohn M.D.

Fact 37: Due to weaken immunity caused by toxic foods and environment people 25 years old and younger can die from mild diseases such as asthma, etc.

Blood Letting

The Caucasian bloodletting (making a person bleed by cutting the skin), superstitions, ceremonies, and rituals of their primitive Ice Age culture still genetically influence their behaviors. The Christians, in their celebration called Christmas, use a white sugar candy cane with red stripe on it that symbolizes the dripping of blood on the shepherd's cane (candy cane). In the past, they used a bloodletting symbol called a barbers pole because early barber's performed bloodletting to cure headaches, "colds and flu," sex problems and to do physic readings (fortune telling). Today, they center their scientific studies, preventive medicines (pus peddlers use vaccinations and inoculations), laboratory values, tests for venereal disease or other diseases on blood.

It is a characteristic of sick people to use bloodletting or to make blood in the bones while healthy Africans make blood in the spleen and digestive tract (i.e., stomach villi). In African sciences such as those of Dr. Imhotep, they used hair, skin, breathing, pulses, eyes, acupuncture, water, crystals, colors, metals, magnets, body sounds (auscultation) and other modalities to diagnose and treat diseases. Blood can indicate personality type such as A+ blood type person is impulsive, B+ is emotional, AB+ is introverted, A+ and O+ are outgoing or socially gregarious. However, blood is a crude, primitive form of analysis. But, the Caucasian Ice Age genetics, melanin albino mind and psychotic thought patterns lead them to violence, conflict, sex abuse, group sex, food and drug addiction, White Supremacy and bloodletting.

In the Caucasian history of cannibalism, eating animal flesh, the eating of the raw heart of murdered enemies, butchering one another in violence as well as drinking each others' blood, including menstruation blood to cure diseases, is a psychotic custom. Blood has symbolic meanings. Today, Caucasians use blood-red carpeting, red cars, say a soldier sheds his blood for the government, or that Jesus Christ gave his blood, can put symbolic blood (catsup) on food and Caucasian movies usually have blood and violence. Aside from this, they admire predators who kill and cause blood to spill. The Caucasian woman uses blood-red lipstick, red finger and toenail polish, red underwear or light red (pink) clothing to symbolize a woman captured as prey. They roll out the red carpet to welcome guests; blood is spilled in defeat or if there is an economic loss, a businessman will say he is in the red. They bond relationships by mixing blood from each other's fingers, called a brotherhood bond. Blood means violence to them and red represents a color of action, sex, power, food and excitement. The Caucasian culture is so entrenched in bloodletting and symbols of blood that their mind cannot and will not see it.

Caucasians love each other with the muscle that pumps blood (the heart). They use blood scientifically to indicate their relatives. In African Divine Kinship relatives were related by God. Therefore, when an orphan slave child arrived at the slave quarters on the plantation she was immediately adopted by a family and became a part of that family accentuated by rituals. The child and the adopted parents became related by Divine Kinship through God. However, Caucasians are only related by blood. If Caucasians have a negative relationship with other Caucasians they say there is bad blood between them. It should seem apparent that Caucasian scientists would seek blood usage in their science. If they get sick they put medicine in hypodermic needles and inject it into their blood via veins. To prevent disease they put pus inoculations in their blood via veins. They force feed the sick with sugar and water put in the blood via the veins.

Ironically, if a Caucasian has one drop of African blood in him then other Caucasians will consider him African or a mulatto. The value of blood has any sort of psychotic meaning Caucasians choose to place upon it. Today, in order to get married by Caucasian cultural standards, you have to do a bloodletting (blood test). If you want to attend their public schools or do foreign travel or get some types of jobs you must do a bloodletting (blood test) and/or their pus peddler must give you a vaccination or inoculation into your blood. These are forms of a primitive belief that bloodletting or animal blood or pus in the blood can save a life (vaccination, inoculation) or protect the living from some evil.

An animal's blood cannot make you healthy, spiritual, intelligent or save you from White Supremacy. Africans' blood was used in European (Caucasian) rituals and ceremonies, during slavery and colonialism. Bloodletting in the form of puncturing or cutting open the skin while being hung, using whips to draw blood, castration and other forms of bloodletting for amusement were performed on countless children, pregnant women and young girls as well as men. The book, *Race and Civilization* by Frederick Hertz, can give insight into the cannibalism of Caucasians.

White Racism and superstitions cause Caucasians to discriminate against animal blood. They classify dark red blood as evil (bad) and white blood as good to eat. Consequently, Caucasian health food experts tell Africans to stop eating toxic red blood meat and to eat toxic White blood meat such as fish, poultry and pigs. The blood of any animal is at all times half filled with waste. In an animal's body quarter of the cells are dead, quarter are being created and half are maintaining the body's functions. The half that are maintaining the functions are transporting waste and nutrients at all times. However, in the case of slaughtered animals, a toxic substance called adrenalin is released and this poisons the carcass before death. The animal's blood, pus and adrenalin give animal flesh its taste. If it were protein the dead animal flesh eater wanted then the blood and pus could be soaked out of the flesh. This would leave a bland-tasting-white-grayish meat. The blood could be soaked out of the animal's flesh in salt and water. Whether it is cooked or raw, the blood, pus and waste is delightful to the meat eater's taste buds. The practice by White Racism of labeling red blood evil and White blood pure is a psychotic value connected to bloodletting. Bloodletting practices help make the African mind crazy and Nutricidal.

The Clan's Diseases

Caucasian civilization has not evolved beyond the status of a collection of dysfunctional clans. It has been controlled by clans such as the Duponts, Gettys, Rothschilds, Rockefellers, Krupps, Hesses, Mellons, Hunts, etc. These clans use feudalism to manipulate and control themselves, dysfunctional Caucasian families and Africans. They may label their clans as feudalist, capitalist, socialist or democratic governments, kingdoms and empires or nations. When a few Caucasian families unite they are erroneously called nations. However, they are clans that support and protect each other under the disguise of a nation. Their relationships are built on individualistic clan ownership and power Their relationships range from family to clan (combination of families), to tribe (combination of clans), to kingdoms (combination of tribes) and then to empires (combination of kingdoms).

African people's extended family society, based on spirituality and humanistic relationships (ecology), naturally lends itself to complex human structures such as tribes, kingdoms and empires. Caucasian dysfunctional families are based upon mistrust (backstabbing), selfishness, rape, homosexuality, cannibalism, superstition, individualism, fear, drug addiction and individual ownership. They have not been able to develop beyond governments of clans. This is reflected in the American economy in which six or more families (clans) control over 70% of the wealth resources and power.

Caucasian clans base their definition of clan, tribe, kingdom and empire on ownership of land, not on the Africentric value of contributing the most for the betterment of society. Thus, a British clan that controls major portions of land in Britain is called a government. A government through violence and human destruction that controls land in Europe is called a kingdom. Caucasian kingdoms that control lands in Africa are called an Empire (e.g. the British Empire).

Caucasian civilization has never and can never develop past the clan state. Their psychotic mental illness that created the mental disease of White Supremacy hides from reality. They have not formed a sharing or acceptance with African people, nature or the environment. They have never ecologically shared compassionately with nature and did not adapt to the Ice Age environment. They have failed to adapt to any environment. Caucasians are one of the only races to fail to adapt (ecologically) to nature. They did not develop ways to keep themselves in balance with their cold climate, vegetation or even a rock.

By comparison the Eskimos (Civilization of Man and Woman = Native Americans) mastered their climate and the severe cold climate did not make them thieves, dysfunctional, violent or mentally ill. Caucasians are not maladaptive; they are nonadaptives who are consumed with self-hatred and "nutritional restraints." "Nutritional restraints" are the lack of nutrients caused by nutritionally poor soil, plants and a junk food diet. Nutritional restraints stop the body, mind and spirit from using its full range of actions. It limits the mind's activities. The Caucasian's nutritionally deprived mind is genetically in conflict with itself and their deprived diet malnourishes their dysfunctional families and clan society.

Consequently, they cannot see, accept or understand basic human rights of Africans. For example, it is totally wrong for a White public school (educational plantation) teacher to teach an African boy or girl. White teachers (educational overseers) transfer their cultural values and White Supremacy to the African child. This cultural abuse of the African child also implants the essential ingredients of White Supremacy. A humanistically balanced White teacher would automatically refuse to teach African children and would demand that Africans control their own Africentric curriculum and schools. However, the clan and feudalistic behaviors of Whites will not let them see the harm that their public schools are doing to Africans.

Aside from this, over $5-Billion-a-year Special Education business has introduced over 20,000 psychologists with their immoral and unethical "lifestyle choice" ideas. These ideas about homosexuality, drug use, and free sex as a lifestyle choice have caused an increase in violence, homosexuality, suicide, imprisonment and drug addiction plus only one out of 10 Special Education students graduates. The teachers and psychologists have classified children who react to oppression, White supremacy and malnutrition as mentally ill and made them into drug addicts (i.e.). Ritalin causes cancer, cysts and tumors of the liver. The non-addicted children are forced to socialize with addicts. This causes them to develop co-dependency mental illness. If there is to be a change in the Caucasian clan's public schools or diet it will be Africans who directly cause it. (Source: Citizens Commission on Human Rights and FDA).

Africans must change their diet to natural diet and dis-ease treatments to natural remedies instead of using allopathic drugs. Currently, the Caucasian clan's diet has directly and indirectly caused AIDS to be twice as high among African women compared to White women; asthma is three times higher in Africans than in Whites. Breast and lung cancer is higher among Africans. Diabetes is three times higher among African women. Uterine fibroid tumors are an epidemic; seventy-five percent of African women have them as compared to 33% of White women. Infertility is at least twice as high among Africans. Depression is at epidemic proportions. Lupus is highest among African women, and over 50% of African women are overweight. Added to this is the Caucasian melanin-destructive diet that holistically weakens the health of Africans and increases their disease susceptibility to the Caucasian clan's diseases. These facts have been compiled form data supplied by the

Minority AIDS Project Los Angeles, CA, Asthma and Allergy Foundation of America, National Black Leadership Initiative on Cancer, Bethesda, MD, American Diabetes Association National Service Center, Alexandria, VA, Black Psychiatrists of America Association Oakland, CA, Association of Black Psychologists, Washington, DC, America Fertility Society, Birmingham, AL, America Dietetic Association, Lupus Foundation of America.

Aside from this the hoodlums of the medical clans (i.e., organizations, associations, certifying agencies) and public hospitals will classify an African as mentally ill who has Sunlight deficiency, yeast infection, melanin deficiency, food allergy, hypoglycemia or chronic fatigue syndrome and send him to a psychiatrist. They do not help Africans with a disease; they merely prescribe toxic, suppressive drugs that will suppress symptoms until the body heals itself, deteriorates or dies. If you read the obituaries in the newspaper it will reveal that the M.D.S have not cured, controlled or improved the health state of people. Caucasian medicine clans created by dysfunctional family clans continue to ignore the importance of melanin in Africans. Melanin on a natural food diet free of drugs can coordinate and regulate cells, receive, interpret and broadcast messages, destroy free radicals, can act without or with air, feed forward and feedback sympathetic and parasympathetic activity, travel antigravitationally or gravitationally, increase oxygen utilization and act as an enzyme. Melanin bonds toxins and attempts to transport them out of the body or converts them to a harmless state. Junk foods and drugs stop the conversion or transport of toxins, causing Africans to have an increase in diseases and drug addiction. It is the clan nature of Caucasian society and medicine that creates Nutricidal diseases and death among Africans. A book that can be used as resource is *Dirt* by Terance McLaughlin.

Change the Name, Not the Behavior

The improved changes that have occurred in civilization among the various races were of African origin. Africa is the acknowledged cradle of the world's first civilization, scientists and spiritual peoples. It was Africans who introduced the modern developments to the world. For example, in the Americas (before the invasions of Christopher Columbus) the Africans introduced the system of bureaucracy, government, apartments, orchestra, music, pyramids, medicine and kinsmanship to the natives. In China, the African Fu Hsi of the Divine Dynasty introduced Yin and Yang or Horu and Falcon head energy division system. In Japan, Africans introduced the religious system of which Karate is a minor part.

Africans sailed the seas long before Caucasians and introduced astrology, culture, language, science, banking, textiles, architecture, agriculture, chemistry, mercantilism, mathematics, navigation, etc., to other civilizations. Everywhere Africans went they improved societies and helped to uplift people by initiating constructive changes. Perhaps Africans should have continued to guide, monitor and influence those civilizations' reaction to change, but did not. In other words, Africans are the custodians of change and have nurtured change among others. If there is to be another change on this planet it can only be an outgrowth of the initial change that Africans implemented. Change is a melanin and Godly African responsibility.

Early African Trans-Atlantic and Trans-Pacific traders introduced the fruits such as the orange that came from south and Indo China, Grapefruit (Pamelo, Forbidden fruit, Shaddock) from East Indies, Papaya from America, Pineapple from Brazil, Mangoes from Asia, bananas from India, Avocado from central America, Lemons from Himalayas and Burma and Line from Burma.

The Caucasians are not about change and have not been able to change their barbaric behavior. They can only react to the artifacts or material things of change or steal the products of change; they cannot create change. For example, Africans changed the Caucasian diet by introducing different types of foods and tried to change their disease condition by introducing hygienic medicine. Despite the African foods and medicines, the Caucasians remain basically on a meat-and-potatoes diet and are still a sickly race. They are still a clans people with mob violence, mental illness, dysfunctional families and mob sex.

Historically, mob sex and breeding sex orgies were a central focus in their race. Sex/breeding orgies are usually a confused mixture of mothers, daughters, fathers, sons, relatives, male and female casual acquaintances, friends, strangers, homosexuals, married and single people, young and old who may or may not have venereal diseases. This mob sex can be random or scheduled and is usually called free sex, adultery, sex out of wedlock or permissive behavior. It is merely an extended form of mob breeding founded upon Caucasian individualism, not human relationships. It is a dysfunctional characteristic of their clan societies. Selfish, individualistic societies that have not mastered human relationships are sex orgy oriented.

Caucasians have not been able to escape gang sex, the Ice Age mentality, White Supremacy, full moon, sexual activities, honeymoons, romantic moonlight, etc., or their collective mental illness characterized by self-hatred. They used and use bathtubs for sexual purposes and historically related cleanliness to a form of superstition. Caucasians who did bathe used the bathtub for murder, clairvoyance and sex orgies. Others used sheep fat (lanolin), pig, dog or cattle or rotten animal grease to bathe with (*The Bath*, by D. Von Furstenberg).

Mob sex, or permissive sex as the Caucasians call it is a part of their society and has not historically changed and is constant. The name has been changed by them to permissive sex but the group sex activity remains unchanged. In order to change any part of their society they must overcome self-hatred and stop recycling self-hatred. For example, they kink their hair (curl), thicken their lips, tan their skin, shave their legs, buy buttock pads and brassieres, use makeup to add color to their pale skin and imitate African dances, music and slang words in order to resemble Africans because they hate themselves. They cannot change the diseases and deaths that they cause with nutrition and medicine until they make a holistic change.

They changed the names of diseases periodically. However, the human body has not changed nor has its disease reactions changed. God gave you a human life that you live with understanding and a human body that is easily understood. The human body is a small universe. There are plants, bushes and grass (vegetation) on the skin (topsoil) of the earth. There is also vegetation on the skin of the digestive tract except medical people call it flora (which means vegetation) of the earth. There are animals and insects that live around vegetation. There are animals and insects that live around the body's flora except in science they are called bacteria. The evaporation of the waters in oceans and lakes causes water to go up to the sky where the temperature is below freezing. The water vapor turns to negative charged snow, then the fluffy light snow rises higher into the sky and clusters together which forms positive charged hail. The heavy positive charged hail starts to fall and collides into the negative charge snow that makes energy (lighting). The same thing occurs in the body. The negative charged cells collide with positive charged cells, which makes energy for your body to function. The body is not difficult to understand it is the medical practitioners that are difficult to understand. They are into a name change hustle.

They change the names of disease in order to keep the change (money) out of your pocket so they can put your change (money) in their pocket. Why do they change names of your body's functions and organs to Latin or Greek names? You don't speak the languages and they don't speak it. By changing the names you become ignorant and now need them to translate the Latin/Greek name diseases back into English names. You have to pay them to be a translator. These medical hustlers use the name change game to get your change (money). Again, the human body is easy to understand. Feces (waste) than can out your anus must go up and out. Blocked feces liquid backs up to your kidney (causes High Blood Pressure), eyes (glaucoma, cataracts), veins (varicose), muscles (rheumatism), mouth (tartar and bad breath), arteries (atherosclerosis), etc. Whenever the liquid feces changes its location they change its name. Therefore, the ill person has to change medical specialist, change drug prescription, change another type of series of test and x-rays. This keeps the change (money) moving to the medical hustler's pocket.

Caucasians are consumed by their own minds and constantly recycle diseases of body, mind and spirit. They would rather restore (recycle) or rehabilitate trash (waste paper, plastic, glass, aluminum) than rehabilitate the African continent. Caucasian synthetic junk food clans (companies) are not interested in recycling (restoring) Africans, health. They are more interested in recycling trash, drugs, crime and disease addiction. The clans of synthetic food companies are not built to meet the ethnonutritional needs of Africans. Food companies only respond to profit, not nutritional needs. They use the economics of stupidity. Their nutricidal (unhumanistic) economics is of supply (food) and demand (money). If you do not have money you cannot make demands (eat). Therefore, you do not get supply (food). If you do not have money you starve.

Theirs is an unjust economy that has not changed and repeats recycling economic failures (i.e., recession, depression, inflation, bankruptcy, etc.). If the African eat Caucasian synthetic food they nutritionally starve their bodies into a disease state. Caucasians cannot change their diseased minds and White Racism. Caucasians remain unchanged. They recycle their behavior of violence and change the name of their behavior to manifest destiny, exploration, war, slave codes, colonialism, religion, nutrition but remain unchanged.

They pacify themselves and say they have evolved (changed) from a monkey and will continue to evolve (change) to higher heights. However, historically, they evolved to their highest level with Greek civilization and have not changed or improved since that time. Change is melanin mediated. The more melanin a race has the more able they are to change and create change. Melanin electrochemically and biochemically converts or changes energy be it mental, physical or spiritual. Caucasians are melanin albinos and physiologically have the least ability to change.

Change is sometimes related to karma. Karma in simple definition is reaction to an action. It is believed that the Caucasians, previous negative behavior caused them to be barbaric, mentally ill and enslavers of Africans. It is also assumed that Africans' previous negative behavior of thousands of years ago caused them to be enslaved. In other words, everything is paying for a past negative karma. Karma debt includes the polluted waters Karma debt, the polluted air, fertilizer poisoned soil, hybrid and cloned plants, extinct animals, insects, people as well as religions, science, nutrition, medicine and outer space.

Karma is the relationship of all to the many. The ability to improve, establish, understand and create karmic change is a melanin event. Consequently, it is futile to look to melanin albinos to change or relate to change. They can change the name, but not the behavior. There is no historical evidence to indicate that Caucasians have changed their relationship with Africans. The history of the Caucasians' use of food to destroy Africans has been one of Nutricide. It is Africans who must change and use natural foods and medicines, or their bodies will be a tomb that houses the holistically dead.

The Caucasians have controlled Africans though changes in diet or behavior. Caucasians have told Africans what food to eat and not eat. There are many types of edible grasses. However, Africans are told to grow grass they cannot eat in their front lawn and back yards. In fact, Africans grow grass that only cattle can eat and do not have a cow. Africans are taught to believe that the only food worthy to eat is the food the former slave master eats. Consequently, Africans do not grow edible dandelions and/or poke plants in their lawns or yards. They can be eaten in salads or alone. The young leaves of the maple and/or ash trees can be eaten. However, Africans do not grow these trees and if they do will not eat the leaves unless told to by Caucasian food clans.

Caucasians not only control dietary behavior but also social behavior. The ultimate control of Africans has had a change in name but not in results. For example, slave codes, home rule, states rights, Jim Crow (separate but equal); civil rights and curfew laws are designed to keep Africans in a slave and slave master relationship. Curfew laws (new slave codes) such as those in Baltimore, Maryland make it a crime for children to be outside after 10 p.m. without legal guardians. Violations result in arrest and/or fines for the parent and a criminal record for the child and adult. Adults unable to pay fines can be imprisoned. A criminal record eventually leads to violence, underemployrnent, unemployment, crime, drugs, employment as cheap prison labor and the criminalization of African men and women which creates more curfew violations and junk food addicts.

Africans maimed, mutilated, shot or injured in violence become organ harvest candidates. The organ harvesting or taking hearts, kidneys, lungs, corneas of eyes, bone marrow, prostates, genital parts, digestive organs, arteries, veins, etc., is a profitable economic business. The Americans for Medical Progress Educational Foundation indicates that in order to double the profits of human organ harvesting, there are plans to cut kidneys in half. Added to this are ethnic junk food companies that sell harmful, chemicalized, processed black-eyed peas, collards, corn muffins, sweet potatoes, turnip greens, etc., that weaken Africans, health and help them to become unable to survive physical injuries which make them organ harvest candidates. Caucasians have changed the name of their behavior but have remained slave master, colonialists, and maintain Nutricide.

Fight To Pieces or Eat To Pieces

The mental and emotional signs and symptoms of Caucasian cannibalism are still present in their culture. They continue to have "pretend" meals of human and raw animal flesh. For example, they eat the pretend flesh of the gingerbread boy, animal and human shaped cookies and cereals, vitamin shaped people such as Mr. and Mrs. Flintstones and the symbolic blood dripping from the Christmas sugar candy canes. The Caucasian women continue to symbolically use blood to attract a mate by painting their lips (red lipstick) and claws (red fingernail polish). They continue to eat bloody flesh such as half-raw beefsteak and liver and symbolically pour red blood (tomato catsup) on animal flesh. The irony of this is that the White Race is too psychotic to comprehend their mental illness and too defensive of their inferiority to accept any constructive criticism or therapy or discipline. To attempt to reason with cannibalistic psychotic Whites is the same as doing an African dance without the drum or having a logical conversation with a drunk or drug addict in a stupor.

Confrontation dialogue with Caucasians often leads to violence. Violence is the medium of exchange that Caucasians historically have with Africans, Native Americans, Indians, Koreans and other people of color as well as other Caucasians. Historically, Caucasian violence and fighting among each other was very unorganized. Typically, when Caucasian men fought each other, they would bite pieces of flesh from each others arm's, face, legs, stomach and would gouge out each other's eyes. They also would bite off pieces of ears or noses, mutilate testicles, and bite off fingers which basically amounted to mutilation and cannibalism. Usually after fights body parts, pieces of fingers and flesh would be found on the ground. Defeat was often followed by the further mutilation of the defeated.

The French attempted to put some law and order to fighting and the British attempted to use the laws of Kingsbury. However, each clan had its own chaos and victory was honored as the only rule for fighting. Fighting by Caucasian clans amounts to the loss of one's body parts or life. It is the same with their disease-causing allopathic medicine and junk food diet because Africans lose pieces of their body (heart, kidney, uterus, prostate, teeth, liver) or their entire body (death) to Nutricide.

Crazy White Folks

White Racism is a mental illness that is classified as a psychosis. A psychosis is a total break with participation in the real world. African people have been defending their bodies, minds and spirits from White Racism and in some cases have become infected by

White Racism. White Racism means the power to inflict White Supremacy. White Supremacy is the belief that the White Race is superior without any evidence to support the belief except lies and the imagination of a diseased mind. Understanding the nature of the psychotic White mind helps an African defend him/herself against a white-dominated world contaminated by White Supremacy/White psychotics =crazy White folks.

There are nice, kind, caring, sensitive and humane people with diseases (i.e. cancer, fibroid tumors, arthritis). Being nice does not stop the disease. There are nice White people with White Supremacy disease. Being nice does not stop them from being a White racist. Their niceness is mixed consciously and subconsciously with their mental illness. In other words, they are still crazy.

Psychotic Whites do not accept what is real. They accept only what is imagined to be real and believe what their imagination sees not what their eyes see. They believe, then see and only believe what they see. The nature of the crazy White mind dictates that sanity cannot be trusted; only insanity can be trusted because insanity has become a mental parent, friend, marriage and companion. In many ways, insanity gives security because it never abandons Whites.

Historically, the Ice Age Caucasian could not trust nature to supply food. The environment was hostile with animals and people running from attacks. There were icebergs, earthquakes, land collisions making loud thundering sounds, unstable weather with floods and an unstable breast milk supply which disrupted or destroyed the bond of mother and nature. Aside from this, cannibalism was rampant along with rape and orgies compounded by diseases and nutrient deficiencies that caused mental illness to be an accepted way of life. The White mind in the past and present has manufactured superstitions to explain and protect the mind from emotional, psychological and spiritual harm. These superstitions may have been needed during the Ice Age. However, the Ice Age mentality is still genetically part of melanin albino Caucasian civilization. It is reflected in their mental illness combined with the negative mental effects that melanin deficiency causes. Their minds show the signs and symptoms of a person with an untreated mental disease.

A healthy, untreated mind may regress from "anxiety" to "neurosis" and then "psychosis" (insanity). However, the White mind has never been psychologically treated for mental illness and has degrees of psychosis (craziness) that do not lead back to a healthy mind but back to another type of diseased mind. Their mental illness weaves a thought path based upon the mental life of Whites as normal. Sigmund Freud, a European pioneer on the state of the White mind describes the White mind as a mind diseased with sexual conflicts, self-hatred, anger, violence, in conflict with itself and with its parents and siblings and deficient of love. He essentially says the White mind is created to remain constantly in conflict with good and evil or sanity and insanity.

Other White mind scientists basically say that the White mind is evil or the mind is good and must overcome its evil to self actualize (to be good). The basic ingredient of the White mind remains a conflict in a marriage of good against evil or sane against insane. Needless to say, the Caucasian mind scientists never explain the White race's disease of White racism. This means their scientists are too mentally ill to accept or see that they are mentally ill. White folks have episodes of sanity and are superficially sane in many of their mental activities. This sanity collapses if the mental disease of White Racism is forced to be focused on. They have situational sanity that is united to incomplete thoughts combined with fragments of racism psychosis.

The White mind lacks a beginning path. Their mind sees itself as not evolved from a human state but an animal mind state. For example, evolutionist scientist Charles Darwin wrote that Whites did not evolve from the human kingdom but the animal kingdom. Whites believe they started millions of years ago as a one-celled slime creature that lived in the sea, then evolved (changed) into a fish, then a reptile, then crawled or walked to a tree, then climbed up a tree and became a monkey, then climbed or fell out the tree and became a White man. They believe their minds still have the combined thinking ability of a one-celled slime creature, a fish, a reptile, a monkey and a walking ape. To Whites, their minds still have primitive qualities and are evil. Their White mind must be controlled or it will destroy them in order to satisfy the primitive desire to have sex with themselves or their mothers and fathers, kill for food or be in competition with their brothers or sisters over the parents' sexual attention. They believe their minds to have taboos, superstitions or conflicting (competitive nature) desires and see the world and all animals and plants as in conflict or fighting for food to survive. They believe their minds cannot be trusted—this is mental illness.

White mental illness is constantly moving to and from sanity episodes based on insanity. Insanity that runs from a deep belief that the mind will destroy itself in order to satisfy primitive desires. Insanity is a friend, lover, parent and companion of the White race and a marriage between sane and insane thoughts that produces more insane thoughts. Their minds protect their insanity because it is the only thing in life they can trust. The trust of insanity creates more fear and conflict and mistrust of sanity. Mental illness is the one thing they feel superior to. It brings psychological comfort to them because in the real world they are insane and inferior to Africans, Chinese, Indians, Japanese and Natives in North and South Americas. This diseased mind sees conflict (good fighting evil) in harmony and harmony in conflict. This is a disease that consumes its own mental pus in order to live. The degree of White Racism disease follows an order, be it chaotic, psychotic or perverted.

In mental illness there is order and basically three levels. A sane person can move in and out of the levels or degrees, but an insane person gets frozen in a mental state and cannot move out of it. A creative person may use levels of thoughts to write a novel, music or create dance or paint art but knows when to use them, how, why and when to stop. The insane have lost that ability and are trapped in a mental prison. A mild, temporary, mental imbalance is an "anxiety" which is when you get nervous over something real. For example, a person can get anxious about buying a new house. This is a normal stressor and "anxiety" is a normal response.

"Neurosis" is different. A neurotic person imagines unreal dangers about buying a house. They over-amplify the problems of buying a house and get extremely anxious over an unreal association with reality. For example, a drug addict is "neurotic" because he is addicted and has unreal beliefs about the drug and himself. He may believe he is in control and not addicted (can stop when he wants) and at the same time knows he is addicted. A "psychotic" (White supremacist/racist) person imagines that he has bought the imaginary house and believes that he is actually living in the house and will pay the monthly mortgage with imaginary money. This is a psychosis, a total break with the real world. Any attempt by Africans to demonstrate, vote, pray, educate or give healing therapy to a racist Caucasian will cause the white, psychotic, inferiority complex to be stimulated. This can result in their fighting back with abusive mental, spiritual or physical violence and more varieties of craziness. The psychotic White racists/supremacist are no longer capable of solving the psychotic problems that their diseased minds, bodies and spirit have created.

Added to this, the White race experiences pain from a history of self-abuse, the deliberate murder of 200 million Africans, the enslavement and the colonizing of Africans. At the same time, White racists get a pleasing mental sensation from masturbating their craziness on African people. They continue to fornicate all over the world with images of superiority over Africans with movies, violence, chemistry, wars, videos, history, education, biology, politics, medicine, television, radio, colors, music, computers, laws, religion, money, disease, starvation, crime, ecology, nutrition, jails and sex. They create, control and feed their psychosis by using all activities to make Africans appear inferior. Whites are a juvenile civilization of thugs that entertains itself with ignorance, sex, disease and violence. The White supremacist lives in the nation of "imagine-nation." Consequently, they demand African lives to mutilate and sacrifice to their inferiority.

White Racism is a psychotic cancer of the mind built on a deep mistrust of nature, God, self, other races and their own race. The crazy Whites aim their illness at something they can see, weigh and measure, called Africans. The White's crazy mind cannot measure or quantify mental illness. It feeds their craziness with acts of violence, sex and by ruling or ruining (destroying). Africans are put in an inferior posture by an inferior White race.

A race is measured by its products such as art, science and human relationships. Whites have no sane human relationship with Africans. Whites mirror that they cannot own or create peace, love, spirituality or a humanistically valuable relationship with Africans. Whites recreate what they are inside their psychotic minds. For example, Whites make Negroes feel honored or blessed that Caucasians have accumulated vast research and knowledge. Whites never acknowledge that they stole the knowledge from ancient Africans who are not honored.

Their mind is in conflict with itself. Their minds are violent with a superstitious belief that they want to destroy the evil part of their mind, so they commit violence against Africans who they de-

fined as bad, inferior, evil or criminals. They assume that by stealing a statue of God, they have become God. They assume that by
stealing African people's resources, land, knowledge, culture and
religion, that they are somehow superior. Whites are victims of
their own insanity and assume that by stealing a sane people (Africans), they themselves become sane. The whites' psychosis has
them embalmed in a psychotic cloud which could be cured by mental therapy, spiritual therapy, violence or African holistic sanity. It
is a disease that lives on conflict (competition) with nature, people,
God, life and competition with sanity.

The Caucasian-excessive-conflict-and-competition psychosis
justifies their murder of over 200 million Africans with their theory of evolution. The evolutionary myth ignorantly says that
methane gas accidentally collided with lightning and created the
one-celled slime creature that evolved to become monkey-like, and
walked around until it evolved to become the white man. This
evolutionary myth says Caucasians were first very primitive humans that made mistakes while evolving to become the White
race. The mistakes, conflicts, murders, slavery, cannibalism, chican-
ery and exploitation of African land and peoples are explained as a
part of nature's process of Caucasian evolution. Thus, Caucasian
competition with self, nature, God and Africans is merely a step in
their self-actualization and manifest destiny towards the white
race's perfection.

Competition (conflict) requires that one individual wins and
the other individual loses. Competition is not a family, communal
or people-sharing concept. Whites have their insanity in competition with their sanity. So it follows that in this competitive (conflicting) mental state, if sanity wins, it wins insanity and if insanity
loses it loses sanity and remains insane. White Racism is a disease
that must eat a daily meal of sanity to convert to insanity or a meal
of insanity to be in conflict and married to sanity. Whites are in fear

of insanity and hide from insanity in hopes of becoming sane. Sanity causes a fear because it would mean that Whites must accept their cultural inferiority and give up their false claims to African and American land and their claim to the wealth that the resources of those lands produced. In this sane, White state they would no longer be in power.

Whites will hold onto their insanity because it is a safe, secure state for them. They have learned to defend insanity with logic, wars, racism, religion, money, education and the mutilation and destruction of Africa and Africans. To call an insane white race anything other than crazy (insane) is to support and nourish White insanity. Whites make insanity pleasing and attractive by using violence and sex as an attractive cover (package) for the pleasure they derive from being insane. If this sounds crazy, it is because it is crazy. This is White craziness and cannot sound any other way. A conversation about soccer or baseball will sound like a conversation about soccer or baseball. So it follows, a conversation about White insanity will sound insane.

White psychotics think that they can escape White Racism by reading the autobiography of Martin Luther King or Malcolm X or collecting postage stamps of Bishop Tutu, Joe Louis, George Washington Carver or Marian Anderson. This is the same as a drunk alcoholic or high cocaine addict reading a book about a sober or drug free person and thinking that that will somehow make them sober or drug-free. White Racism is a mental disease that must be fed daily or it will consume the carrier. It makes any brief episode of sanity a horrible experience, because the ghosts of millions of murdered Africans and Indians haunt every sane thought. Sanity is worthless because it does not give the White mind any power. Sanity only reinforces a primitive animal mind that is locked in a battle of good against evil, the conscious against the unconscious, love against lute, power against the powerless and insanity against sanity.

It is clear that in order to be a White supremacist/racist, you first must be insane. Africans who want to gain some insight into white insanity must realize that the highly melaninated African brain, nervous system and skin biochemically makes African thought process different from the melanin-deficient, White thought process. Melaninated thinking is highly rhythmical, electromagnetic, spiritual and communal (family or concept). White thought processes lack the biochemical radiation and tend to travel distance at a slow speed without absorbing charges from other thoughts. African brains have 12 melaninated centers while Whites only have 2 melanin centers. This puts Africans in direct connection with ecological systems (stars, sun, moon, water, earth, plants, people, etc.), so they tend to contact seen and unseen energy in a highly spiritual and extrasensory thought process.

The White brain and an African brain may look alike but are anatomically and biochemically different and have electromagnetic operative factors that make them different. Whites usually learn by thought conflict or memorization, while Africans learn in conceptual and spiritual family pictures. African learning is a rhythmical process, while White learning is non-rhythmical and must place pros against cons or good against evil as the main factor for creating ideas.

White mental illness comes from conflict and escalates to conflicts supporting conflicts. Whites are mentally divided and conquered by their insanity. African people who are forced to socialize in White society may become divided and conquered, unless they are Africentric.

Whites are divided as a people. Whites do not trust each other or each other's governments. They maintain police to protect themselves from each other. White countries maintain armies to protect their countries from other White countries. This universal White behavior is a reflection of the condition of the White mind. Historically, whites arrested slaves for stealing themselves. A slave who ran away (escaped) was considered stealing himself. Consequently, they were captured and punished for stealing. Currently, an African who violently fights for his freedom and liberation from White Supremacy is considered as violating the Whites' freedom and is arrested and punished for crimes against freedom and liberty. It is a crazy White mind that can conceive of a crime of stealing yourself or violating your own freedom by wanting your freedom. They have equally and democratically distributed White Racism and Nutricide to all African people.

Food Terrorist

Caucasians use the need for food caused by famines or starvation as a way to intimidate or seize control of a group of people or government. This is called terrorism. When food is used to control a people, it is food terrorism. Food control is called marketing. Marketing is the manipulation and control of food for economic profit. Marketing is taught in all Caucasian colleges. Marketing requires the invasion of the market place. Invasion is a Caucasian word that means to capture, steal, exploit, control or take by force (violence). Invasions give money or capital that means White power. The power of Caucasians to control the food supply of other Caucasians is a Caucasian issue.

The power of Caucasians to control the food of Africans is a racial issue and a violation of human rights. It is a form of White Racism and nutritional terrorism. Food terrorism is another tool of White Supremacy that serves to exploit, dehumanize, disenfranchise, create diseases and destroy Africans for the economic profit of Whites. Whites deliberately attack the African food supply with their gangs of thugs called the United States of America corporations, pharmaceutical cartels, the United Nations and other Caucasian capitalist running dogs such as Britain, France, Russia, Japan, China, etc.

The Caucasian food terrorist invasions of Africa was and is designed to make the continent of Africa and its people food slaves. The terrorist captures the land, then uses the land to grow Caucasian foods. It then switches the African to Caucasian foods that cause Caucasian diseases and dependency on Caucasian foods. African food dependency required the Caucasians to create an African peasant class of landless laborers. The food terrorists learn in college marketing classes that food has no relationship to physical or mental diseases or behavior. They market Caucasian junk food to Africans and maintain that the food is not destructive to mental, physical and spiritual health. Food terrorists use food to control the rate of population growth and African access to power.

Food-dependent Africans are triage. Triage is usually used when large numbers of people, such as sick or injured people, need emergency medical help. It is a socially accepted form of genocide whereby the extremely injured/sick are allowed to die while the slightly injured are saved. However, triage can be used with institutions, the poor, businesses, services or a race of people. In the Caucasian triage system of food terrorism, the Africans who are made weak or diseased from undernutritional Caucasian junk food are left to die while nutritionally stronger Africans live.

The triage disease and death causing system is built into the marketing scheme. The marketing policy of Caucasians causes Africans to stop eating expensive millet, rye, barley, wild rice, manioc, beans and other seeds in favor of cheap wheat. Caucasians sell wheat at cheaper prices than any other grains. This forces poor Africans to avoid other grains. In other words, they no longer buy from Black farmers; they buy from White farmers. The African then becomes wheat-dependent. The African farmer cannot compete with the rich multinational food terrorist corporations. Wheat-dependent Africans do not grow their own wheat. African land is then used and abused by Caucasians who grow "cash crops" such as peanuts, cotton, sugar cane, rubber, cocoa, etc. Wheat is imported. The African's animal livestock industry is also made wheat-dependent. Africa's land becomes enslaved by Caucasians. Africans on the undernourished wheat-(bleached white flour)-dependent diet in cities will fight each other while Africans in rural areas nutritionally starve to death.

It is an institutionalized, nutritional, terrorist tactic to use Food for the Hunger Programs, United Nations Care Packages, food relief agencies and religious food programs to addict Africans to junk foods. The junk food is believed to stop the diseases that it causes. The Caucasians call it helping Africans. Caucasians use food to manipulate social problems, strife, disease, epidemics, conflicts and decrease populations (exterminate). They disguise their food terrorism as "food gifts to the hungry." They are giving a "gift" of disease and death to the hungry.

The food terrorist's processed wheat-(milled white flour)-centered diet increases acidity in the blood. The Caucasian diet of animal flesh, chicken fetuses and milk is highly acidic. The high acid content of the blood is destructive to the bones, nerves, tissues, reproductive system, glands and the brain. It destroys vitamins, minerals and proteins. Eating large amounts of acidic white rice, sugar and processed wheat flour degenerates the pineal gland.

Processed (bleached) wheat flour becomes manure at the beginning of the 30-foot digestive tract. It slowly travels along the digestive tract, spreading pollution throughout the body. Whole wheat becomes manure at the end of the digestive tract—the colon.

The acidic Caucasian junk food diet causes chronic physical, emotional, spiritual and mental fatigue. Acid foods are constipating. Constipation is the leading cause of melanin deficiencies and 90% of all diseases. High acidity causes an increase in bacteria, infections, white blood cells, fibroid tumors, high blood pressure, impotency, high cholesterol, venereal diseases, hyper-sex drive, colds, learning disorders, heart trouble, kidney stones, violence, allergies, cancer, degenerative diseases, anxiety, nervousness, fear, anger, and cravings for junk food, drugs and sugar. Historically, Caucasian food terrorists caused diseases that caused slaves to be physically handicapped.

Physically handicapped prisoners of war (so-called slaves) were sold at cheap prices at "Refuse Slave Sales. Many slaves became physically handicapped or deformed because of undernutrition, nutritionally caused diseases, work related accidents, self-inflicted injuries or severe torture. For example, slaves on slave ships often suffered from Vitamin D or Vitamin C deficiencies which caused blindness. The victim would become blind because the eyeball (cornea) would dry up. Many slaves would arrive to the Americas blind, crippled, crazy or dead.

Additionally, "Refuse Slaves" were sold and used for medical experiments, circuses, or sex experiments with animals. They were also used to demonstrate methods of torture or punishment to plantation slaves and helped to perpetuate a fear of Whites. It was cheaper to use a Refuse Slave.

A slave master's fear-inducing torture demonstrations included tying each leg of a slave to different horses, then making the horses run in different directions, which pulled the legs off the body. Pregnant slaves would have the baby cut from the womb and fed to the dogs. They would scalp the head of a male, or hang him by his penis, or boil a live slave. For a "joke" a slave would be placed in a barrel that had nails driven in the sides then rolled down a hill, causing puncture wounds to his body and eyes. The slave master considered this funny.

In addition to these barbarous acts, slaves were made crippled by the food terrorist diet. Any slave who was too handicapped or diseased to be sold at the Refuse Sale was sold at the "Scramble Sale." The scramble sale was a two for the price of one sale. Today, the Refuse and Scramble sales are called organ harvest companies. These companies sell Africans' kidneys, eyes, livers, genetic cells, aborted baby parts, melanin, bone marrow, and other body parts for experiments or transplants.

People in civilizations are trained from childhood to adulthood to like and dislike certain foods. Food selection is culturally controlled. Each race has a different ability to see, hear, digest food and taste food based on melanin content. Seeing, hearing and tasting food is a different biochemical reaction and action that is based on melanin concentration in the body. In other words, Africans do not hear, see or taste with the low degree of sensitivity as Caucasians. Added to this, culture orientates responses to stimuli so that an additional difference is added among races. The senses are bonded to the culture when the child is bonded to the mother.

In Caucasian society, food tastes are trained and food selection is controlled by food businesses. The food terrorists select the foods that will be eaten and grown. They select the likes and dislikes of foods. In other words, Africans are brainwashed robots who are forced to eat junk food by the combined forces of Caucasian psychologists, chemists, infantile cartoon characters, teachers, religions, color therapists, music therapists, hypnotists and sex therapists. Africans are trained to accept these practices and are trained to eat what they are told to eat.

These sciences and therapists are used to design food containers and packages, food jingles, food tastes, food commercials and subliminal persuasions and behavior controllers. The total effect of food marketing makes the consumer free to choose the wrong foods. The consumer is manipulated and addicted to foodstuffs.

As part of the marketing strategy, illness is blamed on germs, not on junk food. It is part of the terrorists' tactics to ridicule any junk food addicted person who stops eating their chemical garbage. The ridicule and insults can come from friends, family and strangers. The terrorists teach the junk food addict that getting sick, being sick, feeling sick is normal. They make the African ignorant of food warfare.

Foods are loaded with drugs. In an indirect way, drugs are pushed through food. Food drugs have the chemicals that enslave the body in sickness and handicap the mind. It is difficult for the food junkie to understand or accept reality. Food terrorists make food addicting with chemicals and sugar, then claim that African people are freely choosing to eat the food that they want to eat. This is the same as addicting a person to alcohol or crack cocaine, then saying that because the addict keeps choosing to take the drug, they are exercising freedom of choice. The junk food addict is free to keep choosing junk food to eat because the terrorists are constantly creating the addiction. The terrorist will not turn off the addiction. Since the addiction is not turned off, they say the addicts' constant consumption of drugged foods means that they like being addicted.

The Food Chemical Companies say if people did not like junk foods and dead flesh they would not eat them. In other words, an alcoholic drinks alcohol because he likes alcohol, not because he is addicted to alcohol. The chemically controlled mind believes the food drug pushers' brainwashing and advertisements. The food-addicted parents addict their children to food drugs, animal flesh and sugar. There is always a food drug fix available. The sugar addict always has a candy bar, liquid sugar (soda), sugary chewing gum or some other form of sweets available.

The food drug addict and the sugar addict do not know that they are addicted. The terrorist says that if the addict (junk food consumer) is stupid enough to like the addictive foods, then they should have the right to keep selling them the junk.

A food drug addict is a living sacrifice to White Supremacy. They are physical proof that the advertisements are successful. The mind-and behavior-altering drugs (chemicals) in the foods clone the African. The Caucasian government agencies, food relief agencies, Food for the Hungry religious groups give and sell junk food to starving and poor Africans. The government agencies such as the Department of Agriculture, Foreign Agriculture Service, the Food and Drug Administration, the Red Cross and the United Nations give free demonstrations on how to prepare junk food and free samples in order to addict Africans.

If white society seems concerned about African's health, it is merely a method of deceit used to destroy African's health. White terrorists use food to control and keep Africans sick. Sickness drains African people of energy. Sickness is a profitable business controlled and created by the disease industry. Sickness and White Racism are the only things democratically given to all Africans. Human rights and civil rights are not given to African people, only sickness and White Racism.

The terrorists make Africans believe that natural vitamins, minerals, amino acids, herbs or surgery or inoculations can protect the health of the body from diseases caused by junk foods. There is no miracle drug, herb or therapy that can make junk food addicted Africans healthy. Natural foods are the only miracle medicine; medicine is natural foods. Organic natural foods eaten raw or steamed and correct food combinations maintain wellness.

Food terrorists use their Caucasian superstitions and myths to create horrible food concoctions. For example, the ritualistic eating of the grease or pus (essence) of the animal's corpse and the wearing of fur is believed to give the Caucasian the power of the murdered animal. Animal grease was ritualistically rubbed on the body (grease bath) to protect Caucasians from diseases. Today Caucasians use sheep grease (lanolin).

Historically, Caucasians did not believe in taking baths throughout the span of their life. They believed that eating or rubbing boar (pig) grease gave the strength of a pig and deer grease gave one the ability to run like a deer. Rabbit grease was believed to give fertility, grease from cooked Africans gave savage sexual ability, cat grease protects one from mice, etc. They used the animal's rotten grease to make candles. These candles were believed to release the power of the animal's spirit. The candles, when burnt, gave off a foul odor and black smoke that would fill the hut or cave.

The Caucasian believed that a breakfast of chicken fetus (eggs) and plant seeds (wheat, rice, corn, oats) used as cereals regenerated the body. They also believed that cow's milk purified the body. Their breakfast foods were put together out of ignorance, not nutrition.

The Caucasians used herbs on foods out of superstition. The ancient Caucasians believed that the cold season could be changed to a hot or warm season inside the body by using herbs. Their herbs served as irritants to the delicate skin of their constipated digestive tract. They called these herbs "seasonings." Herbal irritants, such as mustard seed and black pepper were popular in food concoctions.

Many of the sauces poured on cooked animal flesh were derived from their ancient past. Historically, Caucasians would use a Sauce made of strigil to season dead corpses. Strigil sauce's main ingredient was the pus from a dead whale's intestine. It was similar to A-1 sauce. They also liked rotten fish oil in sauces such as Worcester Shire Sauce.

Caucasians like to eat the buttocks (behind, ass) or thighs of dead cattle, chickens, turkeys or pigs. They believed that muscle flesh of animals helps to make muscles in their bodies. Added to this, they believed that the hair from pigs (boar's hair) used to make hair brushes could give strength to their hair.

They also conduct spiritual rituals with animals. For example, the head of an animal (goat, pig) was believed to possess intelligence and represent a gate to a higher evil or heaven. Often they would put an apple or fruit on dead flesh to gain the ability to give spiritual rebirth. Consequently, the Caucasian would eat a pig's head with an apple in the mouth or a goat or sheep's head with fruit in the mouth. In order to gain the birth of new strength and muscles, they would put fruit such as pineapple slices on a pig's ass (ham) and then eat it.

They ate food because of superstitions and ignorance and never associated with nutrition, cleanliness or health. Consequently, they did not wash their own bodies, vegetables or the corpse of the animals that they ate. Their idea of cleaning an animal was to drain the blood from the carcass. They would eat dead animals' genitals, semen, ovaries, or cooked African people's sex organs in order to feel sexually aroused. The food terrorists still have insane attachments to foods that are deeply embedded in their subconscious minds and spirits and based on ignorance. The terrorists are predatory in their approach to food and exploit Africans with food.

Predatory animals and predatory Caucasians capture and kill animals. Predatory terrorists capture the land and food supply, then kill the Africans with a junk food supply. Ironically, the Caucasians are the same with food. They capture the food by cultivation farming, then process the food which kills the nutrients, then they embalm the dead food with chemicals (preservatives) and then they eat it. Caucasians captured African people and Africa's land, then they preserved the African culture by imitating it, and then they destroyed the African by "Seasonin," inferiorizing and victimizing the Black race. They then kill Africans with drugged foods. Terrorists have the same behavior towards Africans, land and God as they have within themselves. They do not trust their own bodies and are in fear that their health will fall ill to disease at any moment. They mistrust their natural bodies. They mistrust God. They mistrust the spiritualization of food and totally mistrust Africans. Caucasians have self-hatred.

The food terrorists use the same predatory behavior as they did during invasions of Africa, during slavery and colonialism. During slavery, all foods, clothing, discipline and religion came from the slave master. After slavery, Africans became wage slaves or sharecroppers. Wage slaves earn only enough money to survive and always stay in debt. Sharecroppers bought food, machines and clothing on credit. They paid their debts and rent by giving a large share of their crops to Caucasians. They bought all of their goods from the overpriced company store (former slave master's store).

The Caucasians used the capitalist system. Capitalism is a Caucasian money ritual whereby they steal (sell-overpriced goods) from the consumer. They steal by selling cheap goods, made by exploiting cheap labor, at high prices. They then put high interest rates on credit (loans). Caucasian money rituals and ceremonies are called finance, marketing, economics and business. These money rituals and ceremonies use deceit, stealing, lies, sex, exploitation, homosexuality, cheap labor, drugs, spiritual perversion, immorality and dysfunctional families.

An African who attempts to participate in Caucasian money ceremonies or rituals must follow the unwritten and unspoken rules of dishonesty, mistrust, deception and ungodliness. Caucasian money transactions are exclusive and not inclusive of Africans–White only. An African is an alien in Caucasian money transactions. Africans are a negative drive for Caucasians and are systematically rejected and punished by Caucasians for participating. For example, Africans who accumulate wealth or earn high salaries cannot openly support African rebellions, African revolutions or militant groups. If they do show any support, they will be killed, jailed, have their character assassinated or in some way be punished. African money in Caucasian ceremonies can only be invested or spent on approved Caucasian concerns.

Africans naturally think that money transactions reflect God, the family, and should go to the highest spiritual good. Caucasians view money transactions as separate from spiritual good. Therefore, the Caucasians, destruction of land, life, food and other people's wealth is not considered because it produces a selfish capital gain and profit for a few. All profit (stolen money) is considered good. Profit is merely used as a form of White Supremacy.

Today the slave master's new company store is the multinational corporation. Multinational corporations own the wage slave, the factories, banks, credit cards, prisons, colleges, religions, militaries, governments, media, hospitals, clothing manufactures, farms, pharmaceutical cartels and food stores. They own the taste buds. Addicted taste buds only eat what the multinational companies tell them to eat. Junk food addicted Africans educate themselves to work for the new slave master-multinational corporations.

The African participates in White culture's diet as if it were their own African cultural diet. The African is addicted to the slave plantation's soul food, garbage diet of food such as fried rice, fried okra, fried chicken, greasy overcooked green vegetables, pig's ass (ham) chitterlings (pig guts), pig hoofs (pigs feet), salt, vinegar, deadly food combinations such as milk, grease, vinegar (a drug), salt (a drug) sugar (a drug), chicken fetus, toxic night shade plants (peppers), onions, celery and overcooked demineralized potatoes with nutrientless lettuce called potato salad. This soul food diet, and the Caucasian junk food diet, is deadly. The choices for Africans are to stop eating the soul food and junk foods, or die.

The food terrorist armies used many tactics. They burned food crops, homes, raped (men, women and children) and lynched Africans to make them abandon their farmlands. After the Civil War, the United States government gave land (which meant food control) to Africans. Then President Andrew Jackson declared that the land was illegally given to Africans. He ordered the Africans to move from their land. The Africans armed with guns refused to move. The government declared an unofficial war against Negroes and sent the United States Army in to attack Negroes. The army attacked, murdered, raped, lynched, terrorized, and burnt food crops and homes.

The Africans who were not killed either had to become sharecroppers or buy the land. The Africans who bought land eventually lost it due to taxes. The Africans became landless peasants who had a choice of starving to death as wage slaves or moving to northern ghettoes. The Negro became an exploitable, landless class of peasant wage slave laborers. This same food terrorist tactic was repeated over and over in Africa or anywhere that the Caucasian wants to steal land and labor.

The Food terrorist uses Caucasian-created starvation as a means to market their tactics. It has never been a case of Africans starving due to lack of farmland, lack of food or overpopulation. It has always been a case of Caucasian Food terrorists causing starvation in order to disguise their forced geopolitical control of land and food. Food terrorist thugs such as the United States Department of Agriculture, Foreign Agricultural Services, Department of Commerce and the Agency of International Development, use wheat to destroy African grain farmers. They use Public Law 480 to switch Africans and Africans' livestock to an acidic, wheat-centered diet.

Basically, the Caucasians' laws and agreements with each other, government control agencies, judicial systems, alliances and consumer protection agencies amount to the insane controlling the insane. For example, weather modification agencies are out of control. Weather modification is the process of changing the weather with concentrated heat radiation or chemicals. Chemicals are sprayed into clouds to force them to retain more water which results in rain. However, making rain in one area causes a violent interruption of the natural weather cycles. This causes the negative rebound effects of droughts, hurricanes, forest fires, insect attacks on food crops and people and crop destruction.

Weather modification companies' reactions to bad weather is to chemically change the weather which causes another negative rebound in the weather. They also use the weather in order to destroy each others' crops in order to create food shortages which result in increased profits. The weather modification companies have weather wars among themselves. The National Science Foundation has stated that billions of dollars and an uncertain number of deaths are caused each year by weather modification. These companies are controlled by the out-of-control government, in essence, the insane controlling the insane.

Food terrorists use weather and food as a weapon. This weapon creates diseases and death in the name of "money" or "profit." Profit and paper money (currency) are the Caucasians' way of worshipping White Supremacy. Caucasian paper money (U.S. dollar, British pound etc.) are their governments paper credit cards and represent money stolen from their citizens. Their currency is valueless and they let the citizens pretend that it has value. Caucasians are insane and pretend that they are sane. They do not have any history of sane spiritual behavior with Africans or any colored people. Their terrorist use of food indicts them, and history verifies this indictment.

Historically, European civilization exploited Africans with food The Portuguese (name means stomach people or mouth of eaters) invaded Africa, burnt homes, raped men, women and children and destroyed crops in order to force Africans to work on peanut, coffee, cotton and other quick cash crop plantations. This tactic of "rape pillage and burn" was used in many African countries. The United Nations Environment Program and the International Crop Research Institute for Semi-Arid Tropics stated that the land, crops and food supply are lost forever. Terrorist destruction of farms and farmers forces Africans to be wheat dependent. The combination of this disease-causing diet and the disease-causing chemical pollutants called medicine destroys the so-called immune system. Food has been the most reliable weapon the Caucasian has used to control Africans. The African becomes addicted to junk food and is mentally and physically controlled by the addiction and by diseases until death by Nutricide.

The Caucasian food terrorist uses the Africans' denial of disease to addict them to junk food, drugs, sex, Caucasian religions and White Racism. Food addiction indicates a failure to accept self. Failure to accept self is denial. Africans fail to accept their racial and cultural superiority. This superiority and spiritual obligations to ancestors demand a spiritual revolution for freedom (i.e. race war). Denial is used to hide pain. The emotional pain of being a defeated people, an enslaved and colonized people has never been confronted or resolved.

Denial disease relies upon the continuous inability to face true reality. True reality is substituted with a false reality. Denial allows its victims to victimize self by accepting White reality as an African reality. Denial is a disease forced upon Africans by Caucasians. The Caucasian's psychotic reality denies their physical, mental, cultural and spiritual inferiority by creating a fantasy craziness called White Supremacy. They cannot and will not accept their inferiority and criminal deeds against Africans. If Whites accepted their crimes against Africans, then self-punishment or suicide would be the only logical action for Whites to take. Denial is the basis for the slave and slave master relationship. It is a failure of a people's group personality (culture) to allow their diet and self to be continuously enslaved by primitive Whites. Africans have failed to accept that Caucasians are insane with moments of sanity. Denial of the mental illness of the Caucasian race supports denial of the trauma of slavery which supports junk food addiction. Addiction is the failure to accept reality.

An African free of the emotionally crippling impact of slavery/colonialism realizes that Caucasian foods are an extension of the insane Caucasian worldview. A worldview based on ignorance, superstitions, addiction and a mistrust of nature. Denial is a silent weapon used to destroy the Africans' ability to heal themselves from the pain of slavery/colonialism. Africans in denial use food to satisfy the sensual taste buds and the hurt of slavery. Food not only becomes a form of pleasure, it also can help soothe and pacify the ugly pain of denial.

Food terrorists must maintain the Africans' denial disease in order to maintain White Supremacy. They use nutritional Uncle Toms such as Bill Cosby, Anita Baker, Spike Lee, Herbie Hancock, Whitney Houston, Michael Jordan, B.B. King, or fictitious nutritional Uncle Toms such as Uncle Ben (rice) and Aunt Jemima (pancake), in order to keep Africans addicted to junk food, denial and fear. These nutritional Uncle Toms are victims of the food terrorist.

Fear combined with denial are the psychological devices used to sell food. Caucasian food terrorists believe that the more "rich food" you eat, the more health you will attain. Health is associated with quantity of food, not the natural quality of food. Poor quality processed junk foods, dairy products and animal flesh cause nutritional starvation. They are starvation foods. These foods cause the body to rot. The muscles get hard, the bones get soft and the teeth rot and fall out. The feet, armpits and body stink with foul fumes caused by constipation or pollution. The skin wrinkles, the eyes and ears weaken. Circulation decreases and the physical degeneration caused by drugged foods is called old age.

The "rich foods" are greasy, oily and heavily seasoned with herbal irritants. They also contain high amounts of acidic, cooked meats and various cooked concoctions with stupid combinations of sugar and starch, or starch and protein. They are worshipped as "good food." Caucasians believe that if you miss one of these rich meals, or miss any meal, you will lose energy and evil bacteria or virus will attack your body, causing a disease. They eat in fear of these attacking germs.

Caucasians, and the Africans who nutritionally imitate them, have a compulsive eating disease which is based on a history of famines and starvation from the Ice Age era (10,000 years). Post Ice Age era (5.000 years) and Cold era (2,000 years). During the Cold Age, Caucasians started inhaling the fumes of their own bowel movements (manure) and sleeping with dogs, goats or pigs in order to use the foul odors as a sort of antibiotic evil spirit.

They would drink, have bowel movements and bathe in the same water that they used to cook food. Cleanliness was not related to health, but related to myths and fears of nature and the belief that nature or an evil spirit was always attacking them. Their pagan rituals of fighting evil germs with antibacterial creams, lotions, soaps, mouthwash, toothpaste, deodorants, douches and cleansers is unscientific.

They also kill germs by sanitation. They sterilize cow's milk, pots, surfaces, clothes, dishes and utensils forgetting that sterilization only lasts a few minutes before the germs return. Africans adopt the Caucasian insane notion of killing evil germs and the Caucasian medical rituals and ceremonies and become twice addicted to ignorance. They are attached to the Caucasian insanity by the Caucasian belief system and by the denial of the slavery trauma.

The Caucasian fear and denial of reality makes their medical rituals and ceremonies seem logical. For example, they believe that taking a poison that is against life =anti-biological (antibiotic) is sensible. It is fear that supports denial and denial that supports denial which is the foundation of the addiction to junk foods. The Caucasian marketing tactics and mind do not separate the rich and the poor, slave and slave master, technology and pollution, food and disease, peace and war, sex and love or good and evil. Their mind bonds and mixes ideas and behaviors together that are not related. Food is mixed with politics, wars, economic profit, chemicals, pollutio4 violence, etc.

Africans only see food as a connection to the spirit world and nutrition. Food to Caucasians is a weapon to control and terrorize. The African connection to food has to be a reaction to the food terrorist, White Racism, the race war, White Supremacy and the disease industry as one in the same problem. Caucasians do not and cannot separate tactics or actions with their melanin albino brain. Caucasian food terrorists have to be destroyed because it is part of and not separate from industry, White Racism, White Supremacy and Caucasian civilization.

Food terrorism is part of a chain reaction of subtle terrorist factors that react to each other and support each other. In this chain reaction, Africans are mentally and socially terrorized. Subtle terrorist tactics keep the African's mind crazy. For example, the institution of banking is alien to most Africans. Banks are not a building or business, but a social institution created by a race to support that race exclusively. A bank is a coalition of people who think, feel and behave the same. Institutions require trust, honesty, spirituality and reliance upon each other. Ex-slaves and colonized Africans are "seasonin" to mistrust each other. The terrorists continue to maintain an atmosphere of mistrust or "seasonin."

African people were made crazy by "seasonin" during slavery. "Seasonin" was (is) a conditioning process in which slaves were made to recite positive affirmations about the goodness of slavery and the White race and negative verses about the Black race (catechism) combined with performing the same menial task daily. The "seasonin" could last from a few months to years for chattel slaves. "Seasonin" slaves were indoctrinated constantly to mistrust other slaves and to feel that "niggers ain't no good and cursed by God." Modern "seasonin" occurs when Africans are trained by food commercials to sing positive music jingles and/or recite positive slogans about harmful junk food.

The constant use of "seasonin" by Food terrorists is apparent in banks. Africans are taught to mistrust each other. Consequently, Africans cannot collectively save money and lend money (interest free) to each other, because they do not trust each other. They are "seasonin" to put money in the slave master's bank. It is anti-African to use Caucasian banks. Caucasian banks are White nationalist banks because they support Caucasian businesses that terrorize Blacks. White nationalists share the common disease of White Supremacy. Ironically, during post-chattel slavery, Africans had savings clubs in which each member would contribute part of his pay each month. Each member would get a loan of $1,000 or more every six months. These savings clubs became part of burial societies and churches they no longer exist. However the contemporary "seasonin" process of the terrorist still exists.

Terrorists must continue to make the African insane (crazy). An insane Negro is nutritionally suicidal and an alien to his own culture. Nutritional suicide occurs when Africans pay money for disease and death causing junk foods. A terrorized African sees food terrorism as separate and divided from White Racism, politics, jail, special education and disease. If the African is divided, then he is conquered. A conquered mind is an alien, "seasonin," confused crazy and terrorized mind.

The Caucasian teaches the craziness that an African in a Caucasian controlled society has freedom of choice. Freedom of choice implies that you have "free will." Africans have the freedom to follow Caucasians rituals and ceremonies but no control over them. Results can only be realized by a group. "Free will" requires that a group have ownership and control over resources and the military power to control the group. Therefore, an African can seek justice in the judiciary system by following legal rituals and ceremonies. However, Caucasians as a group control the judiciary system. Therefore, justice can be denied an alien ("seasonin" African). Similarly, Africans are free to choose different types of Caucasian junk foods, but lack the power to insure that it does not contain toxic poisons.

It is a terrorist tactic to maintain "seasonin." Africans are kept "seasonin" by various subtle means. For example, the Ebonics (Ebony =Black phonics) languages of Africans are labeled as Black English Negro Dialect, Gullah or bad English. Ebonics is the language that Africans speak. It may use English words, but it has distinctly African conceptualizations, word order, rhythms and consonant clusters at the end of words (i.e. "I be goin."). The Caucasians speak a German derived language (60% German words) which they call English. They do not label English as a German Dialect, bad German, or White German. English is labeled as a language. Mislabeled and negative connotations applied to Ebonics helps to make the African an alien, confused and terrorized.

Alien properties and stores in the ghetto are owned by Caucasians or their puppet racial groups. However, terrorists blame the creation of the ghetto and poverty on Africans. The terrorists are in the poverty business, junk food business and the disease industry because it is economically and psychologically profitable. Profit is anything that supports White Supremacy. The only way for Caucasians to make a profit from Negroes is to keep them "seasonin." crazy and terrorized.

A pregnant teenager is a tool of the terrorist. Teenage pregnancy is labeled as hypersexual, immoral and a symptom of a dysfunctional Black family. This increases stressors in the African community. Stress, hypertension, violence, fear and denial cause an increase in junk food consumption. Historically, the Caucasian population in America was started by teenage pregnancy; slavery was maintained by teenage pregnancy, unwed mothers and, so called bastard African and mulatto children, child labor, white men (pedophile) raping African girls and boys and the white (pedophile) women's rape of African boys and girls.

In fact, all Africans married by Caucasian ceremonies and religions are "unwed" and have bastard children. Teenage pregnancy is not the problem. It is the social conditions created and maintained by terrorists and aliens that are the problem.

Social terrorism cascades and perpetuates food terrorism. For example, Africans who suffer from "seasonin" stress, hypertension, fear, denial and violence, eat more junk food. They are easily made addicted to the chemicals in food—food drugs. These chemicals not only alter the thinking, but also cause retarded genital growth, infertility and sexual identity problems. This adds to the "seasonin" of the African community, as Blacks fear Blacks. This influences "seasonin," causing Africans to identify with Caucasian culture.

Alien Africans label themselves as Americans (Whites). "American" is a mislabel that denotes slavery, murder, rape, stealing and White nationalism. Caucasians invaded Turtle Island, renamed the island America and themselves Americans. Africans cannot be Americans because they never voluntarily gave up their African citizenship. The mislabeled American assumes that Africans paid for their transportation to America as slaves and voluntarily gave up their African citizenship. "Seasonin" Africans celebrate American holidays, eat American junk foods and contribute to the tension of terrorism.

Africans miseducated in Caucasian schools and colleges become aliens. These institutions support the myths and lies of White supremacy. They fantasize that the European culture's idea of academics is the only type of academics of value. Africans in these Caucasian schools are majoring in White Studies. White Studies alienates the mind of an African from African culture. Aliens believe that health means the absence of obvious diseases. They go to optometrists who wear eyeglasses and dentists who have no teeth. They are trained to be blind to contradictions and confusion.

Aliens believe in the contraction that homosexuals can have sexual intercourse. Only a man and a woman can have sexual intercourse. Homosexuals merely masturbate each other. Aliens believe that sexual intercourse means the same as love. They refer to having intercourse as "making love." These "seasonin" Africans have difficulty adapting holistically to African culture. Their attempts to adapt cause stress, confusion and terrorism to other Africans. Terrorists destroy holistic African sex principles in order to destroy harmonious relationships. Aliens use the terrorist allopathic drugs to correct sexual infertility, reproduction problems and diseases. They are cloned with junk foods, junk medicine, junk religions and junk language.

Aliens use the language they are "seasonin" with by Caucasian media (movies television. books and textbooks). Their language is based on the movie rating categories of Parental Guidance (PG 13) and Restricted (R). Consequently, they believe adult language means the use of curse words, profanity and obscenity. African adult words are "I respect God in you." "I honor your presence," etc. Often, cloned Africans indicate the words "boyfriend and girlfriend" to indicate a sexual relationship. In African culture, a sexual relationship is based upon a mating with God and families (marriage). They refer to each other as a "mate." Caucasian language concepts maintain "seasonin" resulting in a mind too crazy to stop eating junk foods and too crazy to stop "seasonin."

The aliens who victimize African history, ancestors and the raw food diet are "seasonin." These aliens believe that their great ancient culture became weak, had serious social problems, religious conflicts, too much humanity, tribalism and egotism, which caused Africa to self-destruct. It is within the natural cycle that all creations (people. plants. cultures. planets and religions) adjust, readjust and change. The exploitation of a people in their changing process is a crime. Caucasians are guilty of committing crimes against Africans in the process of change. The Caucasians (crazy White people) have committed the crime and then blamed the victim. In other words, a woman who is raped is blamed for being raped =victimizing the victim. Terrorism is a disease trait of Caucasian syphilization (civilization) and sexual intercourse with Caucasians and mixed-up children, help to maintain "seasonin" and Nutricide.

African Ecology
and Caucasian Pollution

The world's first ecologists in recorded history were Africans of the Nile Valley. Ecology is man's relationship to the environment (plants, earth and animals). Humans must relate to their mother and father (the seen) and the spirit (the unseen) before they can relate to the environment (the seen created by the unseen). Africans learned harmony and human relationship, which is called spirituality. Therefore, African ecology is merely an extension of the relationship between their mother and father (seen) and Mother/Father God (unseen). Africans did not pollute or destroy the harmony of nature because to do so is a form of self-destruction.

Pollution of the earth (Ta) is historically an act of Caucasian civilization. In Caucasian cosmology (worldview), the planet earth exists to serve their needs. It is not a give-and–take relationship. It is not a spiritual relationship. Therefore, they treat Mother Earth as a slave. Caucasians rape the land of resources, mutilate (clone) and pollute the air, water, soil, sound (noise pollution), vision (artificial and perverted natural light reflected from buildings, glass, cars, concrete, asphalt, etc.), clone and exterminate plants, insects, animals and people. The earth, outer space and Africans have become polluted garbage dumps of Caucasian technology. African civilization demonstrated the correct holistic behavior relationship to have between Ta (earth), in Ake-Bu-Lan (Africa), in Khuiland (the ancient state of Egypt), in the nation of Khemet (black soil valley areas of the Nile).

The Hyksos (Caucasians from the Oxus Valley area), and other Europeans who invaded or traded with Africans were called vile, primitive and wretched. Caucasians had a limited vocabulary, did not bathe, were flea-infested, practiced group sex, raped, stole, murdered, were bed wetters, drank pus to cure disease, had no religions, were disorganized liars, urinated in the streets, were superstitious and ignorant, believed the earth was flat and were constantly diseased. Their behavior among themselves and negative treatment of the land caused Africans to pity them and want to help them become spiritualized and ecology minded.

The African worldview (cosmology) sees each of us as custodians or servants of God's land. The land is a living spiritual gift from God. Loving the environment and earth is Erapi-hati-a (hereditary) for Africans. Africans' bodies are the Per-o (house) that ecologically resides on Ta. We give to Ta and Ta gives to us. This is the homeostasis (balance) that African culture has taught human beings (hue =black, man =thinking). The Ta is viewed as a spaceship (mothership) that carries us on our journey by day and by night through the heavens so that we can rise in God's presence. Africans who believed their spirit would resurrect in the West were called Osirians. They were believed to have gone west to be born anew in the Sun God's (Ra) presence. They were called Westerners. The Caucasian ecology is not based on spirituality and a relationship with God. They take all that they can from the earth and Africans for economic profit, giving back pollution. This is contrary to the ecological wisdom of the human body.

Junk food is processed and against the ecological wisdom of the body. For example, vitamins, minerals, fibers and proteins are milled or chemically taken out of whole wheat, brown rice and sugar cane, leaving a pasty, gooey, polluted, poisonous drug (synthetic manure). Basically, the food factories have machines that stimulate the liver, pancreas, stomach and intestine. These machines digest the food (process) and the end result of processing a food is a bowel movement. Technically, a processed food is synthetic manure. Eating processed (machine digested) food is against the body's wisdom, rhythm and ecology. The normal ecology of the body follows a solar and lunar cycle, melanin rhythm and allows each organ to use the food's nutrients. The end product of whole food digestion is manure. Processed junk food starts off in the stomach as manure. This is contrary to the body's natural ecology. A junk food diet causes toxic chemicals, toxic gas, rotten muscles and bones, toxic electromagnetic vibrations and pollution that destroys the body, resulting in disease and death.

The spiritual nature of foods is alive in whole foods and is destroyed by polluted junk foods. An African person claims the spiritual nature of life and foods by eating whole foods. The spiritual rights of food as spirit is ignored by Caucasian nutrition, science and medicine. In their nutrition, medicine and science, they use chemical rituals and ceremonies. So-called experiments and scientific methods are also used to justify destroying natural foods and Africans.

Caucasian science reflects the Caucasian world-view and behavior. For example, any human (or vegetable) right that is not claimed by violence is not respected. The spiritual nature of plants does not allow force and violence against people. The Caucasians do not respect the vegetables, spiritual rights. They apply the same human ritual and ceremony behaviors called laws to all aspects of life.

Ignorance of Caucasian dictated rights or laws of human behavior is no excuse for accidentally violating Caucasian laws. Caucasians say that ignorance of their law is no excuse, and do not exempt the perpetrator from punishment.

The individual right of life, liberty and pursuit of happiness is a right that can only be guaranteed by a group. A group must have land, properly and power (military and economic) to guarantee individual rights. This is the psychotic method of bestowing rights to the elite few, enabling them to exploit, manipulate and control the majority of people, the food supply and the planet earth Caucasian relationships to people, science, the body, nutrition, and food is a series of rituals and ceremonies which they call "law" or "Fact." Further, the Caucasian science rituals (experiments) are used to determine what is real and what is unreal. If a Caucasian can perform the same chemical trick or physical ritual twice, then it is considered real. In other words, since God has not made the same person twice exactly, then God is not real. In nature, even identical twins are not exactly the same. Caucasian science rituals are not directly related to nature, spirituality and God. They are related to their rituals. African science is directly related to the spiritual ecology of nature and God. Therefore, Africans did not pollute or disrespect the ecology of the earth or the human body.

The human body is an ecologically perfect system. For example, the liver takes waste from by-products of digestion and turns them into bile salts which are used as digestive enzymes that break down eaten food. The lungs breathe in air, and exhale carbon dioxide. They use the carbon dioxide to regulate breathing in and breathing out (negative drive). The large intestine (colon) recycles electrolytes and water in food by extracting the minerals and water from di-

gested foods. Minerals are recycled and used to make hair and finger and toe nails. The body's ability to recycle nutrients and melanin is hampered and destroyed by synthetic junk foods, polluted
water and air, eating animal flesh, dairy products, alcohol, nicotine,
drugs, White sugar, salt, oils, bleached flour and vaccines.

Vaccines are pollutants that poison the ecology of the body. Pollutants, poison and waste stored in the body cause dis-eases. Vaccines are a superstitious ritual performed by Caucasian medicine in
health treatment ceremonies called medical care. Vaccines (inoculations) are based on the ignorant belief that the human body will not
react, so-called immunity. The body always reacts to stimulants,
food, drugs, rain, the sun, sound, touch, taste, odors, spirituality,
electromagnetic forces and the environment. A body that does not
react to disease either positively or negatively is not immune, but
dead.

The body is never immune to life. Bodily cleansing or so-called
dis-ease reaction is a life function. A living human cannot be immune to living or bodily reactions. In any case, vaccines are made
of the diseased cells of animals and humans. Vaccines use a concoction of pus and unsterilized human or animal blood, Hela cells
(short form of a Black lady's name, Henrietta Lacks, and are uterine
cancer cells), added to diseased kidney cells from the Green Monkey, cells from the pig's stomach called trypsin and toxic poisons.
This Caucasian polluted concoction is injected into the veins of Africans with a hypodermic needle and called medicine.

All vaccines are chemical garbage that destroys health. This includes the "pus soups" called polio, diphtheria, measles, mumps,
rubella, small pox, malaria, tetanus and Influenza vaccines. Caucasians dump pollution into the body to protect the body's natural
ecology. This is in contrast to Africans who merely extend their relationship with God by spiritualizing the body with natural food.

Oddly enough, the ancient African's garbage dumps were spiritualized with plants and treated like living spiritual organisms.

The ancient cities of Africa had city dumps that did not pollute or destroy the ecology. These city dumps were surrounded by plants. Plants served to use the rich compost of the garbage dump, protect from insect overpopulation, keep the soil in balance, maintain moisture, stop soil erosion and provide food, herbs and beauty. The garbage dumps contained plants such as henbane, apricot, flax, acacia, marigold, olive, myrtle, chrysanthemum, plum, fleabane, basil, and pomegranate.

Builders used medicinal herbs, fruits and vegetable plants in designing temples, cities, irrigation channels as well as garbage dumps. Ineni under King Tuthmosis I (1528-1510 BC) was an herbalist who designed gardens and garbage dumps. Sennufa the mayor of Thebes during the rule of Amenophis II (1425 BC) was in charge of the medicinal herbs and vegetables around the city dumps and cemeteries. There were many medicinal herb stores (flower shops) in the Egyptian Empire. They supplied medicinal herbs for private and public dumps, gardens, clothing and food storage, ornaments, wearing apparel and offerings. The herbalist Nekht during the rule Amenophis III (1375 BC) was in charge of the official medicinal herbs and ceremonial usage of herbs for the city.

Africans, in order to prevent the wasteful accumulation of paper packaging, used herbs for packing, storage of food and the protection of food, clothing and household items. Herbal packaging was used to protect cloth and foods that were to be transported by ships, horses, camels or wagons from insect damage. There were herbs pictured in the Theban Tombs of the 18th dynasty. Herbs also gave a pleasant scent to stored items and respected a spiritual energy. Natural, herbal packaging could be brewed as teas or used as poultices in medical care. This is in direct contrast to the Caucasian wastefulness and pollution of Ta.

Ecology of the body and Ta are one. Living with spirituality means respecting the body and eating natural foods and morality for the body is not taking anything that pollutes the body. This belief is built in the African family, diet, medicine and lifestyle (culture). The African lifestyle uses animals and plants in the written language, arts, cyclic laws, astrological science, architecture and fabric designs-as a way to emphasize a spiritual ecology with nature.

In every area of African society a reverence and respect for the environment is evident. For example, the Egyptian kingdoms were named after plants, insects and animals such as Bull Cult, the Bee King (Lower Delta Kingdom) and Papyrus (reed) King (Middle Kingdom). In African ecology, the family technology was used. The African viewed Ta as Mother/Father Earth. Disrespect for the environment was considered disrespect of the privilege to obey God's will. Any destruction of Ta was destruction of God's spirit reflected by your Mother/Father (parents and family). Therefore, any destruction of Ta also destroys your "hue (Black) man (living)" being.

Ecology says with the holistic balance of a person. This human ecology is reflected in the person's relationship with their family, culture, diet and God. The practice of human ecology is learned by a harmonious interaction with other races and nature. Consequently, environmental ecology merely mirrors humanistic ecology. The smallest unit of ecology is the family. There must be harmonious, unconditional love between one race and another or there cannot be ecology with the environment. It is a human imperative that ecology be preserved.

The world has become a garbage can because of Caucasian pollution. The Caucasian race's inability to protect and save themselves from disease and infertility reflects an error in human ecology. For example, the United Nations census of world population indicates that Caucasians are at zero population growth. Africans in Haiti will double their population in 30 years, while the typical Caucasians in Italy may (by mathematical guess) double their population by the year 3000. In order to balance the infertility, ecological disaster of their race, Caucasians constantly promote sex in all types of advertisements such as toothpaste, automobiles, deodorants, toilet paper, soap, chewing gum and hair grease commercials. They use movies, news reports, sports, religions, weight loss, magazines and music as a sex-ploitation tactic to increase their population.

However, their continued abuse of nature and Africans dooms them to be unhealthy. It must be remembered that they had a population decline of between 8th and $1/100^{th}$ of the world population before they started the race wars with Africans and the Natives on Turtle Island (America). It was after the invasions of Africa that they had an increase to $1/6^{th}$ of the world population. The current decrease in population is viewed by them as another cycle of the decrease/increase/decrease population pattern. The decreases were usually caused by pollution of the environment, the absence of hygiene or by diet, diseases and war. Their destructive human ecology causes the new types of destruction to the environment. It is totally insane to ask the Caucasian people to be ecology minded without military enforcement.

Caucasian's new types of businesses use genetics to clone vegetables, microbes and people. These freak species of vegetables, animals and microbes do not fit into the natural ecology. Nature does not have a method of control to keep these freaks (clones) in balance with the environment. This results in a new type of pollution heaped onto the current pollution. A freak ecology is required to balance these freak "life forms."

The businesses that create these clones do so to maximize profits. Cloned microbes are used to accelerate food animals and vegetable growth, give them a cosmetically healthy appearance and allow poor quality produce to live until sale time. Cloning companies use massive bioreactor tanks to grow genetically altered microbes such as E. coli, bacillus, thuringiensis, methylococcus, thiobacillus, bdel-lovibrio, etc. These microbes are used in copper mining, to make plastic, treat telephone poles, prevent frost on oranges, in therapeutic baths, public water, etc. There is no agency policing, the military or any legal power to make Caucasian' freak users behave.

The ecology of planet earth is on a death course. African children are being terrorized with cloned vegetables, meat and dairy products, vaccines, environmental pollutants and synthetic drugs. They are chemical children that think, feel, behave and react under chemical freak influences. They are chemical freaks (hyperactive, learning disorders etc.,) controlled by freaks (junk foods, fairytale, psychologist etc.) Their holistic health degenerates with constant disease. This results in their being placed in Special Education classes (prison holding cells) leading them ultimately to be placed in elderly concentration camps called nursing homes.

It is the moral duty or curse of Africans to save their children and save this planet. There is no compromise with the curse. Either the African will give the planet ecological freedom or the Caucasians will continue to imprison the ecology with pollution and freaks. Africans cannot leave the fate of the planet on Natural, Karmic, Devine, Prana Laws or a Prophet to correct the polluted, off-balanced ecology. It is the responsibility of all African people to collect the Caucasian people because Africans are the living Natural, Karmic, Devine, Prana Laws and the living Prophets. The Africans' duty is to make the earth healthy so that the children can be healthy. Without a healthy planet, we cannot have a healthy culture.

A natural food diet gives us a healthy body which allows us to have a holistically healthy spirit, family and culture. Holistic health is a Blackener (Africanizer), while sickness and pollution of the ecology is a whitener. Health means to protect ourselves and protect our living quarters, called the earth. It is a matter of life or death. It is life of all living forms that is at stake. If Nutricide is not stopped, then Africans will not have the human body needed to live a spiritual life and to save this planet. It is an African Maat duty to stop Nutricide of the children and to confront the diseased Caucasians.

A Diet Without Chemicalized Meat is Healthier

A recent study conducted by several medical doctors, show that Seventh-Day Adventist, who do not eat meat for religious reasons have:

♦ 40% less coronary disease
♦ 400 % less death rate from respiratory diseases
♦ 100% lower mortality rate from all causes
♦ 1000% lower death rate from lung cancer
♦ 50% less dental caries among their children

The Homosexual Plague and Food

The Homosexual Disease is deliberately forced upon Africans by the junk food industry. Homosexuality is at an epidemic and plague level in African communities. Homosexuality is normal for the nature of the Caucasian, but a disease by African standards. Homosexuality and rap music are not an accepted part of hip-hop African culture. This plague is used to maintain male/female problems, spiritual sabotage, conflicts, divorces, single parents, sexually confused children and to destroy African people. The junk food industry is the main creator and promoter of the Homosexual Plague.

The junk food industry uses psychosexual packaging, sexual food shapes, hidden images of subliminal sexual intercourse with animals, homosexuals and children, suggestive images of masturbation and oral sex, erogenous body areas, and embedded sex curse words in advertisements.

They use sexual symbolism such as shadows, tunnels, hairstyles, landscape, hills, clouds, water and sexually suggestive language to sell junk foods. The synthetic chemicals and sex hormones in the foods stimulate the sex organs, body and mind. This causes stimulating, biochemical, addicting foods to be associated with stimulating sex. In other words, the African becomes chemically addicted to sex.

The synthetic junk foods can cause the corpus colostrum (mid brain) to malfunction and degenerate. This denatures and perverts the biochemical ability to harmonize the Left-Brain (Male Principle) and Right Brain (Female Principle). This limits the Africans' ability to bond harmoniously with the opposite sex, which can result in homosexual tendencies. In experiments, the biochemistry of vegetarian gorillas and monkeys was perverted when they were forced to eat junk food and meat. The perverted biochemistry combined with living in a type of European colonialism (science laboratory = ghetto) caused them to become homosexual.

Junk food perverted biochemistry causes physical diseases that can result in emotional/mental diseases which can lead to homosexuality. For example, diseases of the lungs can cause denial and fear, pancreas -lack of control; heart - irregular lifestyle; circulatory, high blood Pressure - mood swings; liver - unstable personality etc. Africans, biochemically perverted, combined with slavery trauma and colonialism, become easy prey for the junk sex (homosexuality) and junk food industry. They are deliberately taught homosexuality is acceptable and systemically seduced by Caucasian heterosexuality into homosexuality by commercials.

The hidden (subliminal) and obvious sex in the commercials is directed at the voluntary brain function, emotional mind and senses. The voluntary brain's intellectual mind may say that there is not sex hidden in the commercials, but the involuntary brain's emotions and senses respond to the sex. The Caucasian culture miseducates, indoctrinates and trains the senses to respond to their sexual nature. The food industry's use of sex hormones in foods, sexually stimulating colors, patterns, music, sex symbolism, masochism, sadism and shapes is selling homosexuality and their culture.

The sex is suggestive as well as sensual, such as penis-shaped hot dogs, candy bars, French fries, fish and breadsticks; the use of circles to symbolize the vagina such as donuts, pizzas, cheerios, round candies, or grapes/cherries for testicles; whip cream (semen) on pies (vagina); ice cream (semen) in a cone (vagina); melted cheese (semen) dripping from a pizza (vagina); liquid caramel or chocolate (semen) dripping on or from a candy bar (penis); a woman's lips (vagina) sucking on a drinking straw (penis); two ice cubes (testicles) and a straw (penis) in a glass (vagina), soda (semen) pouring out the neck (penis) of a bottle or an explosion to symbolize a climax, etc.

The leaf of lettuce on a hamburger sandwich symbolizes the fig leaf. The fig leaf was mythically placed over Adam and Eve's genitals. Lettuce is not put on a sandwich for nutritional reasons but for sexual stimulation. The African scientist's book *Isis Papers* by Frances Cress Welsing and a Caucasian book *Subliminal Seduction* by Wilson Bryan Key can give information on this subject.

The ancient heterosexual Caucasian cultures included homosexuality as part of normal heterosexual life. Today their mind scientists (i.e. psychiatrist, psychologist) classify homosexuality as normal and overeating as an eating disorder disease. Ancient European females/males had four simultaneous mates which were (and are) the (1) breeder - so-called spouse (2) prostitute (3) lover-homosexual mate (4) and concubine (girlfriend or boyfriend sex acquaintance). There are still remnants of these mating type relationships such as love/sex triangles and orgies (i.e. soap opera dramas).

The ancient Greek/Roman heterosexual males/females would attend sex exhibition/wrestling matches in the arenas/gymnasiums. They would select their homosexual partner by a "pat" on the buttocks. The "pat" on the buttocks used in sports activities is a homosexual gesture. In fact, Caucasians are still sexually attached to the buttocks. They measure each other's sexual ability by the movement and/or shape of the buttocks and are constantly looking at each other's buttocks. Caucasians find that in a brassiere the upper portion of the breast/cleavage resembles cleavage (part) in the buttocks. Therefore, the breasts are sexually exciting. Caucasians suck on each other's tongues (French kissing) because the tongue is sexually associated with the clitoris (lesbians) and penis (faggots). Junk food commercials use suggestive and subliminal homosexual symbolism of the buttocks, breast and the mouth to sexually arouse Africans and sell junk foods.

Homosexual behaviors are deeply woven into the fabric of heterosexuality. For example, women with dresses sit with their legs closed because in the past homosexual men in skirts sat with closed legs so that they would not reveal the size of their penis to possible lovers. In fact, Caucasian women basically dress themselves like men so that they can be sexually appealing to Caucasian men. Consequently, they wear G-string panties and bikini underwear and bathing suits because they were worn by homosexual men in ancient times. Caucasian women wear the ear, vaginal, nose, and navel rings as a form of homosexual bondage. They shave their legs and arms and wear lipstick to indicate that they are available for sex. It is the Caucasian involuntary that believes that the highest form of masculinity is male effeminate behavior. Therefore, the more male in dress and behavior the Caucasian woman is the more feministic. In other words, lesbianism is a high form of femininity and is attractive to the Caucasian male. Masters and Johnson's sex research indicates that homosexual fantasies are sexually arousing for Caucasian heterosexuals.

For more information on homosexuality a book such as *Love In Ancient Greece* by Robert Flaceliere can be helpful. Ancient homosexuals would kidnap young boys/girls during full moons and sodomize them as part of mating with them as a lover. This homosexual ritual was called a "honeymoon." Heterosexuals still use moonlight for sexual arousal. The ancient Caucasians, sexuality, rituals, customs, taboos, and ethics are based on their social laws called "The Law Of the Caves" which they erroneously call the "First Laws Of Nature," "Human Nature," "Nature" or "The Laws of the Jungle." There were no jungles in Ice Age Europe just caves. The Caucasian use the word "jungle" in reference to their society in order to inferiorize African culture, which makes their civilization, seem superior. They also get subliminal, perverted sexual stimulation with an imaginary hypersexed African savage by using the word jungle. Imaginary and subliminal homosexual themes surround their behaviors and heterosexuality.

The constant junk food commercialization of homosexuality is nutricidal. An African who eats nutricidal junk food is economically supporting the homosexual plague. The Africans with signs and symptoms of "Homosexual Exposure" are those in constant social contact with a peer, friend, associate or relative with the plague. Those exposed need treatments. Those with the homosexual plague need detoxification and the cure.

It is mandatory for the Homosexual cure that plague victims stop eating junk foods, attend an African Study Group and Female/Male Group regularly, abstain from sexually stimulating movies, songs, books, videos, dancing and games, stop using European sexual curse words, do not masturbate, abstain from heterosex for two to three months, stop all homosexual activities and sex, use an African spiritual system, practice Maat, avoid all personal and social relationships with homosexuals, use melanin-nourishing supplements/herbs, use a stress formula, use herbs to spiritually and physically cleanse the reproductive systems, use female/male herbal formulas, do a fast, be in constant (daily) contact with a detoxed homosexual mentor, take phenylalanine and chickweed (reduces craving), etc.

This Homosexual Plague must be stopped. It has invaded our religious, politics, entertainment fields, social life and children's classrooms. The Homosexual Mafia has developed political and economic power which allows them to force their sexual perversion upon innocent African victims of White Supremacy and Slavery Trauma. It is not the plague but the Caucasian plague carriers and predatory parasite culture that needs to be stopped by all means necessary.

The homosexuality, junk food addiction and control of Africans is based upon debt. Debt is caused by drug or synthetic food malnutrition, income taxes, loans, eating disorders, homosexuality, credit, mortgages, leases, etc. They make the African consumer dependent upon Caucasian society, sex, money or medicine in order to pay a homosexual sex craving, economic debt or nutritional debt. In the position of nutritional, sex or economic need (dependency) the African tax consumer or junk food consumer can be controlled. For example, the Caucasian international banker hoodlums (i.e. privately owned Federal Reserve) create the social conditions which cause the African to borrow money (ATM, credit cards) to buy junk foods and material goods that he is made to want (seasonin) by sex commercials/media debt.

The pharmaceutical cartel's nutrition-robbing drugs and the junk food Cartel's nutritionless junk foods cause the body to be in nutritional need –debt. Debt makes the tax/food consumer a perpetual slave (economic, sexual, biochemical, social) to White Supremacy (control). The African is biochemically controlled by Whites and is therefore an addict. An addict constantly pays for a fix that never fixes anything. The Caucasian drugs, surgery and medical system never restores the health stolen by drugs and junk foods, nor do the international bankers give back monies stolen by loans, taxes, usury, interest rates, and credit.

Africans in actuality do not pay taxes for earning Caucasian money (or property, stocks) but "rent" for using Caucasian money. The Caucasian own the money (backed by stolen gold, silver etc) and can devalue it and/or take it away from Africans illegally or legally any time they choose. Africans rent Caucasian money, the continent of Africa and all resources and goods while the Caucasians have ownership. Caucasian money is a paper credit card. Every time an African uses the debt is paid for by African human and land resources.

The sex, taxes and drugs are a costly, perverted form of a surrogate African family. Historically, the African family controlled food, sex, resources, produced and provided herbal medicine, spirituality, social order, education and protection. The Caucasian Junk Food Cartel and international bankers (White supremacists) take part of the Africans' wages (taxes) and say it is used to sponsor the government (Mother) which provides the resources and health system that the African continent, civilization and family cannot provide. It is the White Supremacists that military, politically, sexually, socially, nutritionally and economically use institutions and media to stop the African holistically governing (mothering) itself and the continent. If an African sees dis-eases, homosexuality and health as separated divided from politics, food commercials, economics and White Racism, then that African is conquered by White Supremacy. It is the creation of nutritional debt (results in dis-eases) and economic debt (taxes, loans, etc.) that causes addiction. Addiction is the alteration of the mind, biochemistry, economics, mood, social life and state of African consciousness that causes Nutricide.

Nutricidal white sugar is the main addicting drug of the sexual commercials. It has many nutritional debt-causing synthetics. White sugar is a psychotic mixture of pig blood, bleach, acids, antibiotics, carbon dioxide and sugar crystals. A combination of cheap, diseased scrap meat (TB, cancer, etc) of pigs and cattle is used to get blood albumin. Contaminated blood albumin is put in sugar to flush protein particles out of sugar beets/ sugar cane. The purpose of the sugar drug is to cause biochemical debt-addiction.

Aside from this, pork is used to make the sweetener aspartame (Nutrasweet, Sweet and Low, Equal). Pork sweeteners such as white sugar and aspartame help to create an unstable personality that can lead to homosexual characteristics. Caucasian commercials use homosexual symbolism, themes, rituals and ceremonies which bond the consumer to debt-causing sugar. The African is simultaneously made addicted to Caucasian society, economics, medicine, drugs sex, science, sugar, taxes and control (White Supremacy).

The junk food/International bankers' cartel's purpose is to addict Africans. Their ritual and ceremonial usage of foods and monies creates an addiction craving for the nutritional and economic debt. They are constantly creating this. Their psychosis, combined with their rituals and ceremonies (cosmology), is the basis for their avaricious dependency upon control. Control is the major symptom of their psychosis. White Supremacy is an outgrowth of the psychosis. A book such as *The Syndrome of Control* by Lindsey Williams can give some information on their psychosis and cosmology (worldview).

An African who attempts to borrow a healthy future with drug medicines is supporting debt-addiction. The food eaten is the only guarantee of health. Drug medicine and/or junk foods kill the body by creating a genetic nutritional debit. Natural food nourishes the body which allows the body to live. Natural vegetarian food is medicine and natural medicine is vegetarian food.

The Caucasian worldview is expressed by their use of nutrition, homosexuality, medicines, media, economics, government, junk food and diseases. Any relationship the African has with the Caucasians' parasite's cosmology is always one where —"the Blacks give and the Whites take." For example, the food/drug/bankers cartel's economic system is exclusively White only and built upon parasiting (i.e. taxes, credit commodities) money from African laborers, businesses, athletes, actors, singers (peasant class). For each dollar the peasant earns, the white nationalist Food/drug/bankers cartel earns at least 250 dollars. Seasonin Africans (Afropeans) believe that they can use the European economic system to gain money to spend on Black Nationalism (freedom for Africa and Africans). However, for each penny that is spent on Black Nationalism the White Nationalist spend indirectly and directly dollars on White Supremacy. The African in the white economic system is used as an indirect way for the whites to earn money for White Supremacy.

The Caucasian parasites' economic system has to be destroyed or Maat Economics (no usury) used in order for Africans to be socially, nutritionally sexually and economically free. An African who participates in their parasitic worldview must be seasonin and ultimately destroyed–Nutricide. Natural foods is a holistic way to get out of nutritional debt and free the body.

The sex stimulating food commercials create and maintain eating disorder dis-eases. Eating disorders are uncontrolled impulse and behavioral disorders that result in biochemical perversion that causes behavioral perversion Eating becomes a vicious cycle of controlled eating (dieting) then relapse into uncontrollable eating. Relapse can be triggered spiritually, mentally, physically, biochemically, socially, sexually and/or by food commercials. Most people with the dis-ease never know that they have it and if they do know, they never can stop eating continuously and/or sporadically. People with eating disorders eat to relieve stress, tension, racism, depression, anger, worry, anxiety, attention deficits and hyperactivity, have eating binges, weight-loss diet binges, have sex hormone attacks, abusively use laxatives, colonics, chewing gum, hide food, constantly eat at movies, sports events, while watching television, riding in cars or planes or subways, busses or trains, playing games at work, constantly eating health or junk food snacks, chewing gum, sucking on breath mints, drinking sodas, etc. They may have all these behaviors or a few and are in denial that they have an eating disorder. The food industry wants people to constantly eat so that they can constantly earn profits. With each craving for snacks and foods is attached the sexual signs and symbolism of homosexuality that is embedded in the subconscious mind (involuntary brain) by the heterosexually stimulating commercials. The commercials keep the diet out of order and the sexuality out of order. The African is simultaneously made addicted to junk food commercials (i.e. songs, phrases), junk foods, junk sex (homosexuality), etc. The combination of the sex commercials, synthetic addicting hormones and chemicals are holistically destructive. The combination of sex arousal stimulation of commercials and synthetic sex hormones in junk food bonded to the radiation in the junk makes homosexuality and heterosexuality and electromagnetic addiction. Food is radiated while being processed and by the price scanning radiation stimulation being associated with food craving, music, sex and colors. People crave radiation and many can not sleep unless their television/radio is on and radiating them. If you turn off the TV while they are asleep they will wake up because you took away their radiation drug. They crave the radiation stimulation due to its association with homosexuality. Psychosexual stimulation, craving and addiction of Africans is aimed towards homosexuality which makes it another aspect of Nutricide. This is Nutricide except it is called homosexuality.

African and Caucasian Sexual Beliefs

Caucasian	African
Surgery and chemicals can change your sex and redefine sexuality	Surgical and chemical sex organ mutilation cannot redefine sexual gender
A male / female that follows the sexual behavior of another gender becomes that gender	A monkey cannot follow the sexual practices of a lion and then call him / herself a lion
A woman's breast cleavage are sexually erotic because it resembles the cleavage of the buttocks	Buttocks are associated with bowel movements (Europeans associate the cleavage of the buttocks with the cleavage of the breast)
The behind (buttocks) are sexually erotic	The buttocks are associated with male homosexuality
Homosexuality is lifestyle choice	European "Seasonin" creates African self, mother, father, relationship and/or Black race hatred
Homosexuality is psycho-social	Homosexuality can be caused by synthetic chemicals or radiation which causes deterioration of corpus colostrum and/or damage to the smaller bundle of nerves in hypothalamus resulting in homomasturbators.
Sex drive	Reproductive drive
Genetic possibility for disease is normal /healthy	Genetic possibility for diseases is not normal. The genetic hybridization of disease is cloning people for disease industry
"Nature" is a non-cultural scientific term	The word "Nature" and "Science" are political and social terms of a culture. They are culturally based.
Evolution	Adaptation

Caucasian	African
Opposites Attract (man attracted to woman means one is opposite in sexuality)	Balance Attracts (man attracted to woman means both seek harmony / balance)
Homosexual	Homomasturbators (Same sex masturbators) antisexuals (the mouth, teeth, tongue and lips are made for eating, the anus is made to pass out manure)
Same sex intercourse	Only a female and male can have sexual intercourse (the penis enters the course (pathway) of the vagina

African Sex Organ, Energy and Movement

Female Sex Organs
> Inside body (Earth element)
>
> Close together
>
> Move East to West (Fallopian Tubes)

Male Sex Organs
> Outside (Testicles) and Inside (Prostate) = Air Element
>
> Far apart
>
> Move South to North (Scrotum and Testicles) move up and down

Caucasian Homosexuality Recruitment Techniques

❏ Homosexuals must constantly recruit or become extinct as a group

❏ Promoting sex change surgery and hormones as normal. It is mutilation of the sex organs with a knife or synthetic sex hormones.

❏ Women dressing in ancient Greek homosexual clothes (i.e. bikini, G-string, high heels, pony tail and pigtail hair styles suggest buttocks

❏ Fashion industry controlled by homosexuals = "Cross Dressing" = "Homosexual Dressing" (Zipper in front of ladies pants, bikini underwear for men - with no front flap, male boots for ladies, "unisex = homosex hair styles," etc.)

❏ Advertisements and commercials that focus on Buttocks (cleavage of breast is symbol of buttocks)

❏ Non-gender specific (cultural) dancing Homosexual

❏ Promoting heterosexual activity as violent or unstable (domestic crimes, rape, divorces, single parents, adultery, etc.)

❏ Sexual symbolic use of guns (penis), ball games (testicles) symbolism of baskets, holes and pool pockets as vaginas to be destroyed

❏ Homosexual themes in elementary school story books (i.e., *I Have Two Mommies*)

❏ Sex words that have no gender that are applied to homosexuality =

"Go to bed" "Make love" "Sleep together"

❏ Homophobia defines people that reject homosexuality as somehow mentally ill

❏ Songs, movies, soap operas, books and sexual crime news reportage used to create hyper sex and homosexuality as an outlet

❏ Heterosexuals presented as having many relationship problems, while presenting harmony in homosexual relationships

❏ Non-gender = Unisex = One Sex = Homosexual deodorant, perfumes (cologne) tattoos, ear and body rings, clothes, hairstyles and sports. (wrestling, boxing, basketball, baseball etc.)

❏ Advertisements and commercials that focus on:

- Non-reproductive sexual behavior projected as normal (masturbation, phone sex, watching sex stimulates homosexual eroticism)

❏ Women being called by Lesbians names = "Guys," "Man"(sexual cross-over language)

❏ Homosexuality explained as acceptable "Lifestyle Choice"

❏ Advertisements and commercials that focus on:

- Exercise equipment marketed with sex poses and homosexual symbols

- "Double Your Pleasure," showing fun between same sex - homosexual theme

- Homosexuals being idolized on TV shows, Talk Shows, etc.

- Drag Queen (Female) dressing by Black man = homosexual subliminals

❑ Job applications and tests for jobs are deliberately designed to cause homosexual ideation to score higher (i.e., The Brain Watchers, Martin L. Gross).

❑ Religious shows used to raise emotions and misdirect emotions by showing homosexuality as spirituality.

❑ Homosexuality pictured as a happy, normal life = GAY

❑ Advertisements and commercials that focus on:

- Beer with white head of foam (semen)

- Sexually shaped foods and candy

- Penis-shaped candy bars with nuts, named after men (i.e., Babe Ruth)

- Lip movements suggesting oral sex

- Hot dogs placed in between buns

Is Your Friend Ma Bell a Lesbian?

• Support of "homosexual marriage": According to *Diversity Digest*, a publication of AT&T's Information Research Center, the Lesbian, Bisexual and Gay United Employees at AT&T (LEAGUE) held a conference in which members were encouraged to "help devise a legal definition of marriage, so the company can work on extending domestic partner benefits to employees in states that do not recognize marriages between same-gender partners" *(Diversity Digest* August 1994, p. 10).

Homosexual activists often use the power of the government and media to try to force society to accept their behavior. But the homosexual lobby is also active in corporate America.

• Support of "The Gay Games": According to *Businessweek* magazine, AT&T helped sponsor a series of sporting events featuring 11,000 athletes and a budget of $6.5 million. *Businessweek* described the "Gay Games" as "less a series of sporting events than a nine-day celebration of culture, complete with parades, plays, music, art shows and food feasts" *(Businessweek* July 4, 1994, p. 38).

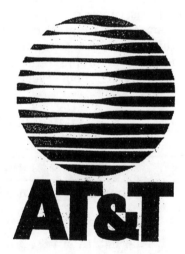

• Indoctrination of Employees: AT&T has held workshops and "diversity training" sessions in an effort to force employees to accept homosexuality. The company has used Brian McNaught's video, *On Being Gay* in these workshops. The video is filled with misleading claims and presents homosexuality as a normal, healthy lifestyle.

McNaught, who has done several workshops for AT&T, shows his bias against those who hold traditional religious values in his book, *Gay Issues in the Workplace.* McNaught links religious conviction with hate and bigotry. He suggests that people who hold strong religious convictions need "counseling" (p. 100). He shows contempt for those who hold traditional family values by suggesting that these values fuel "anti-gay bias.

Study Reports that Lesbians May Have a Higher Risk of Getting Breast Cancer

Lesbians may be at a greater risk of getting breast cancer than others, according to a study found in the Journal of the Gay and Lesbian Medical Association.

Three factors contributing to a higher breast cancer risk for lesbians are a lower pregnancy rate, higher weight and greater chance of having a biopsy.

Dr. Stephanie Roberts, the study's lead author, and colleagues examined medical records of 1,019 women at San Francisco woman's health clinic, according to the Chicago Sun-Times. Forty-Two percent were lesbians.

The study found that 63 percent of the lesbians had never been pregnant, compared to 17 percent of heterosexuals. Not having children increases a woman's breast cancer risk by between two to six times,

Lesbians are at a higher risk of getting breast cancer for another reason because higher weight, especially after menopause, increases breast cancer risk. The study, according to the article, found that lesbians weighed. On average 160 pounds, about seven pounds more that heterosexuals.

Homosexual Addiction

TREATMENT

- Must bond to African-defined sexuality (culture)

- Must have basic needs of spirituality, family, shelter, foods, health, and job met

- Must provide personality and sexual adjustment

- Counseling must be at arms length and not allow homosexual flirting, erotic gestures, jokes, and body movements must not be allowed.

- Abstinence from all homosexual-related activities, friends, and heterosexual intercourse

Homosexual Addiction

Steps In Treatment

1. Bond to Maat, African culture, and natural foods

2. Confront issues of sexual abuse of others, rape, incest, etc.

3. Identify activities, feelings, and thoughts that trigger homosexual feelings and sex activities

4. Confront emotional and spiritual issues concerning sperm abortion, child abortion, infertility, fibroids, and prostate disease

5. Heal relationship with self, family, friends, culture, etc.

6. Design method to change negatives to positives

7. Evaluate achievements (rewards, punishment, etc.)

8. Follow treatment schedule, goals, relapse therapy, etc.

9. Stay in constant contact with mentor (advisor) detox homosexual, study group, female/male group, etc.

Withdrawal Crisis

- Craving Addictor
  (Social, Emotional, Biochemical Triggers)
- Depression
  (Death of a behavior, Lifestyle, Friendship, etc.)
- Denial of Addiction/Disease
  (Alternative lifestyle, Genetic, Don't like opposite sex, etc.)
- Stressor Can Cause Relapse (Death, Out of work, Money problems, Alcohol, Drugs, White sugar, White supremacy)

Withdrawal Steps

Anxiety
Fear
**(Won't get better, Challenge of
heterosexual life, Rejection, etc.)**
Anger

Self Hatred   **Race Hatred**

Analyze Self   **Analyze Addiction**

Bond to Culture   **Co-Dependency**
(Reclaim African Life)   **(Reclaim European Sex Life)**

African Centered   **European Centered Alien Sexuality**

Life   **Death**

Homosexual Treatment / Detoxification

• **Diet**
No junk foods, alcohol, drugs
 • **Supplement**

Beta Carotene
DHEA
Evening Primrose Oil Cap-
sules Histidine
GABA
Glutamine
Manganese
Melatonin

Phenylalanine
Pumpkin Seed Oil Capsules
Glycine
Selenium
Serotonin
Tyrosine
Vanadium and Chromium
Vitamins A, C, E, B$_6$

Psycho social Treatment

Abstinence from heterosexual and/or homosexual intercourse
❑ Abstinence from sexual-related dancing, movies, songs, etc.
❑ Participation in African spirituality group, women's group,
    men's group, cultural group, study group
❑ Mentor (Sponsor): talk with daily. Mentor must have empathy
    and/or detox from homosexuality
❑ Positive support from family and/or peers
❑ Abstinence from socializing and/or activities with active homo-
    sexuals
❑ Meditation, Egyptian Yoga
❑ Abstinence from sexual-related "words" and clothes

Herbs

Bilberry	False Unicorn	Milk Thistle
Catnip	Feverfew	Pau d'Arco
Chamomile	Gingko	Sarsaparilla
Chaste Tree Berry	Golden Seal	Saw Palmetto
Chickweed	Gotu Kola	St. John's Wort
Echinacea	Ibogaine	
Elder	Kudzu	

Juice

Alfalfa	Cherry	Papaya
Beet	Currant	Pineapple
Burdock	Kelp	
Celery	Lemon	

Factors

❑ In recorded history is a practice of European civilization
❑ Is directly and indirectly (sublime) a part of European heterosexual activities
❑ Social conditions (engineering) creates homosexuality
(schoolbooks, movies, television, clothes, organizations, etc.)
❑ Is a sign and symptom of European caused
- Slavery Trauma
- Cultural Stress
- Population Control (Genocide)
- Dysfunctional Genders, Relationships and Families
❑ Is part of Africans trying to be accepted by Whites a form of self-hatred and hatred of Africa co-dependency psychosis
❑ Homosexuality is a disease for Africans but normal for Europeans

Science and Addiction

Chemistry is the science of studying the activity of chemicals called elements which are the building blocks for living and so-called "non-living" things. Elements such as carbon, hydrogen, sulfur and phosphorus form atoms which join together to form molecules. Each element is a universe within itself that has a type of family structure. The way the chemist's kinship group sees the world and the family is reflected in his group's science of chemistry. The Caucasian scientist, in order to understand chemicals, first destroys the elemental family with heat or another form of energy. He does not study elements in their natural environment. Instead he studies them in an artificial environment called a laboratory.

The Caucasian scientist can only gain knowledge by destruction of Afrika and Afrikan people. The more destruction the Caucasians produce, the more "scientific" and wealthy they become. Scientists act out their superstitious rituals, ceremonies and world in a laboratory by exploiting chemicals. No scientist can divorce himself from his group's worldview. They cannot become "objective." This is a human impossibility. The Caucasian labels his destructive biochemical alterations, rituals and ceremonies as science.

In the food industry, Caucasians use the science of chemistry to destroy the natural nutrients of food by processing foods into biochemically-altered food "stuffs." Food "stuffs" (drugs) are sold by fast-"food" chains, sugar refineries, dairy, meat, fish, soda, snack and flour mill industries. The destruction of food creates diseases. Diseases create wealth for the Disease Industry (i.e. hospitals, pharmaceuticals, doctors, laboratories, etc). The "food"/disease industries cannot be separated anymore than can technology/pollution. You cannot have one without the other.

In order to change the food industry or any part of Caucasian society, the foundation has to be changed. Caucasian rituals, ceremonies, theories and myths would have to be changed. African victims are addicted to Caucasian rituals, ceremonies, theories and myths which are erroneously called science, law, economics, nutrition and culture. Caucasian-based thought and behavior are hazardous to African people.

Alimentary canal   food processing plant

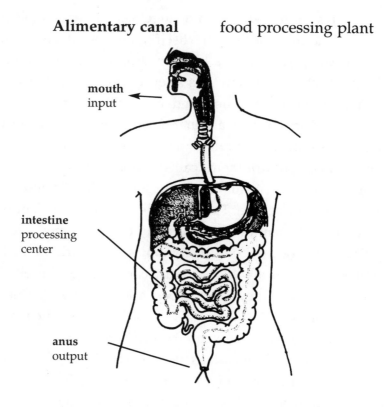

Processed food is synthetic manure dirt. The machines and synthetic chemicals in the food-processing factory imitate the liver, pancreas, digestive enzymes, stomach, intestine, colon and rectum. These machines chemically and mechanically chew and digest (process) the food which means they take away the foods nutrients and fiber. The end result of your body digesting (processing) and eaten apple is a processed food called feces, manure, a bowel movement or scat (also named given to a type of jazz singing). A processed food by definition is a bowel movement. Bleach White flour, White rice, white sugar, oil and white grits are a processed bowel movement of a factory. These are waste by products of a factories digestion-a foodstuff, food contraband, starvation food, etc.

Alimentary canal   food processing plant

mouth
input

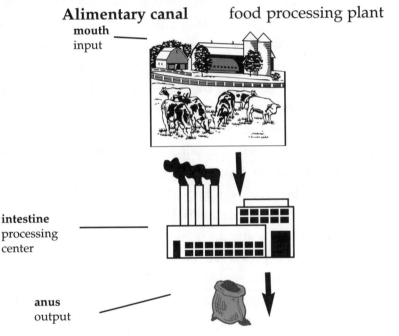

intestine
processing
center

anus
output

Caucasians have been a historically toxic people. For ages they have turned natural foods into synthetic chemicals, chemically altering them. They use chemistry to invade countries and to control people. They used alcohol on the Native "Americans," opium on the Chinese and alcohol, marijuana, heroin and cocaine on Afrikans. Caucasians have been (and are) addicted to synthetic chemicals such as sugar, nicotine, caffeine, salt, cocaine, vinegar, oil, opium, valium, amphetamines, etc. They are addicted to the taste of burnt dirt as in Bar-B-Q. They are addicted to rotten food such as cheese, yogurt, buttermilk, beef jerky, rancid oil salad dressing and sauces, hardtack (dried fish), beer (fermented-rotten hops), wine (fermented-rotten grapes) as well as the rotten cooked blood and pus of juicy steaks, chicken, pork, etc. Historically, Caucasians ate many foods based upon them smelling like urine and/or feces (manure). For example cucumbers were eaten because they smell like semen, roasted animals smell like rotten decomposing human bodies, asafetida smells like farts, cabbage smells like salted fish, some cheeses and onions smell like human feces, tobacco resembled the smell like rotten urine, vinegar similar to sweat or an unclean vagina (sexually erotic to Caucasian), fish similar to vaginal yeast infection etc. The more food is corrupted, i.e. made rotten, processed, synthesized, burnt or smoked, the more they like it.

Ironically, the more the Afrikan is destroyed (Europeanized), the more the Caucasians like them. A likeable Afropean (Negro) is mentally and behaviorally processed (seasoned). They are drugged and fermented (rotten Afrikans). Negroes live on **junk** "foods." Negroes are biochemically altered slaves serving White slave masters or searching for White masters to serve. Most of them worship Caucasian **junk** science i.e. biology, chemistry, nutrition, etc.

Synthesized "foodstuffs" (**junk**) cause mental and physical changes in children and babies. Babies have undeveloped immune systems while the elderly have deteriorated immune systems. This causes synthetic chemicals to be twice as harmful and addicting to these age groups. Biochemically altered newborn babies are born with diseased bodies because their parents' sperm, uterus, ovaries, and bodies were cesspools of synthetic chemical waste as a result of eating **junk** "foods," taking drugs and being vaccinated. Many babies are born as sugar addicts, alcoholics, sex hormone drunkards, and cocaine addicts and are severely biochemically altered.

They can be addicted to toxic substances because of the biochemical trauma of Cesarean section (C-section/birthing interrupts). Biochemically altered and C-section/interrupts babies are prone to have emotional problems, allergies, learning problems, asthma, self-control deficiencies, suffer hyper-sex and lack the ability to bond to parents and to Afrikan culture. Biochemically-altered "foods" processed into **junk** food "stuff" are starvation "foods." They lack over 90% of their natural vitamins, minerals, proteins and fibers. They are especially low in a B vitamin called thiamin. Thiamin, along with the B complex (family), is needed to control moods, violence, aggression etc.

Junk food "stuff" has synthetic toxic dyes such as red and yellow food coloring. Food coloring irritates the brain and causes allergic reactions. Meats (including fish) are biochemically altered with nitrates. Nitrates cause mental illness, hyperactivity and violent moods. Biochemically altered "foods" are addicting and cause a craving for the same synthetic chemical (drug) eaten. For example, an alcoholic craves alcohol. The biochemically-altered child is addicted to and craves sugar, hormones, salt, nitrates, carbon and other synthetic chemicals. A child in a state of craving will be illogical in thought, emotion and spirit. They are going through food "stuff" withdrawal and need another synthetic chemical fix.

Biochemically altered children are usually raised by biochemically altered parents who live for the next synthetic chemical fix. They are continuously getting high off food, in withdrawal, or between fixes. They and their children have junk "food" eating binges (Mac attacks). They are driven to take synthetic chemicals for headaches, pain, stress, constipation, energy, weight, fatigue, birth control, sleep, rashes, indigestion, colds, etc. It is these chemical people who decide that say it does not matter whether you eat junk food or not cause you're gonna die from "something." Then they proceed to die from a "something" disease. Some synthetic, chemically caused addictions and diseases are less obvious but just as deadly.

Irradiation of food is dangerous. Irradiation is the use of toxic radiation chemicals to "preserve" foods. Radiation causes disease such as cancer. Radiation-sprayed foods store low level radiation. Irradiation destroys electrically positive charged protein amino acids such as arginine and lysine. Lysine is used to help stop infections and arginine is used in reproduction. Radiation halts the cell's ability to live, protect itself and reproduce. Radiation, coloring and preservatives create deadly combinations. Preservatives are tasty forms of embalming fluids used on dead bodies (corpses). They retard cell and brain activity. Preserved (embalmed) Afrikans move from chattel slavery to synthetic, chemical slavery.

Biochemically altered people are "seasoned." They sing or rap junk food jingles that praise the tasty goodness of poisonous chemicals such as carbonated sodas. This is ironic, because the lungs exhale in order to get rid of carbon waste produced by the digestion of foods. Afrikans are "seasoned" to drink carbon waste. Their minds and behavior are "seasoned" by commercials to practice the direct opposite of health, i.e. disease. The slaves were "seasoned" to like the White man and the instruments he used to destroy their women, children, culture and country.

A "seasoned" biochemically altered Afrikan has thoughts that take a chemical chain reaction response to ideas spoken by others. The synthetic chemicals in the body and brain cause reception of stimuli to be misdirected, misreceived, misinterpreted, refracted or blocked. For example, the sound of music may cause sex stimulation, sex may cause violence, violence may trigger a euphoric high, a high may trigger homosexuality, and the sight of the elderly may trigger hate.

Afrikan culture may trigger fear, fear may trigger denial of slavery, learning may trigger self-hate, etc. The nerves are saturated with synthetic chemicals in the food that is craved. The biochemically altered Afrikan reacts to artificiality and not to reality. Synthetic chemicals stop melanin usage. This causes Afrikans to mimic Caucasian thinking and behavior. In other words, they act unnatural, unreal and crazy in normal social situations. They get chemical stimulation from many sources.

The biochemically altered African is a walking time bomb of diseases and mental confusion who may have illogical, emotional, spiritual, mental and/or disease outbursts from the cyclic behavior of synthetic chemicals. Even water can be biochemically altered. Public drinking water is basically chemically deodorized, ammonia treated, bleached and fluoridated toilet water. Fluoride stimulates passive, docile behavior. It also destroys teeth and irritates nerves. Chemicals in antiperspirant deodorants stop the glands from working normally (i.e. pineal, uterus, prostate, adrenals, eyes, etc).

Toothpaste contains bleach (peroxide) or salt (baking soda) which denatures the nerves, bones, digestion, etc. Aside from this, the toothpaste does not protect the teeth. The chemical additives in digestive "aids" stop digestion. Therefore, they cause toxins to build, accumulate and contribute to mood swings and constipation. Additives in cold, cough, asthma and antihistamine "remedies" slow down and retard glands and the normal mucus secretion of the uterus, prostate, etc.

Any chemical that stops, slows down, or builds waste constipates the brain. Afrikans get negative chemical stimulation from the toxic chemicals of microwaves, cellular phones, low frequency radio stations, lasers, computers, television screens etc. *No "benefit" of Caucasian "science" come without destruction.* The "benefit" and "destruction" of biochemical alteration and Caucasian "civilization" cannot be separated. You cannot have one without the other. For example, a "seasoned" Afrikan who learns to obey Caucasian rules simultaneously learns to disobey Afrikan rules, especially of nutrition culture. A "seasoned" Afrikan who is taught and supervised by Whites is simultaneously being taught not to be supervised by Blacks. It is built into Caucasian rituals and ceremonies. You cannot have one without the other. However, there is an alternative.

Whole foods (health foods, natural foods) should be the diet of Afrikans. Natural foods establish the nutritional foundation for a healthy mind, spirit and body. Before slavery and colonialism, America-born Afrikans ate natural foods, thought about natural foods, talked about natural foods and imaged them.

Natural foods are central to freedom. Afrikans must be able to image and talk about the natural foods they should eat. Afrikans image by thinking in pictures. A whole picture image gives mental, spiritual and cultural meaning to ideas, events, food, herbs and history. Afrikan written language is a whole picture image language which includes a spiritual symbol, action symbol and phonic (sound) symbol. The foods that ancient Afrikans ate were whole foods and their whole picture language described the food. The American-born Afrikans should be able to image the preparation of natural foods. These foods must be imaged with delight.

Others in the family such as babies, pregnant women, the sick or the elderly must be able to eat without harm. Therefore, the family should be the first consideration in Afrikan food technology. The traditional Afrikan family did not eat foods that could harm a baby, i.e. alcohol, salt, vinegar, grease, sugar, rotten food, animal blood, pus and flesh, as well as cooked concoctions. These foods "stuffs" harm God's Temple–the human body. The ability to image natural foods in a natural environment was destroyed by the institution of slavery and colonialism. This started the perversion of the taste buds. "Seasoning" perverted our appetites and television images of "food" continue the process.

A natural foods diet can stop the chain of synthetic chemical addictions and disease. Afrikans who eat whole foods free of synthetics will no longer be a biochemical altered people who serve the slave masters synthesized food, and disease. Afrikans on a natural food diet will bring an end to genocidal nutrition (Nutricide) and regain control of their community, country and culture.

European Medical Superstition versus African Truth

European Lie	African Truth
◆ Energy is *transformed*	= Living things grow and then die, they are not physically transformed, spirit energy never transforms
◆ Salt (Baking Soda)– is a deodorant and good for teeth	= Salt weakens skin and teeth
◆ Science is racially neutral, non-cultural	= Science and Art are political and social languages of a culture.
◆ Disease is caused by old age and bacteria	= There are old people with diseases
◆ Body attacks itself–(autoimmune)	= Body cleanses itself of impurities (so-called attack)
◆ Heart attack	= Poor health destroys the heart, the heart does not destroy itself.
◆ Catch a Cold	= You cannot catch the weather (i.e. catch hot, catch partly cloudy etc.)
◆ Ritalin—improves intelligence and attention	= Proven to deteriorate intelligence.
◆ Virus (dead cell particle) is alive causes diseases	= Synthetic chemicals and nutritional deficiency causes disease.

European Lie	African Truth
◆ Weight loss—exercise muscles will reduces fat	= Diet reduces fat.
◆ Plants eat dirt	= Plants gain electromagnetic and chemical stimulation from dirt not food.
◆ Homosexuals can have sex	= Only male and female have sex intercourse.
◆ Free radicals causes diseases which can be prevented by antioxidants	= Both are theories (science fantasy)
◆ High Blood Pressure medicine can grow hair	= Dilates pores of scalp.
◆ Synthetic Dirt (Drugs) can cure disease by poisoning the body	= Healthy foods and herbs cure.
◆ Plant cell can become human cell	= Plants cells stimulates human cells and corpuscles.
◆ Body is a slave to serve man	= Body is a holy temple, you serve it.
◆ Cross-linkage	= A dead cell can unite with a healthy cell. (cross link)
◆ Cell division	= Corpuscles divide cells have a nerve attached and blood supply attached to nerve. They grow from a melanin template called a stole.
◆ Modern technology improves health and civilization	= Family structure improves civilization.
◆ Teeth are white	= Teeth are yellow bones, all bones are yellow.
◆ Disease is a mechanical body process	= Disease is holistic cleaning.
◆ Blood brain barrier	= Blood does not have a liquid floating barrier wall

European Lie	African Truth
◆ Vaccination kills germs	= **Vaccination fluids cause germs to grow**
◆ Inertia	= **All things in motion.**
◆ Law and Balance	= **Nothing is in balance (oceans of the world, vegetation distribution, left and right side of the body).**
◆ Sex drive	= **Reproductive drive (instinct)**
◆ Evolution	= **A physical characteristic must already be present in the body before it can be adopted. It does not evolve.**
◆ Law of Conservation	= **Animals, plants, and people are destroyed (extinct) not conserved.**
◆ Theory of relativity—Living things move uniform and rectilinear motion and on the same plane	= **There is no uniform movement, only rhythmic cyclic type.**
◆ Lotion makes skin smooth	= **Skin becomes smooth to touch from oil in lotion.**
◆ Sheep fat (lanolin) makes hair curly	= **Fantasy belief.**
◆ Chewing gum can save teeth	= **Good nutrition saves teeth, people with cavities, chew gum.**
◆ Antacid helps digestion by stopping digestion	= **Contradiction in logic.**
◆ Race (Melanin) is not important in treatment	= **Contradicts field of Ethnomedicine.**
◆ Eat muscle to grow muscles	= **Eat amino acids and build muscle by stimulation.**
◆ Transplanted organs and bones solve medical failures	= **If medicine were successful transplantation would not be necessary.**

	African Truth
♦ Miscarriage and birth defects are caused solely by women	= **Both parents create and/or defect a child.**
♦ Diagnosis of women and children are the same as men	= **Symptoms vary with gender and age.**
♦ Human growing is same	= **Hair, teeth and bones grow the same. The root, center is alive while outer part is dead. Cells replace themselves, build a new Melanin template called a Stole and then cell Mass.**

Weight, Over Waste (Overweight) And Lies

Another lie in health is the Caucasian worldwide-distributed normal body weight chart formulated in 1959 by insurance companies. The Caucasian false standard of normal weight is racistly applied to Africans. This is in direct contradiction to the facts that Caucasians generally have more muscle mass (big calves, big thighs and flat buttocks muscles) while Africans tend to have less muscle mass and more skin surface (due to longer arms and legs). This means Africans have a greater ability to cool themselves in hot weather. Caucasians as compared to other races have the least amount of skin pores, the most bodily hair added to a larger muscle mass tend to have more bodily heat and lack the ability to be cool in hot weather.

An overweight person can have excess water retention (edema) or an overwaste (overweight) person can have 7 to 15 pounds of feces, caked, impacted or coated in the digestive tract. An obese person has excess bodily fat. Therefore, a person can be overweight and have obesity.

The insurance companies set the normal weight tables at a low weight per height ration. This causes many people to be declared over weight, an overweight person's insurance rate is higher. It was to the insurance companies economic advantage to falsify weight tables.

The normal weight table was reformulated in 1990 to reflect the true weight for height of Caucasians. However, the vast majority of Caucasian health practitioners and drug companies still use the 1959 tables. This helps them to classify more people as ill and helps them to increase the amount and strength of drugs prescribed to a person.

Comparison between the 1959 and 1990 tables
Weight Chart

Height (no shoes)	1959 Ages (25 and older)		Weight (no clothes) (19-34)	1990 Ages (35 and up)
	Women	Men		
5'0"	103-115 -		97-128	108-138
5'1"	106-118	111-122	101-132	111-143
5'2"	109-122	114-126	104-137	115-148
5'3"	112-126	117-129	107-141	118-152
5'4"	116-131	120-132	111-146	122-157
5'5"	120-135	123-136	114-150	126-162
5'6"	124-139	127-140	118-155	130-167
5'7"	128-143	131-145	121-160	134-172
5'8"	132-147	135-149	125-164	138-178
5'9"	136-151	139-153	129-169	142-183
5'10"	140-155	143-158	132-174	146-188
5'11"	143-158	147-163	136-179	151-194
6'0"	147-162	151-168	140-184	155-199
6'1"	152-167	155-173	144-189	159-205
6'2"	156-171	160-178	148-195	164-210
6'3"	160-176	165-183	152-200	168-216

Cancer Foods

National Academy of Sciences, the following 15 pesticide, herbicide and chemically contaminated foods were found to cause the greatest cancer risk

1. tomatoes (catsup, salsa and tomato sauces in Italian and Mexican dishes)
2. beef (burgers, steaks, roasts and processed meat)
3. potatoes (potato chips, fries and baked potatoes)
4. oranges (orange juice and marmalade)
5. lettuce (salads)
6. apples (apple juice, sauces, dried apples and apple butter)
7. peaches (jams and sweetener)
8. pork (chops, bacon links, lunch meat and sausages)
9. wheat (most breads, bakery goods and crackers)
10. soybeans (tofu, dressing, soy oil, lecithin, mayonnaise and most bakery items with soy oil)
11. pinto beans (refried beans, soups and Mexican dishes)
12. carrots (carrots juice, salads, soups and baby food)
13. chicken (fried chicken, soups, chicken sandwiches and baked chicken.
14. corn (fresh, frozen, canned, cornmeal, corn tortillas, cornbread and corn chips)
15. grapes (fresh raisins, jellies and fruit concentrates widely being used in natural foods)

Food Medicine

Healing Ingredient	Benefit	Foods that contain it are:
Allylic sulfides	*dissolves cholesterol, protects against carcinogens*	Garlic
Allphalinolenic acid	*Reduces inflammation and enhances the immune system*	Flaxseed, soy products, purslane walnut
Carotenoids	*fights cancer, reduce plaque*	Parsley, carrots, winter squash, sweet potatoes, yams, cantaloupe, apricots, spinach, kale, turnip greens, citrus fruits
Catechins	*fights gastrointestinal cancer*	lower cholesterol, Green tea, berries
Coumarins	*prevents blood clotting, helps High Blood Pressure, anticancer activity,*	Parsley, carrots, citrus fruits
Flavonoids	*decreases cancer*	Parsley, carrots, citrus fruits, broccoli, cabbage, cucumbers, squash, yams, tomatoes, eggplant, peppers, soy products, berries
Gamma-glutamyl allyic cysteines	*lowers High Blood Pressure and enhances immune system*	Garlic
Indoles	*normalizes estrogen action PMS*	Cabbage, brussel sprouts, kale
Isothiniocyanates	*stimulates liver, helps blood pressure*	Mustard, horseradish, radishes
Limonoids	*alkalines, has enzyme action*	Citrus fruits
Lycopene	*fights cancer and its progression*	Tomatoes, red grapefruit

Healing Ingredient	Benefit	Foods that contain it are:
Monoterpenes	*fights cancer fighting antioxidants that inhibit cholesterol production and aid protective enzyme activity*	Parsley, carrots, broccoli, cabbage, cucumbers, squash, yams, tomatoes, eggplant, peppers, citrus fruits
Phenolic acids	*fights cancer, blood cleanser*	Parsley, carrots, broccoli, cabbage, tomatoes, peppers, citrus fruits, whole grains, berries
Phthalides	*detoxify carcinogens, blood cleanser*	Parsley, carrots, celery
Plant sterols	*block estrogen promotion of breast cancer activity decreases cholesterol*	Broccoli, cabbage, cucumbers, squash, yams, tomatoes, eggplant, peppers, soy products, whole grains
Polyacetylenes	*fights carcinogens help regulate prostaaglandin production*	Parsley, carrots, celery
Triterpenoids	*prevents decay; fights cancer*	Citrus fruits, licorice-root extract, soy products

Seasoning For Food

You can use your seasonings as a medicine and taste.

Use about one-eight to one-quarter teaspoon of herbal spices for every 4 servings. For a combination of herbs and spices, approximately one-quarter teaspoon of each herb and one-quarter to one-eight teaspoon of spice for every 4 servings. For example, you may try quarter teaspoon dill seed and quarter teaspoon dry mustard on vegetables, or you may try quarter teaspoon basil, and one-eight teaspoon of garlic powder in soy burgers/meat substitutes.

The following is an example of seasonings which that can be used on foods.

Asparagus	-Lemon juice, dry mustard, marjoram, sesame seed, tarragon, pepper, thyme.
Beef-	-Bay leaf, basil, dry mustard, nutmeg, green pepper, sage, marjoram, onion, pepper, thyme, dill seed, oregano, caraway, garlic, parsley, rosemary, savory, tumeric, allspice, celery seed.
Beets-	-lemon juice, dill, cloves, allspice, ginger, savory, thyme, pepper.
Broccoli-	-Lemon juice, pepper, caraway seed, dry mustard, nutmeg, basil, curry, oregano, garlic.
Cabbage and Cauliflower-	-Lemon juice, caraway seed, dill seed, cumin, allspice, celery, seed, mace, mint, dry mustard, savory, tarragon, oregano, parsley, rosemary, pepper.
Carrots-	-parsley, cinnamon, lemon juice, allspice, nutmeg, mint, bay leaf, caraway seed, dill seed, ginger, mace, thyme, marjoram, pepper.
Corn-	-Green pepper, onion, paprika, pepper, curry.

Eggplant-   -Lemon juice, onion, bay leaf, pepper.

Eggs-   -Basil, curry, dry mustard, green pepper, onion, paprika, parsley, nutmeg, cardamon, pepper.

Fish-   -Bay leaf, basil, curry, cumin, dry mustard, green pepper, lemon juice, paprika, marjoram, allspice, fennel, mace, onion, nutmeg, tumeric, parsley, sesame seed.

Fruits and Fruit Desserts -Allspice, cinnamon, cloves, ginger, mace, mint, nutmeg, vanilla, or herbal extracts.

Greens-   - Lemon juice, onion, allspice, pepper.

Lima Beans-   -Sage, lemon juice, chives, pepper, onion.

Oira-   -Lemon juice, pepper, onion.

Onion-   -Caraway seed, nutmeg, oregano, sage, thyme, pepper, basil, marjoram.

Macaroni and Noodles- -Allspice, onion, poppy seed, dill seed, whole grain, green pepper.

Peas, Green- -Onion, mint, sage, rosemary, parsley, savory, green pepper, basil, oregano, poppy seed, lettuce leaf, pepper, garlic.

Potatoes-   -Onion, basil, mace, parsley, paprika, bay leaf, green pepper, chives, celery seed, oregano, poppy seed, rosemary, thyme, pepper, garlic, mint nutmeg.

Poultry-   -Bay leaf, cranberries, thyme, paprika, parsley, green peppers, sage, curry, dill seed, pepper, ginger, marjoram, nutmeg, tarragon.

Rice-   -Tumeric, cumin, allspice, nutmeg, cinnamon, onion, green pepper, pepper.

Spinach-   -Lemon juice, onion, allspice, basil, mace, oregano, pepper.

Squash-   -Ginger, mace, allspice, onion, basil, cinnamon, cloves, nutmeg, fennel, rosemary, pepper.

String Beans- -Marjoram, lemon juice, nutmeg, savory, dill seed, thyme, dry mustard, oregano, onion, caraway seed, sage, garlic, pepper.

Tomatoes-   -Basil, marjoram, thyme, onion, lemon juice, oregano, green pepper, pepper, caraway seed, sage, sesame seed.

Herb Seasoning for Dis-ease

Allspice   - digestion gas, diabetes, stimulant

Anise   - digestion, liver, colic, tonic, colds, spasm

Basil   - rheumatism, cramps, vomiting, mucous

Chervil   - swellings, edema, diuretic, eczema, gout

Cinnamon - diarrhea, poliomyetis, upset stomach

Coriander - stomach tonic, digestion problems, rheumatism, joint pain

Dill   - indigestion, gastritis croup, nausea

Fennel   - laxative, diuertic, digestion, sores

Garlic   - hypertension, infections, High Blood Pressure, worms

Ginger   - nausea, cramps, meningitis, edema

Horseradish - dysmenorrhea, High Blood Pressure, diuretic, arthritis

Kelp   - thyroid, goiter

Marjoram - headaches, acidity, colds, measles, nervousness

Mustard - gastritis, liver, rheumatism, digestion

Oregano   - leukorrhea, colds, headaches, asthma, tonic

Paprika   - sinus trouble, colds

Parsley   - diuretic, dropsy, edema, colds

Pepper   - neuralgia (nerve pain)

Rosemary - colds, arthritis, memory, digestion, spasm

Sage   -sores, bleeding wounds, depression, stops sweating, sore throat

Savory   - ear trouble, colds, digestion, stimulant

Thyme   - headaches, colds, hypothyroidism, worms, loss of appetite, diarrhea

Turmeric - fever, colds, skin problems, diuretic, high blood pressure

Vanilla   - digestion, gas, neurasthenia (sooth nerves)

Nutritional Approach

- Eat raw whole food, such as fruits, vegetables, grains, beans.
- Food should be eaten FRESH and RAW.
- Eat whole grains and lightly steamed vegetables.
- Dark green leafy vegetables and the juice of dark green leafs should be eaten generously.
- No dairy products. No fried food.
- No animals. No fish. No fowl. Dead food produces dead cells.
- Use fresh, raw, organically grown garlic if possible.
- Do not take drugs of any kind. No prescribed, over - the counter or street drugs.
- Drugs destroy the immune system.
- Herbal extracts and teas go directly to your bloodstream and work better and faster than pills and capsules.

Blood Cleansers

Burdock

Dandelion Root

Elecampane (lung congestion and blood)

Garlic (for white blood cells)

Green vegetables

Milk Thistle (protect liver and blood)

Pleurisy (lung congestion and blood)

Red Clover

Wheat grass juice (for red blood cells) Spirulina

Wormwood (parasites, worms)

Immune System Builders

Spirituality = helps utilize Gods help

Exercise - the best immune system builder

Garlic (antibiotic, parasites)

Vitamin C (-25,000-60,000mg (300/2hrs.) (infection)

Echinecea extract (infection)

Grape Seed Extract (infection)

Pine Bark extract (colds, infection)

Yohimble extract (energy reproductive organs, female use with Diamiana)

Goldenseal extract (good for all types diseases)

Vitamin E -up to 800 I.U./day

Ginseng (energy)

Lecithin - for the nerves

Lysine 1000mg (infection, herpes)

Fotin (energy)

Ginger (digestion, edema)

Glutathione (removes cellular waste)

Creatine (build healthy tissue)

Skin
MSM tablets and lotion
Lysine creme
Zinc creme
Yeast Infection
Pau D Arco

Sleep

Valerian	Kava
Catnip	Passion Flower
Chamomile	Hops

Digestive Enzyme
Tablets =improves metabolism of supplements, herbs and food.

Medicine Food

White Folks Thinking

The African peoples have been taught an unreal idea of how the Caucasian mind is psychologically structured. In psychology Africans must follow the Maat principle which clearly states that we must know and separate the real from the unreal. A children's story be it in English (fairy tale) or Latin (myths) is not real it is unreal (Fantasy, fiction, decorated lie).

Sigmund (Sickman) Freud helped to establish the unreal idea of the Caucasian mind. He used a Caucasian children's fairy tale/folktale for the foundation of their mind. He decided that each character in a story represented a fragment of their mind (i.e. Oedipus, conscious, subconscious, ego, id, superego etc.) This is similar to watching an animated children's cartoon or movie and saying the cartoon characters represent the true and pure psychological aspects of the mind and entire races mind-way of thinking.

A Caucasian Greek/Roman myth is a story in which the characters have Latin/Greek names. If the characters in the myth (story) had English names the myth would be called a children's fairy tale or folk tale. The Caucasian mind does not function like a fairy tale. A fairy tale does not explain the Caucasian mind.

Sigmund (Sickman) Freud made up the idea of a Caucasian mind. Therefore, the Caucasians idea of their mind and how their mind functions is totally unreal. It is a fantasy. An idea or scientific fact based on a fantasy is a fantasy. If you use a lie to explain a lie then what you are saying is a lie. A real idea of the Caucasian mind and how it functions can be obtained by a historical examination of their past behavior, family structure and the way they treat each other and African peoples. History more than anything reveal the real mind of the Caucasian.

If I were to tell you that the African mind is based upon and functions the same way as the characters in Cinderella or Goldilocks and Three Bears you would clearly see the absurdity of their psychology. The Caucasian mind structure based on a fairy tale/myth is in itself crazy. It is from this Freudian Psychological construct (foundation) of craziness (mental illness) that the Caucasian explains their mind and their mental illness (craziness). Their mental illnesses are in itself a craziness based upon a craziness which maintains a level of craziness. The absurdity of this situation is that African peoples use Caucasian fairy tale psychology to understand the psychology of the Black mind. They use it to find the solution to their own problems as well as their problems with the Caucasian peoples. This means that any solution Africans derive for overthrowing White Supremacy, Oppression, Colonialism, White Domination and White Racism will fail. Build into any solution that uses Caucasian fairy tale psychology will be the craziness of the unreal (fairy tale). A real problem (White Supremacy) cannot be solved with an unreal psychological solution (fairy tale craziness).

Chapter Five
Chemical Madness

"At some point—like right away—we are going to have to deal with the destructive effects of fast food, TV, integration and village breakdown…"

Kiarri T-H. Cheatwood

Chemical Madness

Deficient Junk Food Diet Increase
Life Expectancy Decrease

Average Life Expectancies at Birth

The maps show countries where the average life expectancy at birth is within the age limits stated below. The graph show the percentage of the total world population born in countries belonging to the different groups.

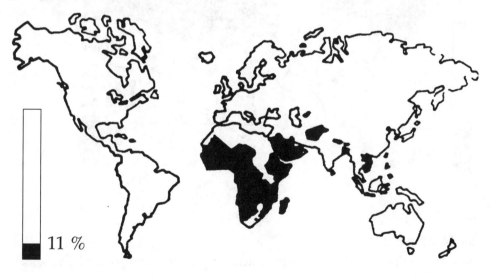

11 %

38-46 years

Developing countries in Africa and Southeast Asia have the lowest average life expectancy figures. This is related to the nutrient poor diets, synthetic chemicalized food and Caucasian land control in Africa.

List of some African countries in the 38 to 46 years Life Expectancy Group

Mauritania, Senegal, Mali, Guinea, Sierra Leone, Liberia, Ivory Coast, Upper Volta, Ghana, Togo, Niger, Zambia, Malawi, Nigeria, Chad, Cameroon, Gabon, Congo, Zaire, Angola, Namibia, Botswania, Zimbabwe, Equatorial Guinea, Mozambique, Somalia, Ethiopia and Madagascar

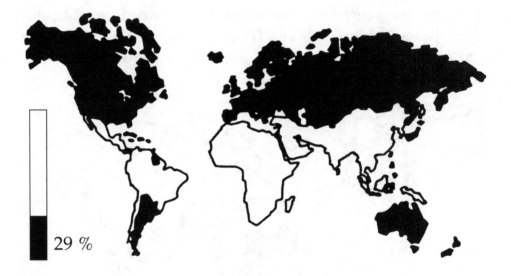

29 %

66-74 years

North America and European countries are in this group. Denmark, Iceland, Norway, and the Netherlands all have the highest figure of 74 years. This verifies the Caucasians' deliberate attempt to exterminate Africans.

The EPA estimates that Chemicalized Indoor Air is 1,000 Times Worse than Chemicalized Outdoor Air

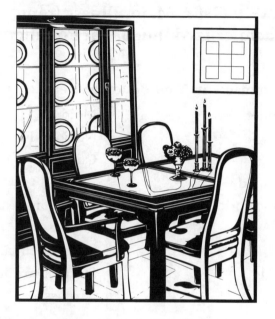

Some of the Possible Effects of Indoor Air Pollution are...

Bronchial Constriction	Headaches
Cancer	Memory Loss
Depression	Pulmonary Irritation
Dizziness	Gynecological Problems
Drowsiness	Respiratory Irritation
Eye, Skin and Nasal Irritation	Shortness of Breath
Fatigue	Slow Poisoning

The EPA Estimates That 20% of All Workers Will Get A Major Illness from Chemicalized Indoor Air Pollution

Common Contaminants in Your Building Are:

Animal Dander	Mold
Bacteria	Noxious Fumes
Benzene	Odors
Carbon Monoxide	Pollen
Carbon Tetrachloride	Radiation toxins.
Dust	Smoke
Dust Mites	Static Electricity
Formaldehyde	Sulfur Dioxide
Mildew	Viruses

Contaminants can originate from:

Adhesives	New Fabrics and Carpets
Air Dust	Paint, Glues
Appliances	Particle Board
Cleaning Supplies	Particle Boards
Cleaning Supplies	Pets
Concrete	Plywood
Construction Materials	Wall Paper
Drapes	
Dry-Cleaned Clothing	
Electric cables	
Furnaces	
Gas Burners	

Do You Live
In A Sick home?

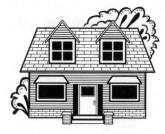

Do You Work
In A Sick home?

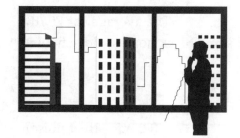

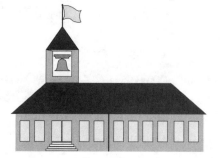

Do You Attend
A Sick school?

Noise Pollution

Noise Pollution

Noise above 60 decibels is toxic, drains Melanin and can cause mental fatigue. Research has shown that performance errors can occur within 10 minutes of exposure to 100 decibels. Some common noise levels:

(decibel)

Whisper 20 dB

The average home 40 dB

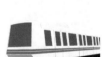

The average car 70 dB
(and some Black homes and schools)

The average airliner cabin 85 dB
(Ghetto street noise)

Subway Station 105 dB

12 lb. cannon blast 300 dB

100 decibels is considered very noisy, while 140 is painful. Go up to 160 decibels and deafness occurs. Another 40 - to 200 decibels - can kill.

70 decibels. Loud radio in an average house. A noisy restaurant. Ghetto traffic. This type of noise makes it difficult to hear telephone conversations.

80 decibels. Road construction site. This sounds twice as loud as 70 decibels.

90 decibels. Loud shout. Busy city street. This sounds four times as loud as 70 decibels, is annoying and causes neurological damage after eight hours of continuous exposure.

100 decibels. Subway station. Running printing press. Train horn 33 yards away. This noise is eight times as loud as 70 decibels.

110 decibels. Sheet metal grinding. Loud music. This is 16 times as loud as 70 decibels and requires shouting to be heard.

130 decibels. Pneumatic chipping and riveting, machines from the operator's position. This is 64 times as loud as 70 decibels. Shouts can't be heard. This noise level is considered intolerable.

Toxic noise sound levels can damage the ear over time.

RITALIN

(a type of crack-cocaine)

Stimulant Medication Side Effects

Common Initial Side Effects (*try dose reduction*)

Abdominal pain   Headaches
Anorexia   Irritability
Easy crying   Weight Loss
Emotional
oversensitivity

Less Common Side Effects

Anxiety
Decreased social interest.
Depression (*rare*)
Dysphoria or exaggerated feelings of depression and unrest
    without apparent cause (*especially at higher doses*)
Hypersensitivity rash, conjunctivitis or hives
Impaired cognitive test performance (*especially at higher
    doses*).
Insomnia
Insomnia
Less than expected weight gain.
Nervous habits (*such as picking at skin, hair, etc.*)
Rebound attention deficit hyperactivity disorder (*ADHD*)
Rebound overactivity and irritability (*as dose wears off*)
Withdrawal effects.

Rare but Potentially Serious Side Effects

Depression
Growth retardation
Hypertension
Motor tics
Psychosis with hallucinations
Tachycardia
Tourette's disorder
Stereotyped activities or compulsions

Side Effects Reported With Cylert (Pemoline) *Only*

Chemical hepatitis (elevated liver enzymes, jaundice, epigastric pains).

Choreiform movements (nervous condition marked by involuntary muscular twitching)

Dyskinesias (defect in voluntary movements)

Lip licking or biting

Night terrors

Behavior Symptoms of Hyperactivity or Attention Deficit Disorder

Aggressive Behavior (Male principle expression of dis-ease	Passive Behavior (Female principle expression of dis-ease
Aggressiveness	Accident prone
Angry outbursts	Anxious
Bully	Daydreams
Clumsiness	Depressed moods
Compulsive aggression	Distractibility
Eats lots of sugar and drinks a lot of caffeine	Eating problems
Inability to concentrate	Emotional instability
Inability to make and keep friends	Fearful
Junk-food eater	Hyperventilates
Lying	Insecurity
Not good in sports	Lying
Poor handwriting, drawing, and reading skills	Mood swings
Poor muscle coordination	Poor math calculations
Poor sleep habits	Poor muscle coordination
Quarrelsomeness	Poor reading skills
Resentment of punishments	Poorly developed musculo-skeletal system
Restlessness	Reasoning difficulty
Self-mutilation	Show off
Show off	Skin problems such as rash or hives
Stealing	Sleep problems
Temper tantrums	Slow reader
Unable to complete projects	Stays close to mother
Unaware of danger	Temper tantrums
	Withdrawn

Psychiatric Terms/Meanings

Psychological terms are political and social tools used to manipulate and control Blacks. They define Blacks as dysfunctional. This makes Blacks beneficial for Caucasian society.

Aggressive Tantrum = aimless, thrashing, flailing limbs, wiggles legs

Attention Deficit = easily distracted, loses things, fails to Finish Task, Doesn't Listen

Dementia = forgetful, memory problems

Developmental Arithmetic Disorder = difficulty understanding and solving mathematical problems

Drapetomania = a mental illness which causes a slave to think about running away from the plantation or attempt to escape from freedom.

Dysaethesia Aethiops = a mental illness which causes a slave to be disrespectful or disobedient to Slave Master

Dyslexia = fails literacy test misspells words, cannot read, puts letters backwards

Hereditary Violent Genetic Disease = protesting, acting militant or confronting White Supremacy or expressing doubt about White authorities, at risk social conditions (ghetto, poor education) which genetically makes you inferior

Hyperactivity - impulsive, constantly moving, excess talking, impatient, makes excessive mistakes, excessive running and/or climbing

Hypoactivity = withdrawn, passive, plays alone, talks very little, seems lost

Oppositional Defiance Disorder = acting independent, having self identity

Pain Disorder = having headaches, backaches

Passive Tantrum = frown, cries, grimaces, beats on objects/furniture, throws and/or breaks objects

Persecution Complex = getting into confrontations with authorities, getting into fights

The above terms are political and social and are used to manipulate and control Black Folks in order to make them dysfunctional and an economical benefit to Caucasians.

HYPERACTIVITY / Attention Deficit Disorder SUPPLEMENTS

B Vitamins = Nervousness, stress, mood swings, fear, depression, anxiety, concentration, tantrums

Calcium = Nervous stomach, tingling arms and legs, cramps, inattentive, irritable, angry, sleep disturbance

GABA (Gamma Amino Butyric Acid) = Anxiety, Stress, pain, depression

Gingko or Gotu Kola = Memory, concentration

Glutamine = Memory, concentration

Glycine = Reduces aggression, manic depression, sugar substitute

Magnesium = Irritability, confusion, nervousness, jerking muscles, noise sensitivity, constant eye twitching, muscle spasms, tremors, pain

Niacinamide (B3) = Calmative, improves circulation

Phenylalanine = Turns into Tyrosine and Dopamine

Pyridoxine (B6) = Calmative, irritated nerves (Carpal tunnel)

Taurine = Anticonvulsant, antianxiety, eye problems

Tyrosine = Stress, anxiety, depression

Vitamin E = Slowly enhances learning

Zinc = Fatigue, lost taste, alertness, decreased appetite, healing

Hyperactivity and ADD Misconceptions

Misconception 1
He'll outgrow it. This is often stated when the child is young. It's a lifelong behavioral and thought process, which the child can adjust to in a positive manner.

Misconception 2
The ADD child just needs a "good spanking" and "firm discipline." Many parents have failed trying this and few have been successful. There are specific appropriate behavioral techniques which are consistent nonpunitive punishments that works over 80% percent of the time.

Misconception 3
The ADD behavior and thought patterns causes a dysfunctional lifestyle. There are adults who have ADD who adapted to it and have developed ways to coping with effect.

Chemically Induced Teen Suicide

**Blacks in the U.S.A. are #1 in the world
in Black teen suicide.**

**The below Vitamin deficiency causes suicide and
behavioral problems in school**

1. Low Vitamin B intake causes mental and emotional imbalances in teen.

2. Teens junk food diets are deficient in vitamin B content.

3. They addictively consume sodas, junk foods, and alcohol, which biochemically reduce already critically low levels of Vitamin B in the body, dehydrate the cells and cause nutritional starvation

4. The signs of vitamin B deficiency are characterized by *delusions, disorientation, mood swings, and depression.* These symptoms are consistent with early **Beri Beri,** a thiamine, and Vitamin B deficiency disease.

5. The major symptoms of B Vitamin deficiency are anxiety, fear, depression, hostility, rage, vagueness, forgetfulness, instability, craving for sweets, mental confusion, vague fear, mindless sex, irritability, and **a constant feeling that something dreadful is about to happen.**

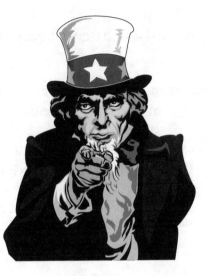

Black Children and Adults
I WANT YOU IN PRISON

Blacks nutritionally deficient, consuming chemicalized junk foods, and legal and illegal drugs are at a higher risk for crimes and prison. Court is where the negative behaviors caused by mal-nourishment from junk food goes on trial. The food industry is found innocent while the Black consumer of junk is found guilty and sent to jail. The food Industry's nutritional crime is turned into a misdemeanor or felony crime.

McDonalds uses addictive synthetic chemicals, sex hormones that stimulate hypersex, sublime sex connotations. Their commercials create self-hatred in Black folks by using minstrel clown character (negative image of the Blacks).

Commercials that psychologically help Black consumers to hate themselves have an increase in sales.

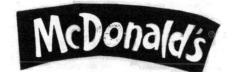

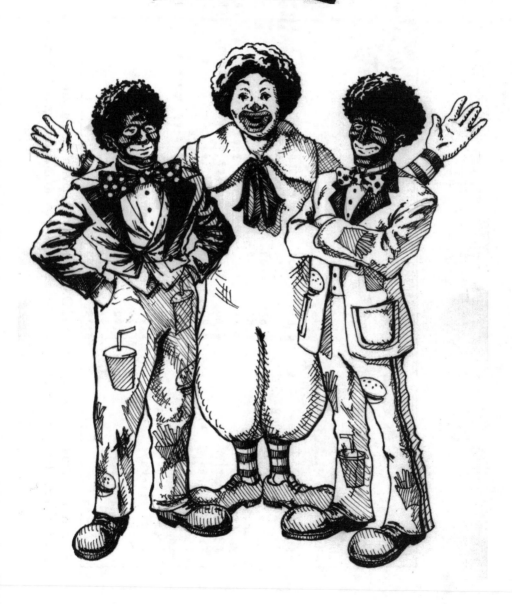

Industries Black Slaves

```
DATE:                    INMATE EARNING STATEMENT      PAGE:
INMATE-PAYROLL              PAY DATE: 12/31/97          USER ID: annler

INST:   FACT:      GROUP:                CREW:
Name                                     Grade:
Reg-Hurs

                  Amount   Hours              Date Computed        01/05/98
Standard Pay      $ 44.05  191:30            Anniversary Date     12/01/97
Group Incentive Pay  0.00    0:00            Longevity Months            1
Indiv. Incentive Pay 0.00    0:00            UNICOR Work Months          1
Overtime Premium Pay 8.05   35:00            Accrued Vacation Hours   003:45
Holiday Pay          3.46   15:00            Prev Yrs Vacation Hours  000:00
Administrative Pay   0.23    1:00            Unpaid Call-out Hours      0:00
Vacation Taken Pay   0.00    0:00            Rework Hours               0:00
Vacation Cashed Pay  0.00    0:00            Unpaid Off-std Hours       0:00
Lost Time Wage       0.00    0:00            Final Pay?                   NO
Premium Pay          0.00
Longevity Pay        0.00
Gross Pay           55.79
Adjustments          0.00
                  -------  -------
Net Pay           $ 55.79  242:30
```

Reproduced above is a copy of a UNICOR pay statement with the inmates's identity blacked out. This worker has a base pay of 23 cents per hour and received a total of $ 55.79 for 242.5 hours of work

Prisoners for Profit

The Corporate Prison System
The private prison industry has boomed in recent years

Capacity on the rise
Actual and predicted capacity
of private prisons in the United States:

1996	77,584
1997	111,588
1998	142,799
1999	179,884
2000	223,002
2001	276,455

Slicing up the market
Two companies dominate the industry.
Percentage of the market share based
on U.S. contracts:

Corrections Corp of America	52.03 %
Wackenhut Corrections Corp	25.11 %
U.S. Corrections Corp	5.20 %
Management & Training Corp.	3.84 %
Cornell Corrections Inc:	3.37 %

Source: Private Adult
Correctional Facilities Census,
10th edition, prepared by the
Private Corrections Project
Center for Studies in
Criminology and Law,
University of Florida

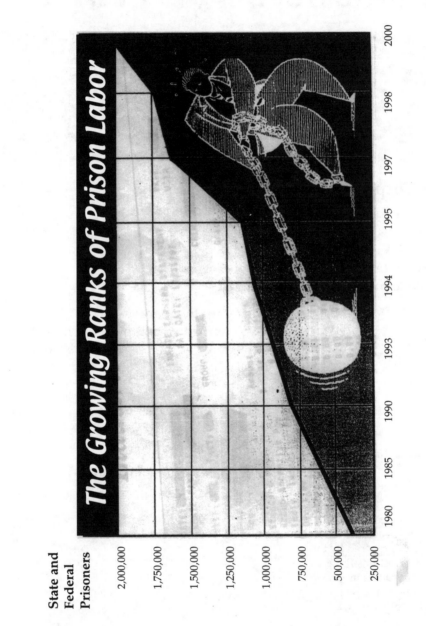

The Growing Ranks of Prison Labor

State and Federal Prisoners

Chewing Gum

(Commercial Toothpaste has the same ingredients as)

Ingredient	Harmful Effect
BHA (Butylated Hydroxyanisole)	Cancer
BHT (Butylated Hydroxy toluene)	Cancer
Plasticizers	Solvent (Dissolves Skin), Digestive Problems
Aspartame	Nerve Damage, Cancer, Cysts, Tumors
Polysobutylene	Solvent, Skin Irritant, Suffocation
Polyterpene	Respiratory Failure (Death) Skin Irritant
Aluminum	Brain Damage, Clogs Glands
Propyl Gallate	Skin Irritant
Polyvinyl Acetate	Damages lungs and kidney, Tumors
Coal Tar	Cancer, Degenerative Diseases
Wood Tar	Cancer, Insanity
Petroleum Tar	Cancer, Degenerative Disease
Paraffin	Cancer, Degenerative Disease
Approved Non-food Dirt(Dead insects, Rat manure Filth)	Unknown
Unspecified Ingredients (Over 20 not listed)	Unknown
White Sugar	Kidney failure, Diabetes, Blindness, Addiction, Cancer
Dyes	Cancer

White Spots on Black Folks' Skin

The effect of junk foods, meat, drugs, sunlight deficiency, synthetic chemicals and nutritional deficiencies causes

❑ Melanin Deficiency (Internal organs use external melanin).
❑ Cellular and food waste constipation.
❑ Sunlight Deficiency (sunlight helps retain minerals, pH level, electrolytes, produce Melanin).
❑ Retention of waste in body due to salt addiction.
❑ Radiation toxicity (i.e., computers, X ray, TV, appliances).
❑ Lymph gland congestion.
❑ Excessive sex or sex stimulation.
❑ Loud sounds (noise pollution).
❑ Toxic liver.
❑ Unable to metabolize food properly (digestion too fast, stomach skin thick, colitis, etc.).
❑ Body too acidic to use nutrients.
❑ Fungus infections (Athletes foot, Yeast).
❑ Severe Vitamin C and D deficiency.
❑ Potassium deficiency.
❑ Micronage of cells.
❑ Vitamin A_1 B_{12} and/or Iron Anemia

Symptoms

◆ Deterioration of cartilage, cell glue, bones.
◆ High blood pressure, stress, cyst, tumors.
◆ Cracking, ridged and/or splitting fingernails.
◆ Waste in uterus, waste in prostate.
◆ Menstruation problems.
◆ Mood and thought problems.
◆ Urine alkaline and saliva alkaline.
◆ Micronage of cells.

Partial-birth Abortions

The murder of late term Unborn babies by sucking out brain (D&X)
The Black mother is drugged and the murdered baby parts are sold.

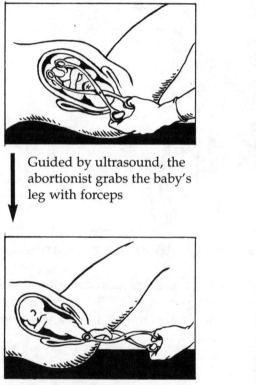

Guided by ultrasound, the
abortionist grabs the baby's
leg with forceps

The abortionist delivers the
baby's entire body, except for
the head.

The baby's leg is pulled out
into the birth canal.

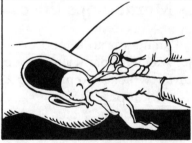

The abortionist jams scissors
into the baby's skull. The scissors are opened to enlarge hole

"The abortionist punches a hole into the base of the skull with a scissor...
[H]e spreads the scissors to enlarge the opening. The abortionist removes
the scissors and puts a suction catheter into this hole and sucks out the
brain. With the cathether still in place, he pulls the fetus out to he uterus
of the mother

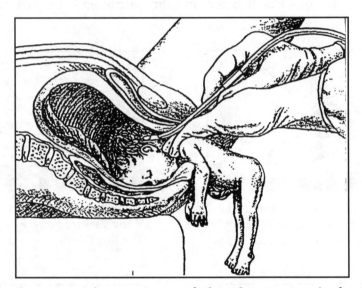

Murder tops the causes of death among infants

Parents on junk food and legal drugs murder more infants. 10,370
injury-related infant deaths were reported between 1983 and 1991. After
murder, which accounted for **23%** of the deaths, the leading causes were

suffocation, ... **18 %**;
car accidents, ... **15 %**;
fires, ... **9 %**;
drowning;, ... **7%**,
choking on food, ... **7 %**;
choking on objects, ... **6 %**;
other intentional injuries, ...   **11%**; and
injuries undetermined intent, . . . **4 %**.

Infants were more likely to die of injuries including murder, if their
mothers were young, unmarried, had little education and their diets
tended to be junk foods—nutrient deficient

Hair Relaxer Chemicals

(Absorb into skin and gets into blood)

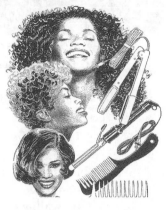

Relaxer Protection Pre-Treatment	
Ingredients	**Effects**
Dicetyldimonium Chloride	∞ Poison ∞ Deadly if swallowed ∞ Breaks hair ∞ If inhaled - damages lungs ∞ Used in explosives batteries, freezing mixtures ∞ Diuretic ∞ Damages kidney, liver, skin and glands

TEA
(Triethanonlamine)
	∞ Tannic Acid
	  - Irritates
	  - Inflames skin (blisters)
	  - Alters skin color
	∞ Caffeine
	  - Decreases blood flow to uterus and prostate
	  - Alters blood sugar, influences Diabetes
	  - Stresses heart, lungs and nerves

Relaxer Protection Pre-Treatment	
Ingredients	Effects
Propylene Glycol	⌘ Moisturizes ⌘ Transports chemicals into hair, blood, nerves ⌘ Causes skin disease
Polyquarternium	⌘ Poison ⌘ Type of Lye ⌘ Hair, skin, and Melanin bleaching agent (destroys melanin) ⌘ If swallowed - causes death ⌘ Causes nausea, burns, hives, swelling of face, allergic reactions ⌘ Irritates eyes
Hydroxyethyl Cellulose	⌘ Made from contaminated cotton and wood with Lye ⌘ Holds poisonous chemicals together for better effect
TEA Cocyl	⌘ Same as above ⌘ Detergent ⌘ Dehydrates skin
Lactic Acid	⌘ Decreases oxygen to brain, bones, skin, nerves ⌘ Destroys skin
Methylchlorol-Sothiazolimone	⌘ Alcohol ⌘ Preservative ⌘ Damages liver, kidney, nerves and brain ⌘ Eye damage (sensitivity to light)
Polysorbate	⌘ Irritant ⌘ Helps skin and hair absorb toxic chemicals ⌘ Emulsifier

No-Lye Conditioner / Relaxer	
Ingredients	**Effects**
Petroleum/Mineral Oil	∾ Destroys Vitamin A, D, E, and K. Drys skin and cloggs tissue
Calcium Hydroxide	∾ Poison ∾ Type of Lye ∾ Destroys hair (depilatory), skin, nerves, bones, blood, and glands ∾ Burns skin, eyes, throat ∾ Can die from shock if swallowed ∾ Used to make cement, plaster and fireproof ∾ Pesticides
Polyquarternium	∾ Lye
Nonyl Phenyl Ether	∾ Poison ∾ Damages liver, kidney, skin, and hair ∾ Causes Cancer
Carboxylic Acid	∾ Poison ∾ Causes high blood pressure, mental confusion, lung problems
Phosphate	∾ Skin irritant ∾ Preservative ∾ Causes liver damage
DEA **(Diethanolamine)**	∾Poison ∾ Irritates skin, lungs, uterus, prostrate ∾ Damages liver, kidney, and nerves

No-Lye Conditioner / Relaxer	
Ingredients	**Effects**
PEG **(Polyethylene Glycol** **/ Polyoxyethylene)**	↣ Poison ↣ Damages kidney, liver, glands ↣ Destroys hair (relaxes), skin ↣ Dissolves skin oil and skin tissue ↣ Used in antifreeze

Relaxer Activator	
Ingredients	**Effects**
Guanidine Carbonate	↣ Used to make rubber ↣ Muscle poison ↣ Holds toxic chemicals in skin, hair, and blood ↣ Moisturizer
Methylparaben	↣ Irritates skin and blood ↣ Kills cells and microbes Preservative
Xanthan Gum **(Corn Sugar Gum)**	↣ Made from rotten starch

Relaxer Neutralizing Shampoo	
Ingredients	**Effects**
Sodium Laureth Sulfate	↣ Lye ↣ Stabilizes color ↣ Prevents growth ↣ Destroys and dissolves nerves skin, bones, cells, and hair ↣ Alcohol (damages liver, kidney, brain, nerve cells

Relaxer Neutralizing Shampoo	
Ingredients	**Effects**
Disodium Cocoampho-Dipropionate	☞ Stain remover, oven cleaner ☞ Reduces friction ☞ Helps chemical to get absorbed into hair, skin, blood, etc.
Lauramide	☞ Makes bubbles ☞ Skin irritant
Citric Acid	☞ Preservative ☞ Astringent ☞ Decreases circulation
Tetrasodium Edta *(Ethylenediamine Tetra Acetic Acid)*	☞ Causes cyst, tumors, fibriods ☞ Alters ability of muscles to function and Calcium usage ☞ Causes errors in laboratory tests for diseases
Diazolidinyl Urea	☞ Disinfectant ☞ Slows down brain and nerve function ☞ Skin irritation ☞ Causes convulsions, paralysis, nerve damage and Cancer
Phenolsulfon-Phthalein	☞ Type of Lye ☞ Disinfectant _ Destroys hair (depilatory) and breakage _ Irritates eyes, skin, nerves _ Causes Cancer _ Machine lubricant _ Wood / roof water proofer

Conditioner / Relaxer (Leave-In Hair)	
Ingredients	**Effects**
Polyquarternium	_ Lye
Dimethicone Copolyol	_ Transport chemical into skin Poison

| Conditioner / Relaxer (Leave-In Hair) ||
Ingredients	Effects
Glycerin	_ Keeps moisture and chemicals Solvent Soap
Acetamide Mea (Monoethanolamine)	_ Type of Lye _ Cancer- liver _ Skin irritant _ Poison
Dicetyldimonium Chloride	_ Lye
Amino Acid	_ Helps toxic poisonous chemicals to get absorbed into hair, skin, blood, etc.
Panthenal - DL	_ Breaks down fats and proteins in the body _ Destroys skin and hair (relaxes)
Hydrolyzed Collagen	_ Animal waste _ Connective tissue destroyed by water
Diazolidinyl Urea	
Polysorbate	

| Oil Moisturizing Lotion ||
Ingredients	Effects
Petrolatum/Mineral Oil	_ Destroys Vitamin A, D, E, and K _ Causes dandruff _ Fossilized oil does is not metabolized into body causes cells to stick together _ Drys skin

Oil Moisturizing Lotion	
Ingredients	Effects
Lanolin	_ Causes dry skin, hair, and dandruff _ Sheep fat _ No nutritional value _ Destroys Vitamin A, D, E, and K
Essential Oil	_ Mixture of sheep, pork, goat, fish, cattle and synthetic oil
Benzoate	_ Irritates eyes, skin _ Kills human cells and bacteria _ Preservative
Borax	_ Poison _ Antiseptic _ Kills cells _ Alters digestion

Dandruff Treatment and/or Shampoo	
Ingredients	Effects
Salicylic Acid	Stomach Pain Ulcers Mental Problems Rapid Heart Beats Used in Aspirin Bleeding
Salicylanilde	Same as Above Irritates eyes, uterus, prostate, lungs and stomach Combined with sunlight, causes rashes, inflammations swelling
Resorcinol	Stimulant (speed) Irritates lungs, uterus, prostate, skin Anti-itching (stops blood flow) Poison

| Dandruff Treatment and/or Shampoo ||
Ingredients	Effects
Hexachlorophene	Kills cells, nerves, blood Causes dark spots on face and coma Kills bacteria
Quaternary Ammonium	Lye Poison Destroys hair, skin, blood and cells Irritates eyes, lungs Preservative
Sulfur	Skin irritant Antiseptic
Allantoin	Made with Uric Acid (Urine Waste), and Dichloroascetic Acid Destroys liver, kidney, nerves and brain cells Diuretic Fertilizer
Zinc Pyrithione	Damages nerves
Anionic Detergent	Type of lye
Coal Tar	Causes Cancer
Petrolatum	Destroys Vitamin A, D, E, and K Drys skin Clogs pores Causes dandruff and scalp irritation Dissolves and Destroys Cells, Oil and Skin Makes Skin Dry

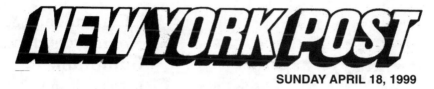

SUNDAY APRIL 18, 1999

LOOKS TO DIE FOR

Methyl methacrylate (MMA) can rip nails off fingers, cause nerve problems and severe rashes —and over the long term hurt kidneys, livers and fetuses

Federal Food and Drug Administration officials ruled in the early 1970's that MMA is poisonous when used on nails.

■ Acrylic nails — often called sculptured nails — should cost $ 35 - $ 40 a set.
■ MMA nails usually $20 or less. MMA has a superstrong, sweet fruity smell that's distinct from other acrylics.

■ The manicurist has to severely abrade the surface of the nail until it is very rough—called the "shag carpet" look — to get MMA to stick.

■ Fake nails made with MMA are almost impossible to get off, even after soaking them in acetone for hours.

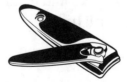

Vaccination/inoculation (Chemical, pus and filth)

Carcinogens &
Toxic Substances
Aluminium
(a Neuro-toxin)

germs

Live Viruses

Thimerosal
(a Mercury Derivative)

Bacteria

Formaldehyde
(a major component
of embalming fluid)

Animal RNA and DNA

Monkey Kidneys

Foreign proteins

Chick Embryo

Calf Serum

undetected
Animal Viruses

Hyperdermic needle

Causes Diseases and death in
**Healthy
Babies**

AFFIDAVIT
DECLARATION OF VACCINATION EXEMPTION

"EXEMPTION FROM IMMUNIZATION", I hereby declare that I as guardian/parent/adult having responsibility for my self/child named herein _____
withhold my consent and let it be known that said adult/minor is exempted from any and all vaccinations on the grounds that such is contrary to my personal beliefs.

IMMUNIZATIONS OF A PERSON SHALL NOT BE REQUIRED FOR EMPLOYMENT, ADMISSION TO A SCHOOL OR OTHER INSTITUTION...IF THE GUARDIAN, PARENT, OR ADULT WHO HAS ASSUMED RESPONSIBILITY FOR HIS OR HER CUSTODY AND CARE IN THE CASE OF A MINOR, THE PERSON MUST FILE WITH THE GOVERNMENT AUTHORITY, A LETTER OR AFFIDAVIT STATING THAT SUCH VACCINATION IS CONTRARY TO HIS/HER BELIEFS...

Any institution, school or medical authority which tries to enforce vaccination on children or anyone else is in violation of the laws of the United States, and may be subject to prosecution.

Amendment 14 of the United States Constitution:
"No state shall make or impose any law which shall abridge the privileges or immunities of the citizens of the United States, nor shall any state deprive any person of life, liberty, or property."

Amendment 4 of the United States Constitution:
"The right of the people to be secure in their persons shall not be violated."

INTERNATIONAL (TRAVEL) VACCINATION EXEMPTION
Exemption has been ratified and approved by all United Nations members under WORLD HEALTH ORGANIZATION International Sanitary Regulations Article 83, Chapter IV; "each individual has the right of vaccination exemption".

SUBSCRIBED AND AFFIRMED TO BEFORE ME ON THIS _____ DAY OF
_____, 19_____.

_____
SIGNATURE AND DATE

_____
NOTARY PUBLIC
COMMISSION EXPIRES

_____

(Your Address)
Date

Dear *(School Nurse or whoever it has to go to)*:

RE: Religious Exemption from Immunization Requirements

Please be advised that I am hereby requesting a religious exemption for my *(daughter/son),* ____*(name)*____. *(Select and continue here with (A), (B) or (C).*

(A:)   Our family follows the tenets and practices of a religion which strictly forbids....

(B:)   Our family are members of *(or: have recently joined a)* religion whose tenets and practices strictly forbid.....

(C:)   Although my *(daughter/son)* previously received some immunizations, our family are now members of a religion whose tenets and practices strictly forbid.....

...immunizations of any type, including those injected, ingested or infused into the body.

Kindly enter this religious exemption into my *(daughter's/son's)* school records.

Thank you very much.

Sincerely,

(Your Name)

Orange Chemical Liquid—Orange Juice
Commercial orange juice can have dangerous amounts of the following:

1. Water–extracted soluble orange solids.
2. Dehydrated water-extracted soluble orange solids
3. Commuted (pulverized) oranges.
4. Dehydrated commuted oranges.
5. Dehydrated extract of comminuted oranges.
6. Juicy orange pulp for manufacturing.
7. Dehydrated juicy orange pulp for manufacturing
8. Noncarbonated flavored beverage
9. Concentrate for flavored beverage
10. Powered flavored beverage.
11. Orange drinks and diluted orange drinks
12. Concentrates for orange drinks.
13. Powered orange drinks
14. Orange-flavored drinks
15. Concentrates for orange-flavored drinks.
16. Powered orange-flavored drinks.
17. Concentrated water-extracted orange juice.
18. Orange blend.
19. Orange juice drink
20. Orange drink
21. Concentrate for diluted orange juice beverages.
22. Orange juice drink and blended orange juice drink
23. Concentrate for orange juice drink and for blended orange juice drink.
24. Powered orange juice drink and powered blended orange juice drink
25. Concentrate for orange drink.
26. Concentrate for orange-flavored drink.
27. Powered orange-flavored drink.

Condom—Rubber coffins (Latex and Chemical poisons)

- Condoms cannot prevent emotional pain.
- Condom failure rate for pregnancy prevention is 13-31%[1]
- Condom Research: Latex condoms may have voids (holes) approximately 5 microns in size that occur naturally during the manufacturing process.[2]
- The powder in condoms cause cyst and tumors
- The spermicide causes cancer
- The condoms fail to prevent nearly 1 in every 3 HIV infections.[3]
- Sexually transmitted viruses and bacteria can pass through the voids in a latex condom.[4]
- The latex condoms causes Chlamydia, Pelvic inflammatory dis-ease – PID and cancer of the female reproductive system.

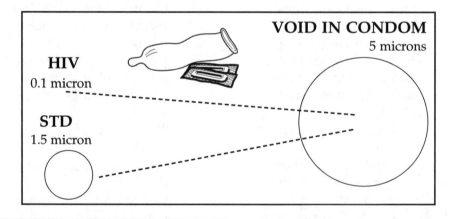

[1] Family Planning Perspectives, V. 24, 1992.
[2] Roland, C. M., Rubber Chemistry & Technology, June 1992.
[3] Weller, Susan, Ph.D., University of Texas, June 1993.
[4] Carey, R. F., et al, Sexually Transmitted Diseases, July/August, 1992.
[5] Manual of Clinical Microbiology, 4th edition.

Disease by Blood Type.

Africans are higher in Type A and B with a normal level of Type O

Have a moderate RH—(negative) level, very rare RH$^+$ (positive) and RHO. The body's low melanin content White Blood Cells (WBC) sacrifice themselves in order to protect the high melanin content Red Blood Cells (RBC)

The synthetic, chemicalized junk food diet causes specific diseases amongst blood types.

TYPE A				
Supplements	Exercise	Positives	Risk	Personality
Vitamin B, B$_{12}$, C, E, Folic Acid	Moderate	Digestive system highly responsive, long and high fermentative bacteria	heart disease, Cancer, Anemia, Diabetes, Liver and Gall Bladder Disease	Humanitarian, Organized, Harmonious, Intelligent, Spiritual
TYPE B				
Magnesium, Zinc, Lecithin, Echinacea Gotu Kola	Moderate	Digestive system highly responsive, long and high fermentative bacteria	Lupus, Diabetes, Fatigue, Multiple Sclerosis, Stress Digestive	Adaptable, Empathetic. Aggressive, Sensitive
TYPE O				
Vitamin B, K Calcium	Intense	Digestive system highly responsive, long and high fermentative bacteria	Arthritis Endometriosis, Ulcers, Allergy, Hypothyroid	Determined, Constructive, Leader type, Communicator
TYPE AB				
Vitamin C, K Manganese, Potassium	Challenging	Digestive system highly responsive, long and high fermentative bacteria	Prone to Anemia, Cancer, Heart Disease	Spiritual, Diplomatic, Charismatic, Emotional

Chemical Malt liquor and beer

Methanol
(wood alcohol, poison, mental illness, cancer, liver, kidney and sex organ damage

Ethanol
(narcotic,starch alcohol, poison, narcotic explosive, liver, kidney and sex organ damage)

Butanol
(poison, narcotic, explosive, cancer, petroleum alcohol, liver, kidney and sex organ damage

Isobutanol
(poison, natural gas, alcohol, eye, lung skin, liver, kidney and sex organ damage)

White Sugar
(nitroglycerin, diabetes, blindness, gangrene, addiction)

Acetaldehyde
(poison, paralysis, nerve, brain, lung, skin, digestion and sex organ damage)

Histamine
(shock, swelling, skin rash, headache, low blood pressure, digestive problems)

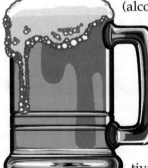

Phenol
(carbolic acid, poison, convulsions cancer, circulatory collapse, paralysis, coma, numbness, burns, digestive problems, skin rash)

Propanol
(poison, narcotic, toxic gas, disinfectant, cancer)

Isopentanol
(alcohol, poison, irritates eyes, lungs, liver, kidney and sex organs)

Cobalt
(metal, digestive problems)

Lead
(poison, nerve and brain damage, digestive problems)

Iron
(poison, skin disease, coma, hypotension, restlessness)

Carbon Dioxide
(high blood pressure, mental confusion, lung disease, digestive problems)

Viagra:

Citrate Salt of Sildenafil.

Increase and disturbs blood inflow to brain, glands, eyes, lungs heart, lover, kidney, prostrate

Chemical
Nitric (Nitrous) Oxide
(Laughing gas, causes psychotic Illusions)

Viagra cause abnormal increase in Nitric oxide
High concentration is narcotic
Burns and irritates skin
Decreases oxygen
Explodes cells
Used in explosives and fertilizers Nitric (Nitrous) Oxide
(Laughing gas

Side Effects[6]

Headaches	Weakens immunity
Infections	Lung and nasal congestion
Urinary tract infections	Blurred vision
Peptic ulcers	Dizziness
Arthritis	Back pain
Chest pain	Heart problems
Mood swings	Depression
Frequent urination	Thirst
Incontinence	Increases breast size
Multiple myeloma	Colds and influenza
Blood Cancer (Leukemia)	Sickle cell
Hypotension	Flushing
Diabetic problems	Nerve problems
Hypertension	Bleeding disorder

---

[6] Pfizer info sheet

The Untold Caucasian History
(Dirt, Fart, Feces, Fun and Sex)

The European relationship to health is reflected in their relation-ship to the soil (Mother Earth) which they call dirt. The soil pro-vides the plants that we eat. A healthy relationship with dirt (soil) indicates a healthy relationship with your body. However, many factors helped to create a negative, hostile and, in many ways, dis-torted relationship between the Caucasian and dirt.

The Ice Age and Cold Age that followed created nutrient-poor soil. The many mud slides, floods, thunder storms and subsequent forest fires stripped the land of valuable topsoil. This caused good dirt (topsoil) to be scarce. This inadvertently caused famines, food shortages and starvation. The ancient European population con-sisted of gangs, thieves, roaming bandits, cannibal gangs, wild dogs which ate humans, people attacking each other, diseases, violence, water shortage, rape, looting, filthy, unlighted homes and cities, dead bodies and manure hills, and people who stayed dirty in fear of water.

Because the dirt (soil) was unable to provide adequate food and the many taboos about cleanliness the Caucasian developed many myths and superstitions about dirt. The Caucasian's language refers to dirt in many ways, such as dirty shame, filthy rich, dirty dancing, dirty lie, dirty words, dirty dog, dirty nigger, dirt poor, dirty sex, etc. They believe the human race evolved from dirt and that humans are made from dust (dirt). In reality, humans are approximately 80% water which means they may have been made from water and not dirt. Caucasians use dirt as money, such as, yellow dirt (gold) or crystallized dirt (diamonds). Today, they make synthetic, tasty dirt called bleached white flour, sugar, etc. In their past it was believed that dirty children were healthy. Women's dirty faces were believed to block out the sun. If the Caucasian woman was unwashed and had a foul body odor and a foul smelling, vagina, then she was considered sexy.

Other people were considered dirty. Sartre wrote in *Huis Clos* that hell is full of dirty people. Dirty people were believed to contaminate society and needed to be murdered. In their genocide against each other they refer to it as "racial cleansing." This is an expression for getting rid of dirt (genetically inferior, dirty people).

The original reason why the Khazars (so-called Jews) and Caucasian Moslems did not eat pigs had nothing to do with the bacteriology or worm infestation of the pigs. The Khazars worshipped the pig and thought the pig was sacred not dirty. If cleanliness were truly the reason, then cats would be eaten as food instead of cattle and fish (they swim in their own feces and urine). On the early explorations (invasions) of Africa and the Americas, the Caucasian sailors would eat the dogs, then the cats, then the rats, then their leather boots, shoes, hats, ropes, etc. Since the leather items were not made from pig, it was considered clean flesh food to eat. They would eat bone meal cooked in fat and insects and the food found in a dead animal's stomach along with the animal's feces. This indicates confusion about what is and is not dirty.

The ancient Caucasians' behaviors indicate a mixed and at the same time confused relationship between dirt, food, sex, medicine, health and disease. In primitive Caucasian rituals, feces (manure) is symbolic of gifts, death, money, babies, the penis, art, spirits, sex, poison, foreigners, disorder, gold, the vagina, golden eggs, candy, food, etc. In books such as *The Ontogenesis in the Interest of Money* by Sandor Ferenczi (1914), *Studies in Psychology of Sex* by Havelock Ellis (1906) and *Character and Anal Eroticism* by Sigmund Freud (1908) it is reported that anal sexual ideas of Caucasians begin in childhood when weird feces associations are made by Caucasian babies playing with their own feces in the diaper. The babies play with mud, sand, pebbles, hair, buttons, fingers, lips and coins because it is associated with feces. The coins (money) are seen as an extension of feces and the sex organs. Therefore, buying sex from prostitutes is emotionally an extension of feces. In the Caucasian subconscious mind the need for economic control (power) over others is an extension of their sexuality and sex is an extension of feces and urine.

Historically, Caucasians used human feces in religious ceremonies. Ancient Greeks rubbed feces on their bodies to atone sin. Urine and feces were used during funeral ceremonies in rituals. Joshua used feces in the Bible's Zechariah 3:3-4. Books such as *Scatalogic Rites of All Nations* by John G. Bourke (1891) Caucasian customs with feces is indicate this.

A German harvest festival game involved farm laborers covering each other with feces and then being throwing each other on a hill of feces. A harvest game in Netherlands and Zealand allowed farm workers to run and catch each other, then bury the caught person in dirt up to his waist and then defecate in front of and on the caught victim's face.

Historically Caucasian criminals in the act of a crime would have a bowel movement on the floor at the crime scene. This was considered a spiritual way to prevent from being caught. If caught the English prisoners were given bread and drinking water with chicken feces in it.

The "Feast of the Fools" which dates back to the Roman Saturnalia Festival used feces in the worship ceremony. The naked participants would eat sausages (sexual, erotic penis symbol) at the church altar, paint their bodies, cross dress, and throw feces on each other.

The Caucasian historical figures involved in feces-related behaviors are plentiful. Robert Boyle (1627-1691) physicist/chemist recommended human feces be used as an eyewash. King James I (1566-1625) of England, Scotland and Ireland constantly had bowel movements on himself rather than stop hunting. He was a homosexual and authorized the famous King James Version of the Bible.

Martin Luther (1483-1546) said he got his spiritual inspiration while having a bowel movement. Luther believed that Satan had an anus face and farted on him. Richard III (1452-1485) of England decided to murder his nephew Terril while having a bowel movement. It seems that Caucasians believed that feces had some psychic ability. Psychologist Carl Jung (1875-1961) was obsessed with the idea that God sat on a toilet in heaven, and had a big bowel movement, which fell down to earth and broke the cathedral roof. This, he said, was God's way of telling him that his thoughts had no boundaries. Elizabeth Charlotte (1652-1722) in the court of Louis XIV in a letter to her Aunt Hanover (1694) said that during the day ladies constantly had bowel movements on themselves and would wait until evening to clean off the day load of feces. Francois Voltaire (1694-1778) while dying in bed ate his own bowel movement as a cure for his disease. Sigmund Freud (1856-1939) had erotic, sexual associations about his feces and his penis. He had constant constipation probably due to his diet and got sexual arousal from feces in his anus.

The Caucasian nutrient poor soil (dirt) produces nutrient poor vegetables, which cause diseases and mixed emotions about dirt. Added to this they have disease-causing behaviors with feces. Their methods for wiping feces from their anus after bowel movements caused diseases.

Ancient Romans kept a bucket of salt water with a sponge attached to a stick soaking in it. The sponge-on-a-stick was used to wipe off the feces from a bowel movement. Seneca's Epistle No 70 told of the sponge-on-a-stick ass wipers being used to choke people to death and to commit suicide. One of the members of the crowd that surrounded the Caucasians' Bible's Jesus at the crucifixion, poked a sponge-on-a-stick in his face (John 19:29), Matthew 27:48 and Mark 16:36). The poor could not afford this luxury, so they used their bare left hand to wipe their behinds and the right hand for eating and shaking another's hand. The African slaves in America's slave colonies used their hands and soil to wipe themselves. The Caucasians thought the Africans had a primitive need for cleanliness. In the Middle Ages some ass-wiper sticks were curved. This modern curved stick would confuse the wipers and often times they would mistakenly grab the wrong end of the stick. This has given rise to the expression "I got the short end of the stick (was wronged)," "this is a stick up" (to take advantage of, to clean out someone's money,) "stick it to him" etc. Before the stick Caucasians such as Louis XIV used prostitutes and flea-infested wool or lace to wipe their behinds. Medieval monks used cloth, rags and/or pottery shards. In France rich folks used grass and grew lawns for wiper use. Aristophanes wrote that the wealthy used onion leeks. In Europe and America people and mailmen use newspapers, letters and magazines. In 1907 crepe paper was invented to be used as toilet paper. In 1910 catalogues were popular as wipers. This caused the Mail Order Catalogue Company to switch to glossy, clay coated paper to stop folks from ordering them for wipers. Most Caucasians and African slaves used leaves and corn cobs as wipers. The Caucasian relationship to their body functions is surrounded by disease producing behaviors and social practices of a dubious nature.

The hands, dirt and grass remained as staple wipers. Diarrhea and constipation could cause scarce wiper items as well as extra wipers items. Enemas were a remedy for the constipating Caucasian diet. *The Essence Gospel of Peace* (3 A.D. Aramaic document) says that constipation was very common and enemas were the solution. In Germany, Dr. Johann Kampf (15 AD) said that enemas could cure all diseases as well as constipation. In 1932 French scientists found that ringing a bell while giving cats an enema caused them to have a bowel movement any time a bell rang. They hoped to use the techniques for constipation and sell anti-constipation bells. Enemas can become just as addicting as a laxative. The colon gets weak and can not function well enough to evacuate the feces due to excess enemas. An enema, colon cleanser, laxative formula, colonic irradiation and laxative stool softener addicts can stay constipated for a week or more if he doesn't get an enema "fix."

Constipation causes flatulence-stomach gas-farts. Farts are a combination of nitrogen, oxygen, carbon dioxide, hydrogen and methane (can burn producing a flame) and hydrogen sulfide (rotten egg smell). Farts have served a social function amongst Caucasians. Many Caucasian fairy tales and stories include character farts. There were many fart performers in literature such as the Greek Aristophane's story *The Clouds*. Farts were edited out of the English version of Chaucer's original *Canterbury Tales* which had farts in it. Joseph Pujol of France, born June 1, 1857 in Marseille, was called Le Petomaine (The Fartiste). He gave fart performances in 1892 at the Moulin Rouge (Red Mill). He was one of the very famous fart performers who amused packed house's of people.

In Britain up until the 1800's landholders had to appear before the feudal kings and had to perform a pagan ritual that included jumping up and farting in mid-air. It is part of the Caucasian belief system that bodily functions such as farts and excrement's (feces, urine) are symbols of life. Therefore, they can be used as sacrifices to appease spirit beasts? They believed good and bad spirits pass from one object into another object called sympathetic powers or magic. Emperor Claudius (41-54.AD) of Rome considered passing a law to allow farting at dinner. In France in the 1400's prostitutes who had to cross a bridge to work had to fart while on the bridge as payment for its use. Crates, (323-324) a stoic philosopher, had a farting contest with the philosopher Metrocles. Adolf Hitler (1889-1945) constantly farted. Consequently, he took small amounts of belladonna and strychnine in unsuccessful attempts to stop farting.

The Bible mentions the Caucasian god of human feces Baal-Peor. Human as well as farts and feces sacrifices were made to BaalPeor (Psalms 106:28, Deuteronomy 29:16, Numbers 5)

The African slaves were fearful of the wilds uncivilized Dutch and other Caucasian because who were unbathed, cannibals, drunkards, violent, homosexual, had a grunt sounding language, were illiterate, foul smelling, flea and lice infested, ate feces and constantly farted. The Caucasians' were a diseased, animalistic, organized mob that had feces and urine in their underwear, had heterosexual and homosexual activities in public, licked and spit on dinner tables and were usually unbathed.

The Caucasian custom of eating human feces and drinking urine appears in the October 1880 "The Lancet" and the Bible's Isaiah 36:16, Proverbs 5:15, Kings 18:31 and in John W. Armstrong's *The Water of Life* and Dr. C. P. Mithal's *Urine Therapy*. Caucasians urinating while having sexual intercourse is considered erotic (*Urodynamics, Principles, Practice and Application* by Mundy Stephenson and Wein, 1984). The Romans used urine as a mouthwash. Women in the city of Versailles urinated during church service. They would pass a urine bucket around to each other as a pagan ritual. In Scotland and France, after a Caucasian woman gave birth, her breasts were wiped with a man's urine. Stale urine was used as a cleanser called "Chamber Lye." Urine was used as a skin softener, shampoo and conditioner. Women used dog urine as an all-purpose beauty lotion.

An ancient European custom was to have married couples urinate on their wedding rings to spiritually protect the marriage from evil. The people who attended weddings were sprinkled with the bride's urine. In England and Ireland the guest would drink the bride's urine. Ancient doctors such as Hippocrates, Paracelsus and Galen recommended urine as medicine. They had a sympathetic belief that urine's medical properties could be transferred to another person. They felt the same about other excrements.

The Roman Empire had public buildings designated for the wealthy to vomit in. It is part of the Caucasian sympathetic belief that the wealthy's vomit smell can carry the spirit of wealth. The poor would smell the rich vomit in order to transfer wealthy ability to them. Later in Caucasian history vomiting became associated with witchcraft and spiritual possession by demons. Therefore, vomiting became disgusting along with other bodily functions.

The scientist, religious men and medical practitioners told people not to bath. Feces foul odor were associated with healthy animals. St. Benedict who founded the Benedictine, monastic order, told people to stay dirty and to very seldom bathe. The early Caucasian Christians did not take baths, marry, drink spirits (wine) or eat flesh. They practiced a life of misery in order to enter heaven.

Hospitals in England and France were staffed with friars and other unbathed, dirty, foul smelling, constipated, farting, rotten teeth and bad breath people. The staff never changed underwear or outer clothing. A bath was considered a medicine and was not to be taken for cleanliness or pleasure. Dr. Russel wrote the book *A Dissertation Concerning the Use of Sea Water in Diseases of the Glands* (1754). He strongly advised against baths for cleanliness.

Queen Elizabeth (ruled 1558) only took one bath a month. Caucasians generally, urinated, had bowel movements, drank and bathed in the same water. This was reported in *New Bath Guide* by Christopher Anstay (1766.) In stories such as *Gulliver's Travels* by Jonathan Swift bathing was reported as not customary. Gulliver and the people called Yahoos stayed dirty and did not take baths and were considered foul, smelly, stupid, violent, had feces and urine in their underwear and were wild. Today, if a Caucasian is having a wild fun time he will often holler "Yahoo." The Caucasian disdain for baths is reflected in phrases such as "you are in a stew," "I am in a stew," etc. "Stew" is the old English word for bath. Since they kept themselves dirty and foul smelling and did not want to bathe, they would refer to a stew as negative. Their health was poor and standards for health reflect it.

Caucasians who lived in old Europe were infested with fleas. The custom of wearing fur coats comes from the abundance of fleas and lice. Fur was worn so that the fleas would get trapped in it instead of getting on the person. This did not work, but fur coats were believed to give relief from the insects. The medieval homes and early ghetto (village homes of Europe) were filled with rats, fleas, human, dog and rat feces, manure, urine, etc.

Fleas and lice were common in beds. Caucasians looked for miracle cures for their living conditions. When the cures did not work they resorted to wearing amulets. They had three types of lice: pediculus capitis (head lice), pediculus curoris (body lice) and phthirus pubis (crab lice). Fevers caused by being bitten by lice were treated with opium. The padding for shoulders in today's Caucasian clothing started as a way to trap fleas and lice and to keep warm. The padding usually acquired a foul odor and flea colonies as revealed in *Pleasant and delightful Dialogues* by Minsheu. Bedbugs were infested in the homes and often fell from the ceilings into the beds. [*The Bed Bugs* British Museum (Natural History) Econ Series No 5 1949]. Bedrooms had foul funky odors, feces, urine, fumes, fleas and lice This added another dimension to the already pervert bedroom sexuality of Caucasians.

The early Caucasians had sex in orgies. Fathers and mothers had sex with their children and animals. Their society had heterosexual and homosexual random rapings, orgy rapes and gang rapes. Caucasian cannibalism adds another dimension to the social atmosphere as the sick, elderly, young strangers were hunted and killed and eaten for food or used for sex orgy feast festivities. King James (known for the King James Version of the Bible) was hyperactive, an alcoholic, constantly drooled at the mouth, was a homosexual and never bathed except for washing his fingertips before eating. He would get involved in homosexual activities in public and during mealtimes (letters and speeches of Oliver Cromwell Carlye). Danish King Christian IV visited England in 1606 got involved in heterosexual and homosexual orgies during feasts (reported by Sir John Harington). Caucasians gained sexual arousal from eating and licking feces. This was a type of coprophilia erotic love of filth (*Psychopathic Sexualis by* Krafft-Ebing). In Elizabethan England sex partners would get sexually aroused by exchanging "love apples." A "love apple" is a peeled apple rubbed with the foul odors of underarm sweat. "Love apples" were carried around by sex partners and sniffed as an aphrodisiac. Students giving apples to a teacher is a leftover fragment of this sex ritual. In a letter written by Napoleon he requested that Josephine not take a bath for two weeks so that they could have erotic sex. James Joyce (1822-1941) in a letter to his wife Nora wrote that he got aroused from her farting in his face, the sight of feces stains in her underwear and seeing her feces come out her anus. The combinations of filth and odors were a delight to the Caucasians. The bacteria on the skin produces a musky odor (androstenol), goat–like –smell (isovaleric acid) and stale urine fumes (androstenone). Funky odors are sexually arousing for pagan and contemporary Caucasians. (i.e. musk perfume).

The body's odors are related to the body's sweat, sex organs, urine and feces. Feces is emotionally connected to "dirt" with its pagan rituals and sexual connotations mixed into the subconscious mind of the Caucasian. Caucasians currently use many of their pagan rituals and ceremonies and still have the same behaviors and thoughts of their ancestors. Many pagan rituals are used in Greek fraternities, sororities, secret societies, Masonic orders, religious initiations, social gatherings, sexual activities and lynchings. They were also used by Caucasians on the African slaves.

Selected Reading for " Farts, Feces, Fun and Sex"

Black Spark White Fire Richard Poe, CA: Prima Pub. 1997

A National History of the Senses Diane Ackerman, NY.: Random House Inc. 1990

The Straight Dope Cecil Adams, N.Y. Ballantine Books 1986

Let Us Now Praise Famous Men James Agee and Walker Evans, N.Y: Houghton Mifflin Co. 1941

Visions of Excess Georges Bataille Minneapolis: The University of Minnesota Press 1985

"The Sweet Scent of Decomposition" *Forget Baudrillard?"* (ed Chris Rojek and Bryan S. Turner) London: Routledge 1993

Scatalogic Rites of All Nations John G. Bourke, Washington D:C.: W. H. Lowdermilk and Co. 1891. First reprint: N. Y.: Johnson Reprint Corp. 1968

Through the Alimentary Canal With a Gun and a Camera George Chappell N. Y: Frederick A. Stokes Co. 1955

Sputum Mauricio Dulfano, Springfield, IL: Charles C. Thomas Pub. 1973

Studies in the Psychology of Sex Ellis Havelock N.Y.: Random House; The Modern Library. Inc. 1936

Colon Hygiene John H. Kellogg, Battle Creek, MI: Good Health Pub. 1917

"The Ontogenesis of the Interest in Money" *Contributions to Psycho-Analysis* Sandor Ferenczi, Boston: R. G. Badger 1916

The Standard Edition of The Complete Psychological Works of Sigmund Freud (tr. James Strachey), London: The Hogarth Press and The Institute of Psycho-Analysis 1959

Memories, Dreams, Reflections Jung, Carl (ed. Aniela Jaffe; tr. Richard and Clara Winston), NY.: Vintage Books, A division of Random House 1965

"On Farting" CO Evolution Quarterly No. 34, Michael Kimball, Sausalito CA: POINT, a California non print corp. 1982

"The Fantasy of Dirt" Lawrence Kubie, The Psychoanalytic Quarterly, Vol. 6. Albany N. Y.: The Psychoanalytic Quarterly, Inc. 1937

End Product: The First Taboo Dan Sabbath, NY. Urizen Books 1977

Le Petomane 1857-1945 Jean Nohain and F. Caradec (tr. Warren Tute), London: Souvenir Press Ltd. 1967

The Foul and the Fragrant Alain Corbin, Cambridge, MA: Harvard University Press 1986

Chapter Six
Once Upon A Time

"Our people must learn to make the analysis of
what is good and healthy."

Del Jones
(The War Correspondent)

Harmful Effects of white Fairy tales on Black Children

Caucasian fairy tales/children's stories were written by Caucasians for Caucasians. The purpose of the fairy tales is to emotionally attach the child to the culture. Fairy tales program the child with Caucasian logic, morals, ethics, social and sexual behaviors and violence. Once the child is psychologically hardwired, a new program (African culture) will be hard to understand, difficult to accept, be questioned, and given less respect and distorted. The first program, (Caucasian thought and behavior program) will be the norm standard and used to understand and measure the validity of African culture.

The fairy tales are a way to program the Black child into having a White consciousness and subconsciousness. They "seasonin" the child into a Caucasian mind set. Fairy tales are basically ancient Greek and Roman myths in which the characters have English and German names. The Black child learns the Caucasian worldview (cosmology), rituals, ceremonies, rewards, punishments, how to act and react and begins to distort and modify their African character logic so that it will fit into a Caucasian personality. Thus, she gradually becomes a dysfunctional personality.

The fairy tales are written oral stories that were originally told about almost primitive Caucasian clans and tribes. Their folk writers lore scientists (social engineers), philologists and mythologists who collected various Caucasian fairy tales and put them in books. Jakob Ludwig Grimm (1785-1863) and Wilhelm Karl Grimm (1786-1859) collected stories that barbaric clans told to each other and compiled the book *Grimms Fairy* tales. Basil (1637 in Italy) compiled various primitive tribes, stories and called them *Mother Goose* which was transliterated by Charles Perault (1697, France) and these stories were revised, modified and changed and put into English in 1729. *The Three Bears* (1834) by Robert Southey is another pagan Caucasian story that engineers the Black Children's mind and behavior. The stories teach the child how to manipulate others, to steal, be disobedient, how to dream, be superstitions, do rituals, to value winning above morality, used in appropriate parenting skills, to be liars, to want and eat junk food and sweets, that killing animals is sport, and to run away from home.

The fairy tales have a story pattern and the child learns to act out his/her life according to the life of the fairy tale. If you have ever wondered why some adults act like they are immature or don't want to grow up and be responsible, look at the fairy tales. This type of dysfunctional adult has the Peter Pan syndrome or the Alice In Wonderland syndrome (never, never land-never, never grow up). The pattern of the stories are;

1) Fall of Character–character has a problem that has caused a change and/or failure in their life.

2) Atonement–character seeks a solution to the problem and has obstacles, to overcome or an enemy, to defeat.

3) Need supernatural Miracle–character seeks special person or item, magic, (i.e. Moses, Jesus, Muhammad), money, good fairy or witch, and/or magic to become happy, successful, rich and normal.

The fairy tales have common ingredients such as
❏ -single women have children
❏ -magic (words, coins, etc.) will save you (i.e. lottery, psychic hotline)
❏ -poor people/poor elves live to serve the rich
❏ -have sex with someone if they dress good (i.e. prince, princess, designer clothes and expensive shoes)
❏ -married couples are miserable, childless (it is best to be single)

❑ -woman want men for their money (king's gold)

❑ -stay in bad relationships (widower married to stepmother who abuses his children)

❑ -no extended families

❑ -black is evil, white is good

❑ -God does not exist for happy people (stories never mention God)

❑ -spirits are evil (spirituality is bad =African centeredness is bad)

❑ -sex symbolism

❑ -evil is successful without magic and goodness/good needs magic to be successful.

❑ -marry a stranger for money not character

❑ -candy, cake and sweets are rewards and make you happy

❑ -meat eating is normal

❑ -man's deceased first wife is resurrected as evil stepmother (true nature of women is evil)

❑ -sacrifice children for wealth (successful career)

❑ -men are sexually wolves

❑ -child abuse is normal

❑ -poor parenting skills are normal

❑ -thieves and liars are successful

❑ -ancestors are not part of the family

❑ -straight hair and Caucasian facial features are beautiful

❑ -beautiful people are good and ugly people are evil (buy expensive jewelry and clothes to make yourself beautiful =good)

❑ -women are not interested in sex =men always want sex because women have charm and beauty

❑ -dysfunctional families are normal

❑ -violence is normal

❑ -no music, singing, dancing or elderly relatives

Fairy tales use a story pattern called "The Chase." In "The Chase" the character is chasing after success or the perfect life (self-actualization). The cartoons (animated fairy tales) such as the Road Runner and Wally Coyote, Tom and Jerry (cat and mouse), Flintstones, Bugs Bunny, Woody the Wood Pecker, Scooby Do, Butt Head and Beavis and Daffy Duck use the chase while Batman, Superman and Spiderman focus on a prophet who will save you. Chase themes are in movies such as "Men In Black," "Star Wars," "Tarzan," "Titanic," "Malcolm X," and "The Wild Wild West." "The Chase" theme is the format for Talk Shows (Jerry Springer, etc.), Music videos, professional Wrestling, Soap Operas and Commercials such as Dave of Wendy's Fast Food Restaurant, Ronald McDonald and Breakfast cereal commercials. "The Chase" has a character (hero, TV host) that chases after a solution by overcoming an obstacle (hunger, social problems) with the help of the Talk Show host, clown, character or hero. "The Chase" is fairy tale based.

The breakfast and fast food commercials use clowns and animated characters which appeal to infantilism (Peter Pan syndrome) plus they emotionally take you down memory lane (back to your past life as a child) and satisfy the need to be nurtured or escape adult life. This causes consumers to emotionally live a fantasy life of happiness with the animated characters, food, sex and clowns. Fairy tales are a propaganda (political and social) tool and used in a 'military logic' fashion to reinforce and maintain White Supremacy.

The Caucasian civilization spends more dollars on media than on its military. The military maintains its power and attacks (makes wars to maintains peace) those who are classified by them as an enemy or operating against their peaceful economic interest. However, the new weapon of the Caucasians is fairy tale propaganda which is used to seize the mind of Black children. Caucasians spend 3 to 4 times more money on the media of television shows, commercials and movies that use exclusively fairy tale themes. They invade Africa and other countries and the mind with a fairy tale type media, and then the military comes to the country to complete the take over. Media is the new military of Caucasians. An examination of the overt and hidden messages communicated to Black children in a few fairy tales/children's stories will reveal their true effect on the mind.

The African, African in American and Diaspora Africans have African centered children's stories (fairy tales) teach the child Maat (truth, justice, balance, reciprocity, righteousness, the real from the unreal, right from wrong, respect, etc.) They teach respect for the privilege to love God and the importance of family and respect for ancestors and Mother Earth (nature's balance =ecology). The stories present a variety of problems and the African Maat solution.

The African children, stories usually have major themes

1) a message gets changed and a character has to seek the true message
2) rebirth (rites of passage) of a character teaches various solutions of a problem)
3) a mixture of 1 and 2
4) they use of Maat will solve problems (Ashanti Spider Stories, Aesop's Fables)

An African ethnic group called the Hottentots has many stories. One story is about the moon (unseen heavenly power) giving a message to a rabbit to tell Adam (Osiris) and Eve (Isis). The rabbit forgets the correct message and tells them a lie. The moon learns of the error and throws a stick (Rod of Righteousness) at the rabbit and splits his lip. Therefore, the child is told not to seek wisdom from those who lie.

The Maasai of Botswana, Kalahari Desert and Southern Rhodesia have children stories. In one story a turtle and rabbit are told to tell man he will live forever. The fast moving rabbit runs to man and reaches him before the turtle. The rabbit with his bad memory forgets part of the message and tells man a lie instead of the truth.

The turtle with the correct message gets to man after the rabbit. This caused man to be doomed to solve his earthly problems by himself.

Basically, the African stories and Greek myths and Roman myths are versions of the series of Egyptian mythological stories about the children Osiris and Seth who are brothers and their sisters Isis and Nepthys. It is a long story about how and why these brothers and sisters maintain Maat, family values and Godly values in the face of negative forces outside and inside the family. It also contains the African spirituality construct.

The African American Carolina Sea Island, Upotos of the Congo and Gallas of East Africa have stories about a bird bringing mortal life and immortal life to man. The stories are built upon the Egyptian Osirian stories. African stories have a common connection and that is to demonstrate what is Maat and how to use Maat to be spiritualized with God. They are designed to connect African children to African culture.

The Caucasian stories are totally different and truly harmful psychologically and emotionally. They addict children to white sugary sweets and they do not reflect a Godly relationship with one's soul. For example, in *Little Red Riding Hood* her mother abuses her by sending her into the woods where wild, man-eating wolves live. *Little Red Riding Hood* is openly disobedient to her mother when she goes off the trail which her mother told her to stay on. *Little Red Riding Hood* talks to the wolf (a total stranger) and tells him she is going to her sick grandmother's house. She should not talk to strangers, but does. She wears a red hood the hood represents hiding something and deceit. Red in Caucasian culture means fertile—sexually active. This is why Caucasian women wear red lipstick, red nail polish, red underwear, red shoes (Dorothy in "Wizard of Oz"), areas of prostitution in cities work in areas that are called *red* light (sex) districts, etc.

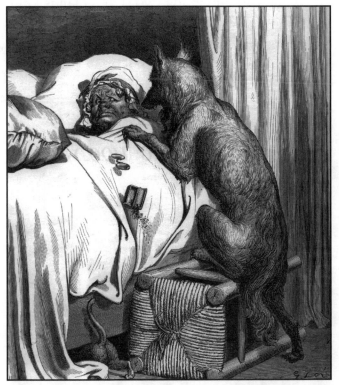

The Grandmother leaves the door open for the wolf

The grandmother obviously is senile as she leaves the door to her house open when she knows wild wolves roam around her house. The grandmother cannot distinguish a wolf's voice from that of Little Red Riding Hood. Then when Little Red Riding Hood arrives at her grandmother's with a basket of food and sweets and a bottle of wine, she cannot recognize (poor eyesight) a wolf from her grandmother.

The story does not seem to make sense to the conscious mind because it is aimed at the subconscious mind. Subconsciously, the wolf is symbolic of men. Men are wolves that seek sex. Men are dogs and want to rape virgin young girls. Girls want a man to be virile and a sex stud =wolf. However, when they get a macho man they are insulted and call him a dog (wolf). If a man is kind and gentle like a sheep, then he is a wolf in sheep's clothing. Men are deceitful. If a man whistles at an attractive lady, then he is acting like a wolf–it's a wolf's whistle.

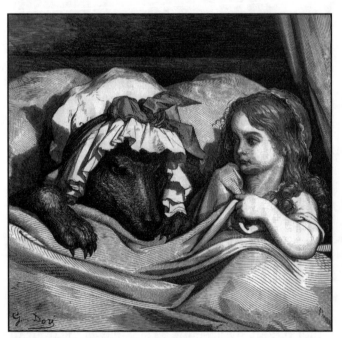

Little Red Riding Hood gets in bed with the wolf

A hunter appears in the story with a rifle. The rifle is symbolically a man's penis. This means that a man's penis will save Little Red Riding Hood from the wolf (whore-like sex urges). Therefore, the idea is promoted that the next man is always better than the last man that the lady was in a sexual relationship with. The wolf dresses up like a drag queen to protect his virginity from hot (red-hot =red hood) Little Red Riding Hood. The hunter impregnates the drag queen (wolf) and the wolf drag queen has rocks (symbolic baby). The hunter skins the wolf and takes his fur. Skinning or scalping people such as the American Indians symbolically means that their soul is stolen because of an evil woman. After the murder of the wolf the grandmother gets drunk (alcohol is called spirits). The wine bottle is symbolically a penis that gives the grandmother her true spirit (sexual awakening).

This story programs Black boys to be wolves and Black girls to be in conflict with their mothers. It can subconsciously cause girls to become sexy hunters of the penis in order to save themselves from the evilness of being a woman with a vagina.

The story Cinderella has many mixed messages and hidden themes. It suggests that dirt (cinder is black ash dirt from burnt wood) poor people can be saved from poverty by the rich, money, expensive clothes, shoes, magic (prophet, lottery), sex and that women, are naturally dirty (evil) etc. Cinderella is a story about child abuse. A father is so in love with his wife's sexuality that he lets her abuse his child. The woman's vagina will get her anything because Cinderella can only be saved from this parental abuse by being dressed in the latest, expensive clothes in order to sell her sexuality. This allows her to marry a man who dresses nice.

The personality and character development of the prince is never an issue. Therefore, if a man dresses nice (expensive clothes, shoes) and has money he can have sex with women. This fairy godmother did not try to correct the father's behavior or put the mother and father in marriage counseling. The story projects the idea that being wealthy will save you from abuse and solve your problems. The story makes ugly people evil with dark hair (Black). The prince picks a wife as if she is a commodity (women do have human rights). Women are valued the same as a slave, horse or ornament. Women are sex candy for men. Women can not truly trust other women (stepmother, female friend or a sister). The stepmother and daughters ask for forgiveness for being abusive to Cinderella. It is denied, which means people should be punished for behavior. This justifies prisons and prisoners.

The children's stories in poem form are harmful. For example, the poem "Pussy Willow," aside from causing the women's vagina to be called pussy, has other hidden: meanings;

Pussy Willow

Verse

Meaning

Pussy Willow wakened
From her winter nap

the vagina is ready for sex barren prepuberty From her winter nap

For the frolic spring
breeze
On her door would tap

sexual intercourse opens her legs so that men can have sex (spring means sex)

Mistress Pussy Willow
Open wide her door

pussy is female =vagina
open the legs and door of vagina

Good morning Pussy
Willow
Welcome to you dear?

men naturally have an erection in the morning which can greet the vagina

Pussy came to town
In a hood of silver gray
And a coat of brown

pussy comes to town for sexual action
pussy with hair

Spring is coming
Pussy Willow out

men will ejaculate (come) in a vagina
that is out the panties the penis will enter

Hickory, Dickery, Dock

Verse	*Meaning*
Hick (Hickory)	unsophisticated, wild a sexual petting bruise
Dick (Dickory)	driver's seat drives it penis makes sex happen dick is a penis picker =penis
Dock	short part of a tail the tail is a penis loads are left on this area of a pier load of semen left in vagina
The mouse ran up the clock	mouse is symbolically a penis, it has a long tail (penis) the clock is a vagina (circle round vagina)
The clock struck one	one o' clock is the hands of clock straight up = erected penis struck is intercourse stroking the vagina
And down he ran	ejaculation penis became flaccid =erection goes down
Hickory, Dickery, Dock	

The earlier you condition a Black child's mind with a fairytale program the better. The earlier the stories are told the more tightly bound the emotional, physical image and behaviors of the characters are imprinted on the mind. The more the stories are repeated the stronger the impression. The adult story teller's voice quality, inflection, voice tone, tension and facial expressions wrap the child into the fairy tale so completely that they will mimic the voice tones associated with anger, sex, joy, stealing, lies, and behavior of fairytale characters all their lives. The fairy tales are hard wired to the electrical circuit of the child and any aggressive attempt to free the child from the Caucasian ideals (cosmology) further bonds them to it. The fairy tales sell them stocks in Caucasian culture that makes them bond to the Caucasian. Fairy tale jingles and songs are repeatedly hummed and song by Black children which makes a negative psychological impression and gives them an emotionally soothing effect. Along with the effect comes the Caucasian mindset. The child becomes possessed by the spirit of Europeans. They became alienated from African culture and aliens. Aliens only serve aliens. The child is created into an Afropean-Black skin, white mind.

The Caucasian fairy tales and children's poems program the future behavior of the child. Consequently, Black women will meet Black men who are either sex hunters, wolves (dogs), Prince Charmings, Peter Pan, men that think they possess magic words (good rappers), men that allow themselves to be dominated (like the husband in Hansel and Gretel or Cinderella), homosexuals (drag queens that are wolves for other men), etc.

Conversely, Black men will meet Black women who are Cinderellas, look for Prince Charmings, princess (dress nicely), submissive (allow men to choose them = Goldilocks), want to rescue the man from childishness and raise Them (Little Red Riding Hoods), gold diggers (marry them because they have a good job not because they themselves are good), or subconsciously chose to be a single female parent that has had a series of bad relationships that have left her with children (Old Lady that lives in a shoe), etc.

The fairy tale programmed adults will follow the fairy tale script to its conclusion. The unreal fairy tale story and their real life story become one and the same. They dress for sexual intercourse like fairy tale characters. The women may wear red *(Little Red Riding Hood)* and the men may wear animal type design underwear (tiger stripes symbolic of being hunters. This fairy tale program influences their sexual positions and erotic sexually arousing areas of the body.

Fairy tales consistently show pictures of white sugary sweets, talk about sweets and use sweets to reward good behavior. The child is programmed to associate white sugar with fun, happiness, family, sex, and love. White sugar, candy, cookies, pies and cakes are in numerous stories such as Hansel and Gretel, Christmas, Halloween and Thanksgiving stories, The Ginger Bread Boy, etc. Sugar Addiction is created by the stories. The only solution to the Black folks having fairy tale syndrome is not to tell Caucasian fairy tales to Black children. Caucasians fairy tales come from a dysfunctional mind created by a dysfunctional culture and have dysfunctional characters, families, behaviors and themes. They will in some way cause an aspect of the child's mind and life to be dysfunctional. "Once upon a time" Black folks only told African stories to African children. Now, is the time to return back to that "Once Upon a Time" so that we can save our children in this time.

SUGGESTED BOOKS

by Afrikan Authors Only

A Healthy Foods and Spiritual Nutrition Handbook—Keith T. Wright

A Holistic Guide To Family Disorders—Ra Un Neter Amen I

African Holistic Health—Llaila Afrika

AIDS, Africa and Racism—Richard Rosalin Chirimunta

Awakening the Natural Genius in Black Children—Amos N. Wilson

Basic Herbs for Health and Healing —Rashan Abdul Hakim

Blueprint for Black Power —Amos N. Wilson

Caribbean Medicine—C. Wolde Kyte

Claim the Victory—Keefa K. Lorraine

Dick Gregory's Natural Diet for Folks Who Eat —Dick Gregory

Forever Young—Dr. Paul Goss

Guyanese Seed of Vegetables, —

Deserts The Vegetarians and Food Lovers Paradise—Yvonne John

Heal Thyself Cookbook for Natural Living —Diana Ciccone

Heal Thyself for Health and Longevity —Queen Afua

Healing, Health and Transformation—Elaine Ferguson, M.D.

Health Teachings of the Ageless Wisdom—R.A. Staughn

Helping Hand (Guide to Healthy Living) —Henry Anderson

How to Eat to Live: Volume I and II—Elijah Muhalrunad

How to Select and Combine, Fruits, Vegetables and Tubers, Through their Color-Powers—Doctor Ignatius

Melanin—Protective Intoxicant Capabilities in the Black Human and Its Influence on Behavior—Carole Barnes

Melanin—The Chemical Key to Great Blackness—Carol Barnes

Message in A Bottle —Alfred "Coach" Powell

Mother Nature—Dick Gregory

Nutrition, Herbal and Homeopathic Guide to Healing -—Ra Un Neter Amen I

Optimizing Health Nutrition—Ra Un Neter Amen I

Organic Wellness (Fasting Technique)—Henry Anderson

Pyramids of Power (Ancient African Centered Approach to Optimum Health) —John T. Chissell, M.D.)—John T. Chissdl, M.D.

Radiant Health Through Nutrition —Alvenia Fulton

Spiritual Nutrition—Doctor Ignatius

The Invasion of the Body Snatchers —Del Jones

Textbook of Black-Related Diseases —Richard Williams

The Conscious Rasta Report by Keidi Obi Awadu

The Harlem Hospital Story by Peter Bailey

The Healers--Ayi Kwesi Arrnah

The Last Great Plague Upon Man, AIDS Related Murder Tools —Georges C. Hatonn

The Rebirth of Gods —Dr. Paul Goss

The Rejuvenating Plants of Tropical Africa —Albert A. Enti

The Science and Romance of Selected Herbs Used In Medicine and Religious Ceremony —Anthony Andoh

The United Independent Compensatory Code/System/Concept: A Textbook/Workbook for Thought, Speech and/or Actions for Victims of Racism (White Supremacy) by Neely Fuller Jr.

To Save the Blood of Black Babies by Kiarri T. H. Cheatwood

Vaccines are Dangerous—Curtis Cost

Vegetarian—Zak A. Kondo

Vitamins and Minerals From A-Z with Ethno-Consciousness—Jewel Pookrum, M.D.

What is Safe in The Age of AIDS-If You Only Know What They Aren't Teaching You—Curtis Cost

Yurugu—Marimba Ani

About the Author

Llaila Oleta Afrika is a health consultant, historian and lecturer. His name Llaila (LA-EE-LA) means, "light of heaven and earth." His last name Afrika is Egyptian in origin and means "land of the Blacks." He is the author of the largest selling Africentric health book in American history African Holistic Health and the African American history book called *The Gullah*.

He has over 17 years of experience in the holistic health field and is one of the pioneers in traditional African ethnomedicine (health care based on the biochemistry of Africans). He conducts history tours of the Sea Islands, does Rites of Passage workshops and children's lectures. He is famous for his in-depth knowledge of diet, health, healing techniques, herbs, supplements, history and culture. He is reluctant to admit that he does have a Caucasian Doctor of Naturopathy diploma and was the first African American naturopath to lecture before the World Vegetarian Congress. He is one of the featured lecturers for the World Melanin Consortium and the Association for the Study of Classical African Civilization. Additionally, Llaila has civilian as well as military work experience as a psychiatric counselor, community organizer and nurse. He is dedicated to educating African people and believes that a healthy body is the temple for building a holistically healthy race. Llaila is a registered drugless therapist.

For lectures, workshops, books, audio and videocassettes contact:

Golden Seal
P. O. Box 2475
Beauford, S. C. 29901

Index